Understanding the Mental Health Problems of Children and Adolescents

D1291565

Understanding the Mental Health Problems of Children and Adolescents

A Guide for Social Workers

Second Edition

KIRSTIN PAINTER
MARIA SCANNAPIECO

OXFORD
UNIVERSITY PRESS

OXFORD
UNIVERSITY PRESS

Oxford University Press is a department of the University of Oxford. It furthers
the University's objective of excellence in research, scholarship, and education
by publishing worldwide. Oxford is a registered trade mark of Oxford University
Press in the UK and certain other countries.

Published in the United States of America by Oxford University Press
198 Madison Avenue, New York, NY 10016, United States of America.

First Edition published in 2015 by Lyceum Books, Inc.
Second Edition published in 2021

Library of Congress Cataloging-in-Publication Data
Names: Painter, Kirstin, 1963– author. | Scannapieco, Maria, author.
Title: Understanding the mental health problems of children and adolescents :
a guide for social workers / Kirstin Painter and Maria Scannapieco.
Description: Second edition. | New York, NY : Oxford University Press, 2021. |
Includes bibliographical references and index.
Identifiers: LCCN 2020037506 (print) | LCCN 2020037507 (ebook) |
ISBN 9780190927844 (paperback) | ISBN 9780190927868 (epub) |
ISBN 9780197554548 (oso)
Subjects: LCSH: Child mental health. | Teenagers—Mental health.
Classification: LCC RJ503 .P35 2021 (print) | LCC RJ503 (ebook) |
DDC 618.92/89—dc23
LC record available at https://lccn.loc.gov/2020037506
LC ebook record available at https://lccn.loc.gov/2020037507

DOI: 10.1093/oso/9780190927844.001.0001

5 7 9 8 6 4

Printed by LSC Communications, United States of America

Dr. Painter completed this work while she was a Program Specialist at the National Institute on Disability, Independent Living, and Rehabilitation Research.

Contents

List of Figure, Tables, and Boxes

List of Figure

List of Tables

List of Boxes

Foreword

Stumbling through the dense forest, the roots of giant trees continually tripped me. One day I tripped on yet another root, but this time I looked up to find the right tree.

This is what it feels like to have a child with mental health problems. If your child has asthma, diabetes, or other illnesses, you can ask around and find resources, physicians, and treatments. But even in the second decade of the 21st century, mental illnesses remain in dark shadows—seldom mentioned in "polite society." Yet one in five children at any given time is experiencing some form of mental illness. Mental illnesses must come out of the shadows, but they have a long way to go.

Imagine, if you will, what it must be like to have a child who is violent, using street drugs, sexually active, or out of control. Because the symptoms of mental illnesses are typically behavioral, parents have a tendency to blame themselves for not teaching their children well. And others blame the parents as well. How often have you heard, "If her parents just spent more time with her," "If his parents didn't let him get away with everything," "If her parents were more involved, they would know where she is and who she is with."

As a parent of a child who was diagnosed with bipolar disorder as an adolescent, I can tell you these remarks sting. Perhaps even more stinging, though, is that you used to say the same things about children and adolescents who seemed "out of control." "What is wrong with the parents? Can't they control that child?"

In the following pages, Dr. Kris Painter and Dr. Maria Scannapieco will present an excellent discussion on mental illnesses in children and adolescents. They have kindly asked me to write a Foreword to give you the perspective of a parent's experiences when a child or adolescent has a mental illness—and ways you can help.

The first thing a social worker can do is avoid guilt-inducing statements, gestures, or eye-rolling when determining a child's background. Yes, the parents might have been responsible in part for triggering their child's symptoms. However, what good does it do to add guilt on top of the guilt? If parents are seeking help for their children, they can't be all bad, can they?

Instead, the therapist can help parents discover their strengths and help them make a better future for themselves and their children.

Second, social workers need to recognize that parents go through all the stages of grief when learning that their child has a mental illness. What would your reaction be if the child you held in your arms as an infant—the child whose future you dreamed—was diagnosed with a lifelong illness that could prevent those dreams from coming true? In the earliest stages, parents are often in denial, no matter how educated or accepting they are of mental illnesses. They do not want this for their children. Social workers can play a role in helping parents recognize and navigate their grief as they work to help their children recover.

It is also common for social workers to become frustrated with parents who will not ensure that their children take prescribed medication. Again, though, put yourself in their place. They have read about children committing suicide after starting antidepressants. The news is big and bold on the front page. Unfortunately, explanations and medical discussions of these issues are buried—if they are included in the news at all. So parents do not always have a wealth of resource information. And they do not turn to their friends because no one ever talks about mental illness, so they feel they must be the only ones grappling with this problem.

It is always important to listen to the parents just as intently as you do the child or adolescent. The children with mental illnesses whom I have encountered are often among the brightest I have ever known. As such, they know what to say to make themselves look good and their parents look bad. In one case, a therapist in a residential treatment center was shocked when my daughter had a full meltdown during family therapy 2 months into her treatment. Her comment was an incredulous, "I've never seen this child before." My response was, "This is the child I live with every day." While there were certain satisfactions in having the therapist see what I had been saying, there was still the wasted 2 months when the behaviors were not addressed because my daughter had never displayed them—in spite of my discussing them.

Another role the social worker can play is mediator/facilitator. Too many therapists see the parent–child relationship as antagonistic. It may appear this way because many parents have no way to understand what has been happening. They have been struggling with discipline and may be at their wits end. There are even some parents who communicate their frustrations to their children, using phrases such as, "I've had enough. I give up." The situation may seem antagonistic, and sometimes it is. Often, though, the parents have no idea how to work with an emotionally disturbed child. They blame themselves, but they keep struggling. And, all too often, social workers present an air of mystery and intrigue. "Thank you for bringing your child to me. Now you just sit out here in the waiting room while we talk." The parent is left totally in the dark, unaware of what is being discussed or—more importantly—what he or she can do to help. The social worker could bring the parent into the room with the child in the last few minutes of the session. This might be a good time to encourage the child to communicate feelings and to discuss the illness openly with the parent and child together. The more parents can be on the same page with the therapist and the child, the more effective the changes at home can be. After all, parents who have been raised a certain way can find it difficult to suddenly change their parenting styles. But if they understand the benefit to their child, they may feel more empowered to make those changes.

Another aspect of the family to assess and counsel is the situation for other children in the home. Mental illnesses do not affect only the child with the illness—or even the child and parents. Often, a child with mental illness will act out against other children in the family. The parents can be so involved in the ill child's care that they cannot find the time they need for the other children, and this can add to the feelings of guilt for the parents. Sometimes a professional can help explain the illness to other children in the family who are old enough to understand. If the family can become more cohesive, it can provide a much better environment for the child struggling with mental illness.

Many social workers have advised me to research parenting tools that could work. It's a good idea to arm parents with whatever you can, but never anticipate that typical parenting programs will work. And when they don't, the parents again feel guilty. They must not have done it correctly or are not capable as parents even when they follow guidelines. For example, many parents try working with privileges. If a child lives up to certain behavioral standards, he receives privileges. If not, privileges are removed. In my own case, my daughter would miss the privileges for a very short period of time and then forget about them. They just didn't matter to her. How do you keep up with privileges to remove when the privileges valued by the child change rapidly? The "behavior contract" is another example of a tool that does not work for every parent. The adolescents you see are often very savvy. They know they just need to sign the contract to move forward, so they do. However, they may have no intention of living up to their promises. Again, the parents feel guilty because they were unable to make the child commit to the terms of the contract.

As you will see in the next few pages, knowledge about mental illnesses is constantly changing. When my adopted daughter was just 6 weeks old— before she came to us—she was physically abused. We knew a little about the abuse when we adopted her, but my thinking was that she would never re- member anything that happened at such an early age. Over the years, research has shown that even early childhood trauma can change the way a child's brain develops. That might seem like common sense to you, but parents con- tinue to be unaware of the nature and impact of early childhood trauma. As a social worker, you can help parents understand the importance of those early childhood experiences. I will always wonder if my daughter's behaviors would have become so out of control if we had addressed the trauma issues.

Finally, social workers often try to help parents deal with their child's situa- tion by encouraging the parents to "take care of themselves." This is good ad- vice, without a doubt. However, parents are often emotionally and financially strapped. Many cannot even afford a movie night out. Single parents may have lost the friends they once had—the parents of their children's friends have busy lives with their healthy children and sometimes they see the parent of a child with mental illness as flawed. So continue to tell parents to take care of themselves for the sake of their children, but give them some ideas on ways they can do that within the limitations they have.

Although I have addressed many issues in this Foreword, I must stress that most of my experiences with social workers have been positive. I consider many of those who worked with my daughter to be life-savers. The ones who cared about my entire family and made that clear have my undying gratitude. I have been fortunate to work with many social workers beyond those who provided therapy for my child, including Dr. Painter and Dr. Scannapieco. I have seen first-hand the help they give to families who struggle every day with a child's mental illness. I thank all of them and encourage you to follow their examples and truly make a difference in lives.

—Kay Barkin, APR, Fellow PRSA

1

Introduction

Mental illness is a serious public health problem that goes largely unrecognized by many Americans. Mental illnesses are among the most pressing public health issues today. The prevalence of mental illnesses in children has increased dramatically, particularly for children and adolescents living in poverty who are vulnerable to experiencing cognitive, socioemotional, and behavioral hindrances (National Academy of Sciences, 2015). Mental illness can be categorized into two distinct types: *situational* and *serious and persistent*. Situational mental illnesses are usually temporary. They can arise in anyone who is experiencing some type of severe stress and has trouble coping with the situation. Serious and persistent mental illnesses (also known as serious mental illness [SMI] for adults and serious emotional disturbance [SED] for youth) are the result of certain psychological, biological, genetic, and/or environmental conditions. Serious and persistent mental illness can include behavioral disorders such as oppositional defiant disorder and conduct disorder or brain disorders such as schizophrenia, schizoaffective disorders, major depression, and bipolar disorder. SMIs and SEDs can be treated and managed effectively if an individual has access to a combination of medication, supportive counseling, and community support services such as education or vocational training. With proper treatment, people experiencing an SMI can return to normal, productive lives.

Mental illnesses are more common than other illnesses such as cancer, heart disease, or diabetes. Anyone, regardless of age, gender, race, ethnicity, and socioeconomic status, can experience a mental health problem. In fact, most of us will experience a mental health problem at some time in our lives. It has been well established that, at any given time, an estimated 1 in 5 children is experiencing some form of mental illness, with 1 in 10 children suffering from an SMI resulting in significant impairments across all aspects of their lives. In 2001, as part of his New Freedom Initiative, President George W. Bush directed members of the New Freedom Commission to study problems in mental health systems and make recommendations for improvement. In 2003, the New

Understanding the Mental Health Problems of Children and Adolescents. Kirstin Painter and Maria Scannapieco,
Oxford University Press (2021). © Oxford University Press. DOI: 10.1093/oso/9780190927844.003.0001

Freedom Commission on Mental Health released a report stating that mental illness was the number one cause of disability and that it cost approximately $79 billion each year in the United States due to loss of productivity, incarcerations, and mortality-related expenses (New Freedom Commission on Mental Health, 2003). The New Freedom Commission also reported children's mental health to be a public health crisis in the United States, noting the existence of many barriers that impede children from receiving appropriate mental health care. Such barriers included a fragmented service delivery system, stigma and stigmatizing behaviors against persons experiencing a mental illness, financial barriers, a lag between discovery of effective treatments and their implementation, lack of early identification and intervention, and lack of adequately trained mental health professionals. Although we know more about the serious consequences of untreated mental illness and what treatments are effective than we did in 2003, many of the barriers to treatment continue to exist today. Fifteen years after the New Freedom Commission released its report, mental illness now costs an estimated $247 billion per year in the United States. Untreated or inadequately treated youth are ending up in the child welfare or juvenile justice systems. The proportion of youth with serious mental health problems in both the child welfare and juvenile justice systems is higher than the national average (Carney & Buttell, 2003; US General Accounting Office, 2003). Of the approximately 2.1 million youth arrested each year in the United States, as many as 75 percent meet the criteria for at least one mental health problem (Grande, Hallman, Caldwell, & Underwood, 2011). Approximately 36 percent of youth in the juvenile justice system nationally become involved due to inadequate or unavailable mental health services, and thousands of families relinquish custody of a child each year in order for the child to receive mental health treatment (Carney & Buttell, 2003; US General Accounting Office, 2003).

In addition to a significantly underfunded mental health system, stigma is another obstacle to children and adolescents receiving appropriate, needed treatment. An increased focus on mental illness has occurred over the past several years due to mass shootings reported in the media. Unfortunately, this media coverage has also increased the stigma associated with mental illness. One needs to keep in perspective that the vast majority of persons with a mental health problem will never harm themselves or others (Phillips, 2012; see also Satcher, 2000). They are far more likely to be victims of a crime than perpetrators. The focus on mass shootings has been both a vehicle to open the conversation on mental illness and treatment and a means of increasing the stigma. In 2009, it was reported that the majority of Americans (nearly 70 percent) would not seek any form of treatment for their own mental health problem or their child's mental health problem because they either did not recognize it as a serious problem or because of the stigma that can be attached to mental illness (US Department of Health and Human Services, 2009). A systematic review of mental health-related stigma found that stigma continues to be a significant contributor to reduced help-seeking (Clement, Schauman, Graham, & Maggioni, 2015). Mental health problems left untreated can cause long-lasting problems. For children, these problems can interfere with their socioemotional and cognitive development (Institute of Medicine, 2009). Left untreated, these problems can follow them into adulthood. Research has found that nearly 50 percent of adults experiencing a mental illness begin experiencing symptoms as early as age 14 and as many as 75 percent experience symptoms by age 20 (Kessler et al., 2005). To compound the problems, youth with a mental illness often have co-occurring chronic health conditions and/or substance abuse problems. The sad realization is that mental health problems can and should be treated. With proper evidence-based treatment, a person can experience recovery and lead a full, happy, healthy life. Unfortunately, current estimates are that only 2 percent of children using public funds receive evidence-based mental health interventions (Public Law 114-255).

In 2016, with the realization that the barriers identified in the 2003 New Freedom Commission continue to persist, the 114th US Congress overwhelmingly passed and President Barrack Obama signed into law an Act to accelerate the discovery, development, and delivery of 21st-century cures (Public Law 114-255, 2016). The law, referred to as the 21st-Century Cures Act, promotes and funds innovative research aimed at preventing or curing serious diseases, responding to the opioid crisis, accelerating the development of drugs and medical devices, and improving mental health service delivery. Included in the law is the Helping Families in Mental Health Crisis Act. This Act authorizes provisions to change or create governmental policies and improve the compliance of group health plans and insurance companies to provide parity coverage for mental health treatment as a means to improve people's access to effective mental health treatment. Specifically, the Helping Families in Mental Health Crisis Act

- Adds an Assistant Secretary for Mental Health and Substance Use Treatment (psychiatrist or psychologist) under Health and Human Services.
- Requires funding of services that are "evidence-based."
- Ensures that states use mental health block grant funds for the purposes of reducing suicides and suicide attempts, substance abuse, emergency hospitalization visits, arrests and incarcerations related to a mental illness, homelessness, and joblessness.
- Increases funding to states for assisted outpatient treatment.
- Changes in the Health Insurance Portability and Accountability Act (HIPAA) and Family Educational Rights and Privacy Act (FERPA) laws to allow, under certain conditions, service providers to share some limited information (diagnoses, treatment plans, appointment scheduling, medications, and medication-related instructions) with "caregivers."
- Changes the Medicaid Institutions for Mental Diseases (IMD) exclusion, which prohibits the use of federal Medicaid financing for care provided to most patients in mental health and substance use disorder residential treatment facilities larger than 16 beds.
- Returns the Protection and Advocacy for Individuals with Mental Illness Program (PAIMI) to its original mission of protecting patients against "abuse and neglect."
- Eliminates the 190-day lifetime cap on inpatient psychiatric hospitalization in Medicare if it is shown to be cost-effective.
- Allows for Medicaid payment for two services received in a single day (e.g., psychiatrist visit and case manager visit on same day).
- Requires formularies to include meds on their Hospital Discharge Procedures.
- Requires Medicare-reimbursed hospitals to prepare discharge plans and facilitate connection with outpatient treatment for patients whom they are discharging.
- Provides $40 million annually for 4 years for the National Institute of Mental Health to study violence to self and others plus the Brain Initiative.
- Authorizes the Minority Mental Health Workforce fellowships to increase the number of culturally competent behavioral health professionals.

- Mandates federal agencies, such as the Veterans Administration, Department of Justice, and Substance Abuse Mental Health Administration, to improve coordination among agencies.

The Helping Families in Mental Health Crisis Act also directed the Secretary of Health and Human Services to establish the Interdepartmental Serious Mental Illness Coordinating Committee (ISMICC). ISMICC membership consists of both federal and non-federal members. Federal members include the Secretary of Health and Human Services (designated as the committee chair), the Assistant Secretary for Mental Health and Substance Use, the Attorney General, the Secretary of Veterans Affairs, the Secretary of Defense, the Secretary of Housing and Urban Development, the Secretary of Education, the Secretary of Labor, the Administrator of the Centers for Medicare and Medicaid Services, and the Commissioner of Social Security. The non-federal, public members include adults treated for SMI, a parent or guardian of an adult child who has an SMI, a peer support specialist, mental illness researchers, mental health practitioners, and other professionals who have extensive experience interfacing with people with SMI or SED. Congress mandated ISMICC to provide two Reports to Congress (RTC). The first RTC, submitted at the end of 2017, reported on the current needs of people with mental illness, key advances in mental health research and strategies to improve services, and current strategies in federal agencies aimed at improving the lives of people living with mental illness. The RTC concludes with a chapter developed by the non-federal members of ISMICC that identifies five focus areas of recommendations.

Focus 1: Strengthen federal coordination to improve care

Focus 2: Access and engagement: make it easier to get good care

Focus 3: Treatment and recovery: close the gap between what works and what is offered

Focus 4: Increase opportunities for diversion and improve care for people with SMI and SED involved in the criminal and juvenile justice systems

Focus 5: Develop finance strategies to increase availability and affordability of care

The full 2017 RTC is available at https://www.samhsa.gov/ismicc. The second RTC is due at the end of 2022. This second RTC will address the progress made since the 2017 report and identify future directions. It will be exciting to see what advances occur as a result of the Cures Act. I hope that, unlike the initiatives of the New Freedom Commission, we will see true progress. The final report is meant to provide an update on all the changes, successes, barriers, and recommendations to continue the work to improve the lives of people with mental health problems.

The objective of *Understanding the Mental Health Problems of Children and Adolescents* is to provide a practical guide for social workers in promoting positive mental health in youth from a bio-socio-ecological systems perspective. Social workers will gain an understanding of the scope of mental health issues in youth to include definitions, etiology, and evidence-based treatments. Furthermore, social workers will understand the importance of partnering with youth and caregivers, addressing issues from a strengths perspective, and engaging in culturally sensitive practice. Social workers will want to take this work and apply it actively in their everyday work with clients.

The mental health scientific community is continually updating current knowledge in the field. On the date that the first edition of this book went to the publisher, the National Institute of Mental Health published a report, "Five Major Mental Disorders Share Same Genes," demonstrating that knowledge is fluid and that what we are presenting in this, the second edition, is the knowledge base at this moment in time. As reported, the largest study yet into genetics and mental health (Cross-Disorder Group, 2013) "reveals that the five most common disorders—autism, attention deficit hyperactivity disorder, bipolar disease, schizophrenia, and major depression—all share similar genetic components. . . . The results suggest that a rethink in how these disorders are defined might be in order. Rather than focusing on symptoms, which can be attributed to one or more disorder, physicians could one day start to rely on specific gene mutations or biologic pathways to make a formal diagnosis" (National Institute of Mental Health, 2013). Since this report in 2013, research on the underlying biology of mental illnesses has continued. In February 2018, a study was published that found mental disorders share a large overlap of genetic risk factors down to the molecular level (Gandal et al., 2018). Research advances in behavioral science and neuroscience have greatly improved our knowledge and understanding of mental illness. Magnetic resonance imaging (MRI) has allowed researchers to gain greater knowledge of brain development and changes in the brain related to mental illness. Brain research has given practitioners the evidence base that they have long been describing in behavioral, emotional, and psychological terms. This knowledge base will continue to grow and influence treatment.

However, despite the advances in research, stigma remains a major barrier that discourages individuals from seeking help. Analysis of consumer and public input has identified stigma as one of seven major categories to be addressed for mental health transformation (Center for Behavioral Health Statistics and Quality, 2011). Stigmatizing attitudes and behaviors toward individuals with mental health problems present multiple barriers that have severe consequences for quality of life. The New Freedom Commission identified stigma as one of three main obstacles that impede individuals with mental illness from receiving appropriate treatment. The consequences of stigma include delays in treatment, challenges to self-esteem, social isolation, discrimination, and lost opportunities in such areas as housing and employment. In addition to mental health stigma, the lack of treatments available to persons in the community is a huge barrier. The research on effective treatments for children with mental health problems has increased dramatically over the past several years, but many children lack access to these treatments for many reasons. And, although there has been an increase in knowledge of effective treatments, child welfare, juvenile justice, and community mental health systems have experienced a lag in adoption and implementation of evidence-based practices (EBPs) and program/treatments (EBTs) due to lack of funding streams and financial constraints, lack of infrastructure in agencies and communities, lack of a trained workforce, and provider resistance (Burns & Hoagwood, 2002; Hoagwood, 2001; Morris et al., 2010).

Compounding the challenge of embracing EBP in these child-serving sectors are organizational structures that are not amenable to adhering to the fidelity of empirically supported treatments (Hoagwood, 2001; Huang, Hepburn, & Espiritu, 2003; Jensen, Weersing, Hoagwood, & Goldman, 2005). Evidence-based practices and treatments have specified practices and processes (fidelity) that must be followed in order to realize the positive outcomes that are reported in the empirical literature (Fixsen, Naoom, Blase, Friedman, & Wallace, 2005). As a result, a vulnerable population of children in high need of these treatments does not receive them or does not receive them as developed. Failure to provide effective treatments to this population results in higher costs to systems. High-risk youth and families repeatedly reenter these systems, or youth end up being placed in more restrictive settings outside of their homes and communities. Not providing effective treatment can also result in long-term costs to these systems as untreated youth often carry their problems into adulthood, resulting in lost wages or repeated cycles of abuse or incarceration, to name a few of the possible consequences (Anderson, Wright, Kelley, & Koorman, 2008).

Diagnosing and the *Diagnostic and Statistical Manual*

In this book, the signs and symptoms of the most commonly diagnosed mental health disorders of childhood and adolescence will be reviewed, followed by a discussion of treatment. The diagnoses that will be the main focus of this book include depression, anxiety, bipolar disorder, attention deficit hyperactivity disorder, oppositional defiant disorder, conduct disorder, and schizophrenia/first-episode psychosis. We include brief discussions of eating disorders in the chapter on depressive disorders due to a high comorbidity of depression with eating disorders and autism spectrum disorders in the chapter on schizophrenia/first-episode psychosis because youth with schizophrenia are sometimes misdiagnosed as having autism. A person is diagnosed with a mental health problem or illness by a professional trained and authorized to make diagnoses following an extensive face-to-face evaluation. Psychiatrists, licensed professional counselors, nurse practitioners, licensed marriage and family counselors, and licensed clinical social workers are all professionals with the training and authority to diagnose mental health problems. During the face-to-face assessment, the clinician must determine if a person meets the diagnostic criteria for a specific mental health disorder. Clinicians in the United States are more likely to use the *Diagnostic and Statistical Manual of Mental Disorders* (DSM) published by the American Psychiatric Association (APA, 1994, 2000, 2013) when making diagnoses; all other countries use the International Classification of Diseases (ICD). The ICD, developed by the World Health Organization (1992), is the official coding system approved under HIPAA. Insurance companies in the United States require a psychiatric evaluation and assignment of a mental health diagnostic code using the ICD for authorization and reimbursement for services rendered. The latest version of the DSM, the DSM-5 (APA, 2013), was restructured from earlier versions that used a multiaxial system for diagnosing. The diagnostic codes of mental health disorders in the DSM are ICD codes.

DSM-5

The DSM provides a common language among mental health professionals and is used as a guide for organizing information and making accurate diagnoses. It also helps guide treatment planning and provides a common language for mental health researchers. The DSM-5 follows a dimensional approach to diagnosing and integrates the latest scientific knowledge of mental disorders throughout its pages. The structure of the DSM-5 is based on evidence that the boundaries between different mental health disorders are less clear-cut than once thought as many of the disorders share similar symptoms and similar genetic and environmental risk factors. Specifiers are used throughout the DSM-5 to document important factors that may have played a role in the development of a disorder. The structure of the DMS-5 takes a lifespan focus by presenting diagnoses on a continuum based on the stage in the life cycle where the disorder most commonly manifests, beginning with disorders thought to begin early in the developmental processes and ending with those that manifest in late adulthood. The diagnostic criteria for each mental health disorder indicate what specific symptoms must be present for each diagnosis and for how long they must have occurred. Exclusionary criteria are also specified for each disorder. Across all disorders, other plausible causes such as a medical condition, substance abuse, or other mental health conditions must be ruled out as the cause of the problems. This can be difficult because people often experience co-occurring problems. The first section of the DSM-5 presents neurodevelopmental disorders, which are those disorders that manifest during childhood development. Examples of neurodevelopmental disorders include intellectual disabilities, autism spectrum disorder, communication disorders, motor disorders, learning disorders, and attention deficit hyperactivity disorder. The next four sections focus on schizophrenia and psychotic disorders, bipolar and related disorders, depressive disorders, and anxiety disorders, respectively. Obsessive-compulsive disorders and related disorders comprise a section that includes disorders characterized by preoccupations and rituals. The final section addresses trauma- and stress-related disorders.

The DSM includes information on and a link to access free, valid, and reliable measurement tools to aid clinicians in making an accurate diagnosis and to use for monitoring a client's progress throughout treatment (APA, 2013). You can access the tools at http://www.psychiatry.org/psychiatrists/practice/dsm/dsm-5/online-assessment-measures.   Included   are   brief measures, called Level 1 Measures, that screen across 12 domains in children and adolescents (depression, anger, irritability, mania, anxiety, somatic symptoms, inattention, suicidal ideation/attempt, psychosis, sleep disturbance, repetitive thoughts and behaviors, and substance use). When a Level 1 domain is found to be elevated, Level 2 Measures allow for a more in-depth assessment of symptoms and facilitate differential diagnosis (APA, 2013).

What Every Child Needs for Good Mental Health

Although mental illness/mental health problems are the focus of this book, it is important to recognize factors important to good mental health. The ingredients needed for a child to develop good mental health are well recognized. Children need to receive unconditional love as well as encouragement, guidance, and appropriate discipline from their caregivers. Providing boundaries for youth, along with encouragement and guidance, allows them to safely explore their world and develop positive self-esteem and self-confidence. Children and adolescents need to live in an environment that is both physically and emotionally safe. Finally, to develop socially, they need to have relationships with peers near their own age with whom they can play, interact, and develop relationships.

A substantial share of children nationwide are estimated to have experienced at least one traumatic event, referred to as an adverse childhood experience (ACE) (Bethell, Davis, Gombojav, Stumbo, & Powers, 2017). Trauma, chaotic homes, violence, neglect, parental mental health problems, biology, and child temperament can all be contributing factors to the development of serious emotional and behavioral problems (Institute of Medicine, 2009). The United States has focused on crisis intervention rather than early identification and intervention. Evidence shows that we can make greater impact on mental health problems by identifying and treating them early on.

Although this book addresses diagnosing mental health disorders and discusses evidence-based practices and interventions specific to each disorder, it is important to consider the individual. The phrase "I am not my mental illness" was used in an anti-stigma campaign commissioned by the Mental Health Connection (MHC) of Tarrant County, a community collaborative of public and private agencies, individuals experiencing mental health problems, and their families with the intent to revolutionize mental health services in their community. It is important to interact with every person as an individual and not to make assumptions based on what we see on the surface or on a label given as a diagnosis. Although providing a diagnosis gives us a common language, the diagnosis should not be the only thing we see. Each person is unique and has strengths. Mental illness is one aspect of a person's life; it is not his or her entire life. Clinical practice should consider each person's uniqueness, strengths, determination, and needs, as well as the climate that surrounds him or her (ecological system model). As you will see in some of the case scenarios provided throughout this book, things are not always as they first appear.

Although we talk about a singular diagnosis, many people experience more than one mental health problem at a time. For example, more than 70 percent of youth diagnosed with depression have also have anxiety (73.3 percent) and nearly 50 percent (47.2 percent) have a behavior disorder (Ghandour et al., 2019). For youth with anxiety, 37.9 percent also have a depressive disorder, and 36.6 percent of youth with a behavior disorder also have depression (Ghandour et al., 2019). This can make determining the appropriate treatment challenging and involve sound clinical judgment. Although there are interventions found to be effective in treating nearly all mental health problems, the improvements are often modest and they are not effective for everyone. In addition, there are many barriers to accessing empirically supported treatments in the community: cost to implement and resistance from providers are among the major impediments. As you read this book, please keep these things in mind and critically assess your role in the provision of services to youth and families.

References

American Psychiatric Association. (1994). *Diagnostic and statistical manual of mental disorders* (4th ed.). Washington, DC: Author.

American Psychiatric Association. (2000). *Diagnostic and statistical manual of mental disorders* (4th ed., text revision). Washington, DC: Author.

American Psychiatric Association. (2013). *Diagnostic and statistical manual of mental disorders* (5th ed.). Washington, DC: Author.

Anderson, J. A., Wright, E. R., Kelley, K., & Koorman, H. (2008). Patterns of clinical functioning over time for young people served in a system of care. *Journal of Emotional and Behavioral Disorders, 16*, 90–104.

Bethell, C. D., Davis, M. B., Gombojav, N., Stumbo, S., & Powers, K. (2017). Issue Brief: A national and across state profile on adverse childhood experiences among children and possibilities to heal and thrive. Johns Hopkins Bloomberg School of Public Health.

Retrieved June 6, 2019, from https://www.cahmi.org/wp-content/uploads/2018/05/aces_brief_final.pdf

Burns, B. J., & Hoagwood, K. (Eds.). (2002). *Community treatment for youth: Evidence-based interventions for severe emotional and behavioral disorders.* New York: Oxford University Press.

Carney, M. M., & Buttell, F. (2003). Reducing juvenile recidivism: Evaluating the wraparound services model. *Research on Social Work Practice, 13,* 551–568.

Center for Behavioral Health Statistics and Quality. (2011). Results from the 2010 National Survey on Drug Use and Health: Summary of national findings (HHS Publication No. SMA 11-4658, NSDUH Series H-41). Rockville, MD: Substance Abuse and Mental Health Services Administration.

Clement, S., Schauman O., Graham, T., & Maggioni, F. (2015). What is the impact of mental health-related stigma on help-seeking? A systematic review of quantitative and qualitative studies. *Psychological Medicine, 45*(1), 11–27.

Cross-Disorder Group of the Psychiatric Genomics Consortium. (2013). Identification of risk loci with shared effects on five major psychiatric disorders: A genome-wide analysis. *Lancet, 381*(9875), 1371–1379. doi:10.1016/S0140-6736(12)62129-1

Fixsen, D. L., Naoom, S. F., Blase, K. A., Friedman, R. M., & Wallace, F. (2005). Implementation research: A synthesis of the literature (FMHI Publication 231). Tampa: University of South Florida, Louis de la Parte Florida Mental Health Institute, The National Implementation Research Network. Retrieved from http://nirn.fpg.unc.edu/sites/nirn.fpg.unc.edu/files/resources/NIRN-MonographFull-01-2005.pdf

Gandal, M. J., Haney, J. R., Parikshak, N. N., Leppa, V., Ramaswami, G., Hartl, C., et al.; CommonMind Consortium, PsychENCODE Consortium, iPSYCH-BROAD Working Group, Horvath, S., & Geschwind, D. H. (2018). Shared molecular neuropathology across major psychiatric disorders parallels polygenic overlap. *Science (New York, N.Y.), 359*(6376), 693–697. https://doi.org/10.1126/science.aad6469

Ghandour, R. M., Sherman, L. J., Vladutiu, C. J., Ali, M. M., Lynch, S. E., Bitsko, R. H., & Blumberg, S. J. (2019). Prevalence and treatment of depression, anxiety, and conduct problems in US children. *Journal of Pediatrics, 206,* 256–267.

Grande T., Hallman J., Caldwell K., & Underwood L. (2011). *Using the BASC-2 to assess mental health needs of incarcerated juveniles: Implications for treatment and release.* Alexandria, VA: Corrections Today.

Hoagwood, K. (2001). Evidence-based practice in children's mental health services: What do we know? Why aren't we putting it to use? *Emotional and Behavioral Disorders in Youth, Fall,* 84–87.

Huang, L. N., Hepburn, K. S., & Espiritu, R. C. (2003). To be or not to be . . . evidence-based? *Data Matters, 6,* 1–3.

Institute of Medicine. (2009). *Preventing mental, emotional, and behavioral disorders among young people: Progress and possibilities.* M. E. O'Connell, T. Boat, & K. E. Warner (Eds.). Washington, DC: National Academies Press.

Jensen, P. S., Weersing, R., Hoagwood, K. E., & Goldman, E. (2005). What is the evidence for evidence-based treatments? A hard look at our soft underbelly. *Mental Health Services Research, 7,* 53–74.

Kessler, R. C., Berglund, P., Demler, O., Jin, R., Merikangas, K. R., & Walters, E. E. (2005). Lifetime prevalence and age-of-onset distributions of DSM-IV disorders in the National Comorbidity Survey Replication. *Archives of General Psychiatry, 62,* 593–602.

Morris, J. A., Day, S., & Schoenwald, S. K. (2010). *Turning Knowledge into Practice, 2nd ed. (revised)*. Boston, MA: The Technical Assistance Collaborative, Inc., 15–16, http://bit.ly/1urQqVM.

National Academies of Sciences, Engineering, and Medicine. (2015). *Mental disorders and disabilities among low-income children*. Washington, DC: National Academies Press.

National Institute of Mental Health. (2013). Five major mental disorders share the same genes. Retrieved from http://www.nimh.nih.gov/news/science-news/2013/five-major-mental-disorders-share-the-same-genes.shtml

New Freedom Commission on Mental Health. (2003). *Achieving the promise: Transforming mental health care in America. Final report (DHHS Publication No. SMA-03-3832)*. Rockville, MD: Department of Health and Human Services.

Phillips, R. T. M. (2012). Health law: Predicting the risk of future dangerousness. *Virtual Mentor, 14*, 472–476.

Public Law 114-255. (2016). Retrieved June 5, 2019, from https://www.congress.gov/114/plaws/publ255/PLAW-114publ255.pdf

Satcher, D. S. (2000). Mental health: A report of the Surgeon General—Executive summary. *Public Health Reports, 115*, 89–101.

US General Accounting Office. (2003). Child welfare and juvenile justice: Federal agencies could play a stronger role in helping states reduce the number of children placed solely to obtain mental health services. Retrieved from http://www.gao.gov/highlights/d03397high.pdf

U.S. Department of Health and Human Services. (2009). Substance Abuse and Mental Health Services Administration: Justification of estimates for Appropriations Committees. Rockville, MD: U.S. Department of Health and Human Services, Substance Abuse and Mental Health Services Administration, Center for Mental Health Services, National Institutes of Health, National Institute of Mental Health. Retrieved from http://beta.samhsa.gov/sites/default/files/samhsa_cj2009.pdf

2

Framework for Understanding and Treating Mental Health Problems

As an overarching framework, this book emphasizes the importance of five components when working with children and families with mental health problems: the ecological systems model, systems of care, evidence-based practices and programs, cultural humility, and engagement and strengths-based practices.

Ecological Systems Model

The ecological systems model provides the wide lens for understanding the multiple layers within the family system. It goes beyond assessing relations and interactions between the parent and youth to look at the effects of all systems in the youth's environment. According to the theory, a developing individual is affected by the environments in which he or she resides as well as by settings in which he or she is not present (Bronfenbrenner, 1979). In effect, the individual affects those environments. A person cannot be studied without including his or her environment in the analysis. The components of ecological systems are the microsystems, mesosystems, exosystems, and macrosystems. The *microsystem* in which a person resides (e.g., a child's family) has the most influence. The *mesosystem* includes settings outside the microsystem in which an individual participates. The child's school and peer group are examples of mesosystems. Individuals are members of multiple social groups, or mesosystems, at the same time.

A setting such as the workplace of a child's parent is an *exosystem* to a child. A child may not have direct contact with the workplace of a parent, yet the workplace affects the child, and the child affects the workplace. For instance, a parent who is overstressed by pressures of employment may lack energy to provide a child adequate attention and care. On the other hand, a parent

Understanding the Mental Health Problems of Children and Adolescents. Kirstin Painter and Maria Scannapieco,
Oxford University Press (2021). © Oxford University Press. DOI: 10.1093/oso/9780190927844.003.0002

may perform poorly at work due to stress resulting from difficult issues with a child or may miss days at work due to the child's mental health problems.

The cultural context of a person's life, including society's dominant beliefs, ideas, social values, laws, resources, and cultural norms lie within the outermost level of the social ecological system, the macrosystem. The macrosystem is the largest and most distant setting of influence. It is within the macrosystem where a person's race, ethnicity, and socioeconomic status reside. The macrosystem influences the interactions of all the other systems in the social ecology, which in turn, influence the child.

People continuously attempt to adapt to their environment. Either they try to improve the fit between themselves and their environment, or they try to sustain a good fit (Germain & Bloom, 1999). Understanding the adaptations a child has developed to fit in his or her environment is a key factor to treating the child. It is also important to identify factors in the ecological system model that either facilitate or impede adaptation. Individuals are usually able to adapt to conventional environments, but they may struggle to adapt during stressful times or in conditions in which they have special needs or limitations.

As life events occur, people deal with them either positively or negatively, depending on their perception of the event. The way in which the person views an event will allow him or her to either cope with it and achieve a successful resolution or prevent him or her from coping with it and lead to an unsuccessful resolution. The response of the individual will affect both the environment and the individual. Successful resolution leads to personal development and/or environmental change.

To understand a life event, one must fully consider all aspects of the person–environment, including all of the systems and subsystems that affect adaptation. These systems and subsystems include a person's cognitive, biological, affective, and behavioral structures, in addition to subsystems of the environment. The relationship between people and the environments in which they are embedded is dynamic. A circular relationship exists in that a change in one area of the system will affect all other levels of the system. Changes in the system will thus affect the individual. We either adapt to our environment or seek to change it. An example of *reciprocation and exchange* can be seen when a child or adolescent is placed in a residential treatment facility to receive mental health treatment aimed at improving problem behaviors. Typically, the child or adolescent fights against the new environment and resists change, yet eventually he or she adapts and problem behaviors improve. If the family does not make changes in the home environment aimed at sustaining the child's or adolescent's behavior changes, the problem behaviors will eventually return. Each element of the system affects another.

Mental health problems develop from multilayered interactions between the youth and the environment. A therapist must consider the dimensions of human temperament and personality in addition to the external environment, culture, and socioeconomic existence of the youth and family. Effective intervention in a youth's mental health problems requires assessment of personal factors (biological, genetic, and psychological) as well as factors across the entire ecology to understand what sustains or diminishes the problem behavior. How does the youth normally react to stressful situations? Does the youth currently have the tools needed to be successful socially and emotionally? Is there a familial genetic predisposition that puts the youth at a higher risk for a certain problem? These are just some of the questions to examine.

The logic of the ecological system model is one of its strengths, allowing it to take into account a larger relationship than do linear models. It allows one to see factors in the environment that may either impede or provide an opportunity for a person's growth. The ecological system model allows for a more complete assessment of a situation and provides more information than general systems theory because it encourages the assessment of interactions between systems. Thus, it expands a social worker's thinking about the causes of problems and allows interventions focused on the total picture rather than only the personal factors.

Systems of Care

Systems of care, initially proposed in the mid-1980s, is a family-centered, strengths-based service delivery model (Stroul, Blau, & Friedman, 2010). Within systems of care, community-based supports and services are organized to meet the challenges of children with serious mental health needs and their families. In 1993, the systems of care movement was enhanced by the development of the Comprehensive Community Mental Health Services for Children and Their Families Program (Center for Mental Health Services, 2006), the most significant federal investment in children's mental health to that date, developed to address the critical problems experienced by youth with serious emotional disturbances (SEDs) and their families. Referrals to systems of care come from a range of child service agencies including schools, and child welfare, state mental health, juvenile justice, and parole and probation agencies. Systems of care seek to remove the silos among juvenile justice, mental health, and child welfare systems and empower families not only to make decisions about their own treatment, but also to affect policy and practice. Developing systems of care is a national movement. A key philosophical underpinning of systems of care is that youth and families are equal partners with equal voice working alongside professionals in the treatment process. Family empowerment has been noted to be a key mediator in improving children's mental health. Treating the youth and family as an equal partner in all decision-making is a major paradigm shift for child welfare, juvenile justice, and mental health systems.

In an effort to provide effective care for children with SEDs consistent with the values and principles of systems of care, many states and communities have adopted the *wraparound process* of mental health care and management (Bruns & Suter, 2010; Burns, Goldman, Faw, & Burchard, 1999; Furman & Jackson, 2002; Suter & Bruns, 2009). Wraparound has been described as a promising practice for treating youth experiencing severe emotional or behavioral problems. It has been identified as both a philosophy and a process of providing supports and services to youth with SEDs and their families and a tool for implementing systems of care. In wraparound, a child and family team is developed based on the desires of the family. Team members may include family members, friends, schoolteachers, pastors, mental health professionals, or any other persons important to the family. A wraparound facilitator guides the team to develop, implement, and monitor a comprehensive service plan. The service plan, developed from the individual needs, strengths, and desires of the family, draws on both formal resources (including evidence-based practices and programs) and informal services and community supports aimed at improving the mental health of the child and keeping him or her in the community.

Evidence-Based Practices and Evidence-Based Programs

The literature is increasingly emphasizing the importance of *evidence-based practice* (EBP) and *evidence-based programs* or *treatment* (EBT). At the same time, there is confusion about what they mean and also controversy about what level of science exists to designate treatments and interventions as evidence-based. How is evidence determined? Many question where clinical experience fits into EBT. So, just exactly what is meant by these terms? These are important issues to understand as we begin to incorporate EBT and EBP into practice with families and children.

The terms "evidence-based practice" and "evidence-based treatment" are often used interchangeably; however, they do not refer to the same things. In mental health treatment, an EBP refers to the provision of clinical practices or techniques that are based on the best available research evidence to achieve the best positive outcomes. The American Psychological Association defines EBP as "the integration of the best available research with clinical expertise in the context of patient characteristics, culture, and preferences" (American Psychological Association Presidential Task Force, 2006).

An evidence-based program (treatment) refers to a multicomponent intervention based on a combination of empirically supported EBPs (core components) that have been highly researched and found to be effective in meeting targeted outcomes. These multicomponent programs are based on the theoretical underpinnings of the ecological system model in conjunction with other theoretical perspectives such as cognitive, behavioral, and social learning theories. Some EBTs follow a more theoretical approach to treatment based on the individual needs of a youth and family, whereas others utilize a manualized approach following a specific protocol. In some instances, mental health providers have been reluctant to use many of the programs or treatments, particularly those that are manualized, feeling that they take their clinical skill and perspective out of the treatment equation. Although most manualized approaches encourage adherence to the treatment, many also encourage integrating the individual clinical skills and uniqueness of the treatment provider into the treatment.

The profession of social work began incorporating EBP models into the professional literature around 2003. Today, the literature is increasingly emphasizing its importance. Although there has been increased emphasis in the literature on the importance of EBT and early identification and treatment of youth with mental health problems, there is a lack of social workers trained in mental health issues of children and EBP and/or EBT. Evidence-based interventions and practices are not being taught in university settings or in community child service settings. Social workers in the workforce are uninformed about EBP/EBT and mental health issues of childhood because of their lack of access to relevant training. A possible contributor to the lack of social worker training is the controversy surrounding EBP and EBT. In particular, most, if not all, EBT models require focused training and ongoing clinical supervision from the developer or organization.

The National Association of Social Workers (NASW) has adopted an approach to EBP that is inclusive of knowledge based on research, clinical skills, and individual determination of those receiving services. Our knowledge is constantly growing, and practices are adapted or new treatments emerge based on the best available research. The onus is on all of us to contribute to this knowledge, to understand what this knowledge is telling us, and to understand the gaps in our knowledge. In past years, excluding empirical evidence from clinical treatment has resulted in practitioners providing treatments that not only lack evidence of effectiveness but that have been, in some instances, found to be ineffective or even harmful. Examples of harmful interventions include *boot camps* for youth experiencing acting-out behaviors and *rebirthing* for children diagnosed with reactive attachment disorder. Empirical research indicates that sending youth to boot camp to manage acting-out behaviors can further exacerbate their problems, for example by increasing anger at caregivers for putting them into harsh conditions away from friends and family, not acknowledging their underlying need for and providing mental health treatment, and exposing them to other youth with similar or worse problems. At least two children have died from rebirthing, in which they are put into a fetal position and swaddled in a wrap such as a blanket to represent the womb. Therapists then simulate labor contractions by putting pressure on the womb and the child fights his or her way out as a way to bond with the caregiver.

Throughout this book, we will refer to and differentiate among existing EBPs and EBTs for different mental health disorders. However, we should remember not to ignore our own clinical judgment, the strengths and needs of the people we work with, or the evidence base as it exists at each moment. Similarly, we should continue to pursue new knowledge and incorporate it into treatment.

Cultural Humility

The disproportionality of minority children, especially African American children, in both the child welfare and criminal justice systems has been well documented over the years. Overrepresentation of minority children and families refers to the difference between their representation at a particular time in the child welfare or juvenile justice system compared to their representation in the general population during the same time period. Minority children account for 15 percent of the US child population; however, they represent 37 percent of the children who are involved in the child welfare system (Wulczyn & Lery, 2007).

Compounding the issue of the disproportionality of minority children in the child welfare and juvenile justice systems is the percentage of youth in these systems needing mental health care. In the United States, nearly 1 million children each year come into contact with the child welfare system because they are victims of child abuse or neglect. Many are at high risk of mental health problems resulting from maltreatment, removal from their homes, and/or the trauma of investigation and intervention by child welfare. The percentages of children with clinically significant emotional or behavioral problems in both systems have been found to be much higher than in the general population. Nationally, it is estimated that 50–80 percent of youth investigated for child maltreatment experience significant mental health problems. In the juvenile justice system, estimates of youths experiencing mental health problems are as high as 65 or 70 percent.

The disparity in the number of minority youth accessing mental health care, the quality of care they receive, and their representation in mental health research has been highly acknowledged in the literature. This disparity is mirrored in the child welfare and juvenile justice systems as well. Minority youth receive fewer services such as birth family visits, developmental and psychological assessments, worker contacts, treatment plans, and mental health services than do white youth.

The National Association of Social Workers Code of Ethics (NASW, 2008) states that

(a) Social workers should understand culture and its function in human behavior and society, recognizing the strengths that exist in all cultures.
(b) Social workers should have a knowledge base of their clients' cultures and be able to demonstrate competence in the provision of services that are sensitive to clients' cultures and to differences among people and cultural groups.
(c) Social workers should obtain education about and seek to understand the nature of social diversity and oppression with respect to race,

ethnicity, national origin, color, sex, sexual orientation, gender identity or expression, age, marital status, political belief, religion, immigration status, and mental or physical disability.

One way of addressing these core values and practice effectively is through *cultural humility*. Ortega and Coulborn Faller (2011) first adopted cultural humility in social work as an approach for working with diverse populations. Cultural humility complements cultural competence by moving away from the notion of understanding similar cultural characteristics within a cultural to understanding individuals and their unique experiences.

Cultural humility embraces a multicultural perspective and an intersectionality approach to understanding behavior, viewing the importance of knowledge, beliefs, values, morals, customs, language, and behaviors in relation to the many cultures one interacts with such as gender identity, class, race, age, occupation, and disability (Hoffman, 2013; Ortega & Coulborn, 2011).

When working with families and children who are experiencing mental health issues, the social worker applying a cultural humility perspective will view the family or child as the expert on their own culture. Cultural humility challenges us to learn from those we work with and to withhold judgment so that we may bridge the cultural divide between different perspectives to promote well-being.

Engagement and Strengths-Based Practice

Many would argue that it is the relationship with the social worker rather than the provision of an EBP or EBT that helps clients reach their goals. Youth and family engagement and strengths-focused problem-solving are critical ingredients in the helping process of social work. Most or all social workers would probably agree. On paper and in theory, these concepts sound good. But what do they really mean, and how does engagement and strengths-focused problem-solving look in practice?

Although we as social workers agree with the values and ethics of social work, we often find ourselves telling our clients what is best for them and what the consequences will be if they choose to ignore our warnings. This can be particularly true of social workers working in juvenile justice, child welfare, and community mental health settings. We get our college degree and enter the workforce armed with the values of our profession, filled with the desire to make a difference in others' lives. In the new work environment, we may start to take on the culture of the agency in which we work, which is made up of persons from many backgrounds and degree programs with varying views. Our intent is good, but we may lose our vision somewhere along the way.

It is important to revisit the practice of social work and our own role and practice. Although research is very clear on the correlation of high levels of engagement and positive outcomes, it is difficult to break out of patterns developed within the culture of an agency. We begin to use phrases such as those stating that the client is "resistant to change" or "resistant to participating in treatment." We even use the social work value of *self-determination* as a reason to discharge youth and families from services, claiming that they have a right to make the choices they make and a right to experience the consequences of those choices. Engaging families requires us to thoroughly examine the situation when a family is not engaging. Lack of engagement is unlikely to occur because a caregiver wants to keep harming his or her child or the youth wants to end up in a detention facility. Problems with engagement can be caused by one condition or a culmination of situations with the family, the individual worker, and the agency.

One possible reason for lack of engagement is that family members have worked with several persons in the helping profession and have not received the help they need. They may feel that you are just another person in a string of people who will not be able to meet their needs. Past experience may have discouraged their belief that things can get better. Alternatively, the family may be experiencing such a large amount of stress or chaos that thinking about trying to add anything into the mix seems daunting, even if you tell them that it will change things in the future. Due to stereotypes in the media and other venues, many people believe that the only role and purpose of social workers is to take away their children. Other reasons may include the family's lack of transportation, long working hours, or focus on daily necessities such as providing food or meeting the rent.

Your own characteristics or situations and/or those of the agency may block engagement. It is easy to get bogged down with heavy caseloads, documentation requirements, and agency rules and regulations. Such distractions may cause us to miss the factors that prevent us from engaging with families. The stress in our lives can engulf us and leave us without the energy needed to engage with families. Engagement requires work on the front end, but it makes the middle and end of our journey with youth and families much more productive and satisfying.

What other reasons can you think of that may cause barriers to engagement? Think through the question and write down as many reasons as you can. Next, think about and write down some tactics you as the social worker can use to overcome each barrier. Be creative in your tactics. Sometimes the smallest of gestures will go far in building relationships. Remember that every individual and family you work with will have unique situations. It is incumbent on you as the social worker to determine the issues that are relevant in each situation. The more things you can identify as possible barriers, the more prepared you will be when you work with families.

Exercise: Barriers and Solutions to Engagement

Barrier 1:
Possible Solution(s):
Barrier 2:
Possible Solution(s):
Barrier 3:
Possible Solution(s):
Barrier 4:
Possible Solution(s):

Case Studies

Following are some real-life examples of things social workers have done to engage families. As you read these scenarios, think about the barriers and solutions you identified. Do these scenarios spark any other ideas?

Jenny is a social worker at a community mental health center. She is having difficulty meeting with a mother to get paperwork signed so that she can start working with Jon, the woman's 6-year-old son. The mother canceled one meeting and was not home when Jenny arrived for a second meeting. When Jenny was able to talk to the mother on the phone later that day, the mother sounded frustrated. She vented about missing the second meeting because she had taken the bus to the food stamp office.

She had to change buses twice to get there, and she missed the second bus. By the time she finally arrived at the food stamp office, she had missed her appointment and had to reschedule for the next week. This left her without the needed food stamps, so she took the bus to a food pantry to get some food, but she wasn't able to get enough to last until her next appointment because she couldn't carry much. Recognizing the situation that the mother was in and the frustration she was experiencing, Jenny offered to drive her to the food pantry the next day and to drive her to the food stamp office for the next appointment. On the way to the food pantry, Jenny was able to chat with the mother. After she took the mother to the food pantry, they sat down and completed the paperwork needed to get Jon into services.

In another situation, a social worker, Otis, was assigned to work with Nguyen and his family, who had been given the option of participating in a diversionary program or sending Nguyen to a detention center. The family chose the program. As part of the program, they were to meet with Otis a couple of times every week. However, both parents worked two jobs and did not have time to meet with Otis. They worked together in the evening cleaning offices. They made Nguyen go to work with them in the evening to keep him out of trouble. Otis asked if he could meet with the family while they cleaned offices. Otis even helped clean offices so the parents had some time to sit and work with him.

Both Jenny and Otis could have said that the family would not or could not meet with them and discharged the family rather than trying to seek a solution. This would have meant that Jon would not have received the needed treatment and Nguyen would have been locked up in detention. Other social workers have done things such as offering to bring pizza to the family for dinner so that they could meet.

References

American Psychological Association Presidential Task Force on Evidence-based Practice. (2006). Evidence-based practice in psychology. *American Psychologist, 61*, 271–285.

Bronfenbrenner, U. (1979). *The ecology of human development: Experiments by nature and design.* Cambridge, MA: Harvard University Press.

Bruns, E. J., & Suter, J. C. (2010). Summary of the wraparound evidence-base. In E. J. Bruns & J. S. Walker (Eds.), *The resource guide to wraparound* (Chapter 3.2, 1–12). Portland, OR: National Wraparound Initiative.

Burns, B. J., Goldman, S. K., Faw, L., & Burchard, J. D. (1999). The wraparound evidence base. In B. J. Burns & S. K. Goldman (Eds.), *Promising practices in wraparound for children with severe emotional disorders and their families* (pp. 77–95). Rockville, MD: Center for Mental Health Services.

Center for Mental Health Services. (2006). *Annual report to Congress on the evaluation of the Comprehensive Community Mental Health Services for Children and Their Families Program, 2001.* Atlanta, GA: ORC Macro.

Furman, R., & Jackson, R. (2002). Wrap-around services: An analysis of community-based mental health services for children. *Journal of Child and Adolescent Psychiatric Nursing, 15,* 124–131.

Germain, C. B., & Bloom, M. (1999). *Human behavior in the social environment: An ecological view* (2nd ed.). New York: Columbia University Press.

Hoffman, M. (2013). Cultural humility: A lifelong practice. Retrieved from https://socialwork.sdsu.edu/insitu/diversity/cultural-humility-a-lifelong-practice/

National Association of Social Workers (NASW). (2008). *Social Workers Code of Ethics.* Washington, DC: Author.

Ortego, R. M., & Coulborn Faller, K. (2011). Training child welfare workers from an intersectional cultural humility perspective: A paradigm shift. *Child Welfare, 90*(5), 27–49.

Stroul, B., Blau, G., & Friedman, R. (2010). Updating the system of care concept and philosophy. Washington, DC: Georgetown University Center for Child and Human Development, National Technical Assistance Center for Children's Mental. Retrieved from Health. https://gucchdtacenter.georgetown.edu/resources/Call%20Docs/2010Calls/SOC_Brief2010.pdf

Suter, J. C., & Bruns, E. J. (2009). Effectiveness of the wraparound process for children with emotional and behavioral disorders: A meta-analysis. *Clinical Child Family Psychological Review, 12,* 336–351.

Wulczyn, F., & Lery, B. (2007). *Racial disparity in foster care admissions.* Chicago: Chapin Hall Center for Children at the University of Chicago.

3

Overview of Child and Youth Development

This book focuses on youth from 6–18 years of age. This chapter is a summary and brief overview of the major developmental milestones and characteristics of the children and youth in this age range. It will exclude infancy-toddlerhood and early childhood and begin with children entering middle childhood. (For a full overview, see Scannapieco & Connell-Carrick, 2005; Hutchison, 2018, 2019.) At the end of the chapter we discuss sound techniques for working with youth.

Middle Childhood

There is great diversity among children and families in the United States, but generally we view middle childhood as a time for education, team play, social activities, and other forms of leisure. Development takes place within the domains of physical, social, and cognitive dimensions (see Table 3.1). Each of these domains will be presented separately, but they occur in an interactive, dynamic fashion.

Middle childhood extends from 6 to 11 years of age. During this time, children enter formal school, and academics and social relationships become increasingly important. Overall, the primary developmental task of middle childhood is the acquisition of new skills—cognitive, social, and physical—and children have school as a new forum for exploration. During what are sometimes called the *school years*, children not only learn the foundations of math, reading, writing, and science, but they also practice their social skills with their peer group.

Understanding the Mental Health Problems of Children and Adolescents. Kirstin Painter and Maria Scannapieco, Oxford University Press (2021). © Oxford University Press. DOI: 10.1093/oso/9780190927844.003.0003

Table 3.1 Middle childhood healthy development (6–11 years)

Psychodynamic

Freud	Erickson
Latency:	*Industry versus inferiority:*

• Sexual instincts decrease. • The superego develops further with more influence from peer relationships and less from family. • Children put their energy into activities, such as school and sports, and their sexual needs become inert.	• Children busily try to master the activities valued by their culture. • The positive resolution of this crisis is the development of industry whereby children feel competent and productive in their ability. • Children continue to master new skills and continue to develop social skills and friendships. • The negative resolution of inferiority manifests as children feel unable to do anything well.

Social

- Children engage in organized games with rules.
- Social cognition develops; children begin to understand their social world.
- Peer groups become increasingly important, which helps develop self-concept and self-competence.
- Acceptance by peer groups is valued, but personal friendships are more important.
- Perspective taking increases.
- Children develop a more realistic level of self-competence and self-esteem.
- Peer interaction becomes more pro-social.

Cognitive (Piaget)

Concrete operational stage: Reasoning and logical thought begin.

- Children are able to conserve and organize objects into hierarchies.
- Children have the ability to interpret experiences objectively rather than intuitively.
- Children understand logical principles and apply them to concrete situations, not hypothetical situations.
- Children understand identity, reversibility, seriation, and spatial reasoning.
- Children still fail to have abstract reasoning.
- Improvement in memory occurs, including an ability to remember facts over a period of days.
- Memory strategies improve: rehearsal, organization, and elaboration.
- Vocabulary at age 6 should be 10,000 words.
- Selective attention develops, which becomes important for school and learning.
- Metacognition develops, which is the ability to evaluate a cognitive task to determine whether it is difficult or not.
- Code switching in language emerges: formal and informal codes are used in communicating with adults and friends, respectively.

(Continued)

Table 3.1 *Continued*

Physical

- Children grow more slowly.
- Children have slimmer bodies with stronger muscles.
- Gross motor skills of running, jumping, batting, and kicking are performed more quickly and with better coordination.
- Reaction time improves in relation to cognitive development.
- Flexibility, hand-eye coordination, balance, force, agility, and judgment of movement improve.
- Fine motor development improves (e.g., building models or weaving on small looms).
- Printing improves from large letters to smaller letters.
- Drawing improves with two-dimensional shapes, depth, and converging lines.

Expected Development over Developmental Domains

Psychodynamic Theories

Freud's Psychosexual Stages of Development. Freud's fourth stage of psychosexual development is called the *latency stage* and occurs between 6 and 11 years of age. During the latency period, sexual instincts subside and become dormant. Instead of putting their energy into psychosexual activities, children focus on more conservative tasks including school and sports. In previous stages, children were influenced primarily by their parents. The latency stage exposes children to formal education and the opportunities that it offers; thus, children are influenced by their peers, their teachers, and the leaders of their organized activities. Their superegos continue to develop as a result of external influences.

Erickson's Psychosocial Stages of Development. During middle childhood, the psychosocial conflict proposed by Erickson is that of *industry versus inferiority.* During the school years, children try to master new cognitive and physical activities. They learn to cooperate, share, and problem-solve with other children, and, as a result, a sense of industry arises. Children with a resolution of industry feel competent at accomplishing tasks alone and with others. However, when children do not acquire the ability to work with others or they have negative experiences in completing solitary activities, they develop a sense of inferiority. Not all children have the same opportunities, and some may be more vulnerable due to poverty, community violence, and school inequities. In these cases, children may have had negative experiences when attempting tasks. Children who do not resolve the psychosocial crisis with inferiority feel incompetent.

Physical Development

Children from 6 to 11 years of age grow more slowly than they do earlier; on average they grow 2–3 inches and gain 3–5 pounds per year. Girls experience their adolescent growth spurt before boys, which may result in girls growing quickly in both height and weight toward the end of this period. Children's bodies become slimmer, and the lower portions of their bodies grow faster. Children may grow out of their jeans faster than their jackets as their legs grow longer. During middle childhood children commonly complain of growing pains, or nighttime aches and pains that occur as their muscles grow and adapt to their changing bodies. They should continue to receive regular medical and dental checkups as primary teeth are gradually replaced by permanent teeth.

Motor Development

During middle childhood children continue both their fine and gross motor development. Gross motor development improves, with children being able to successfully play organized activities and group sports with rules. Throwing, swimming, and climbing improve. These skills are demonstrated with better coordination and more quickly than ever before. Children also become better at bicycle riding, swimming, and ballet, which require good coordination.

Children from 6 to 11 years of age have greater flexibility, balance, agility, and force. The combination of their gross motor developmental changes and their cognitive changes allows children to play sports well; they make quick decisions as they develop skilled movements. As an example, school-aged children play baseball with a strong, quick, and flexible swing, and they demonstrate the ability to abide by the rules.

Fine motor development also continues throughout middle childhood. Children in this period should begin to print letters and learn cursive handwriting. They should be able to print and write stories, and their written words become clearer with age. Similarly, drawing improves so that by the end of this period children can make two- and three-dimensional drawings with attention to detail, depth, and lines. However, girls develop fine motor skills, including drawing and handwriting, faster than boys, and girls outperform boys on gross motor skills that require balance and agility, such as jumping. On the other hand, boys outperform girls in throwing and kicking, primarily due to environmental influences and practice rather than genetics.

Cognitive Development

According to Piaget's theory of cognitive development, children enter the middle childhood years during the second stage—*preoperational thought*—and finish this phase at the third stage—*concrete operational thought*. This stage is marked by the child's ability to distinguish reality from perception. During this period, children are capable of more logical thought; they are able to process operations that require compliance with logical rules. For example, children can pass conservation tasks in which they must focus on more than one aspect of the task in order to solve the problem appropriately. In the early childhood stage, if a child were asked to choose between two beakers with equal amounts of liquid but different shapes, he or she would choose the taller beaker. In this stage, the child would recognize that the beaker being taller does not mean that it has more liquid but that the shape of the glass affects the appearance of the liquid.

Children between 6 and 11 years of age experience an improvement in memory. Children can retrieve stored information for days or longer. They also demonstrate selective attention, whereby they are able to screen out distractions and focus on the important information. For example, during class the 10-year-old will be able to pay attention to the teacher while ignoring and forgetting disruptions from nearby classmates. Thus, the child selectively tunes in to the important information being presented by the teacher. Children also begin to use strategies to improve their memory, such as rehearsal, elaboration, and organization. Rehearsal, or repeating information over and over in an attempt to remember it, begins early in this period. Elaboration involves creating a shared meaning between two or more pieces of information that are not in the same category.

Children in middle childhood focus on both the physical attributes and inner traits of a person. A child may describe a person physically, but add that the person is dull or kind, referring to inner traits. Children at this stage are capable of *perspective taking*, or the ability and capacity to understand what others may be thinking or feeling. They consider the perspective of another person in relation to their own thoughts and those of others, and this helps them to understand consequences, such as getting in trouble or offending a friend. Acquiring a more mature level of perspective-taking is important because without it children risk offending peers and further isolating themselves from social relationships.

Social Development

As indicated by Erickson's psychosocial theory, the acquisition of feelings of self-competence is the major developmental task during this period. Children become more complicated social beings as they enter school and new opportunities arise. Changes in self-esteem, self-concept, and peer relationships occur.

As children mature, they begin to become more interested in peer relationships and they become more independent. Their relationships with their parents is still important; however, school friendships and lifelong friendships emerge. Playing together is no longer the essential measure of friendship, and qualities such as trust and loyalty begin to define true friendships. After children are able to identify friends through more mature characteristics, they use these friendships to practice conflict resolution and joint problem-solving. Consistent with their understanding of internal characteristics and their gains in cognitive development, children also make social comparisons; they begin to more realistically appraise their own behavior and skills compared to those of their peers.

Children understand their proficiency relative to that of another peer, which is influenced by their cognitive development and their expanding social worlds. Friendships during middle childhood tend to be gender-segregated and occur around shared activities.

With more realistic self-appraisal, children adjust their self-esteem to fit their perceptions and evaluations of self. As a result, self-esteem tends to drop during the first years of elementary school but increases again from fourth to sixth grade. By age 6, children have separated their self-esteem into three different domains: academic, social, and physical. They are able to appraise themselves in each of these three areas; for example, a child may have high academic self-esteem but less social self-esteem.

Aggression is still common in middle childhood, but to a lesser degree than in the previous developmental period. By middle childhood, children have learned the cultural and social rules that govern acceptable behavior. Society also expects children to be more able to control their anger by the time they reach middle childhood. At any rate, girls and boys tend to express their anger in different ways. Girls tend to use more *relational aggression*—nonphysical aggression aimed at damaging another's self-esteem or peer relationships. For example, a girl may try to ostracize another child or belittle her among friends. On the other hand, boys tend to use more physical force to express anger. However, both sexes exhibit increased aggression aimed at retaliating against someone who has injured them, called *retaliatory aggression*. Although peers accept retaliatory aggression, it is not accepted by parents, teachers, and coaches.

Peer groups also become an important component of middle childhood. Although true friendships are valued, acceptance by peer groups is also sought. Peer groups tend to be informal, with their own language and vocabulary, and they have a special identity. The peer group has collective goals, leadership, and loyalty. Often it can take the form of a group that engages in organized activities, such as a soccer or basketball team. Another example of the influence of peer groups will be discussed in the section on adolescence. Children switch their language when speaking with adults and peers to reflect the formality of the situation.

Adolescence

Adolescence is a transitional time between childhood and emerging adulthood characterized by profound biological, cognitive, and social changes. According to much of the recent developmental theory, it begins at age 12 and ends roughly around age 24 (Sokol, 2009). Although current developmental theory may extend adolescence until age 20, this chapter will focus on adolescence from 12 to 18, when a child becomes a legal adult in the eyes of the court.

Adolescence is marked by changes in physical, cognitive, and social development (see Table 3.2). The most obvious changes are those that are visible, whereas mood and social changes tend to be the most difficult for adolescents and others to understand. Teens may become sexually active with peers, and they may become pregnant. They are exploring their own identities, trying to find out who they are and what they really believe. They are spending more time away from home with friends, who become even more influential and important than before.

Table 3.2 Adolescent development characteristics

Psychodynamic

Freud	Erickson
Genital:	*Identity versus role confusion*:

- With puberty sexual impulses reemerge.
- The genitals are the focus of pleasure and the young person seeks sexual stimulation and satisfaction.

- Adolescents try to discover a self-identity through political, social, sexual, and career identities.
- The primary job of adolescents is to establish intimate ties with others.

- Adolescents who have had previous negative resolutions have difficulty establishing ties to others and are confused about their identity and roles.

Social

- Parent–adolescent conflict and moodiness increase, but vary depending upon age, gender, and culture.
- Friendships become even more important and influential.
- Peer groups are important and based on similar interests and values.
- Loyalty and intimacy are crucial to friendships.
- Peer pressure has both constructive and destructive abilities.
- Sexual and romantic relationships begin.

Cognitive (Piaget)

Formal operational stage:

- Adolescents have the ability for abstract thought and scientific reasoning.
- Hypothetical reasoning is possible, and problems are approached with logic and reasoning.
- Adolescents can think about ideas rather than only concrete events.
- As a result, ethics and social and moral issues become even more interesting.
- With increases in hypothetical and abstract thought, adolescents have better ability to argue.
- Metacognition and emotional regulation are enhanced.
- With age, adolescents become better at decision making and planning.
- Adolescent egocentrism develops whereby the adolescent focuses on himself or herself, believing that his or her thoughts, beliefs, and feelings are unique experiences.
- The *invincibility fable* emerges: a way of thinking in which adolescents feel immune to the dangers of their behaviors.

Physical

- Puberty begins.
- For girls, puberty sparks the onset of breast growth, initial pubic hair, peak growth spurt, widening of hips, and first menstrual period.

(Continued)

Table 3.2 *Continued*

- For boys, puberty sparks the onset of pubic hair, growth of testes and penis, first ejaculation, growth spurt, voice deepening, and beard development.
- The average age of menarche is 12.5 years.
- For girls, motor performance peaks and then levels off.
- The average age of spermarche is 13.
- Adolescents may have sexual intercourse.

Expected Development over Developmental Domains

Psychodynamic Theories

Freud's Psychosexual Stages of Development. Freud's sixth stage of psychosexual development is the *genital stage*, which begins in adolescence and lasts through adulthood. The adolescent's primary focus is on sexual pleasure and stimulation, coinciding with the onset of puberty. The major developmental task during this period is to achieve mature sexual intimacy. Because much of Freud's genital stage is focused on sexuality, it will be further expanded on in the section on physical development.

Erickson's Psychosocial Stages of Development. Erickson proposed that the major psychosocial crisis of adolescence is *identity versus role confusion*. A major psychosocial task is the development of a self-identity while maintaining some form of group ideals. Teens who resolve this crisis positively leave with a set of self-chosen values, goals, morals, and political ideology. They are not confused about what role to play in various aspects of their life; they may have explored other identities during adolescence, and, by the end of this period, they have settled on a self-chosen one. Individuals who negatively resolve this crisis appear directionless, confused, and shallow. They will be unprepared for the daunting task of adulthood. It is important to mention that previous developmental thought was that the search for an identity was an *identity crisis*, but current thought is that this is not a crisis at all (Grotevant, 1998). It may be difficult for loved ones to adapt to the new changes, ideas, and thoughts of the adolescent, but the teen is not in crisis, but rather in search of an identity.

Adolescents do not initially arrive at a decision; instead they often search for an identity throughout this period. Four identity patterns emerge during adolescence, when teens move in and out of various identities before deciding on one (Marcia, 1966).

- *Identity achievement.* Adolescents who have attained identity achievement have positively resolved the psychosocial crisis of deciding on an identity. These adolescents have explored alternatives and have a set of self-chosen values, goals, and morals. They have critically looked at their belief systems and accepted some parts of them while rejecting others to settle on self-chosen ideals. A sense of psychological peace settles with these teens.
- *Identity moratorium.* Identity moratorium is characterized by a delay in identity achievement. This individual is not making firm commitments to an identity, but rather is exploring various thoughts and activities. Attending college is often thought of as a socially constructed moratorium in which students can try different identities and behaviors until they decide what is appropriate for them.
- *Identity foreclosure.* Identity foreclosure occurs when adolescents fail to question traditional values; they do not take the time to explore various alternatives but prematurely decide on a set of values and goals that others have chosen for them. An example of this is a teen who becomes a preacher because his father and grandfather were both preachers, and this decision is expected of him.
- *Identity diffusion.* Identity diffusion occurs when adolescents are directionless. They are not in search of a self, goals, or values, and they have not committed to any. Many teens find the task of exploring their identity daunting and overwhelming and therefore fail to do so. They appear apathetic and may even have difficulty doing tasks that require thinking about the future. They may fail to commit in friendship or romantic relationships.

Adolescence is marked by decisions concerning an individual's life: college or vocational school, work, personal values, goals, and aspirations. It is important to understand that identity discovery is culture-based. In cultures in which there is virtually universal adhesion to social norms and roles, the transition from adolescence into adulthood is relatively short and easy. When few options exist, deciding on an identity is a short and quick decision. This is a time of great self-exploration for many teens, and it is an important one. Teens who are able to fully explore the challenges ahead are prepared for adulthood.

Physical Development

Physical change is greater during adolescence than at any time other than infancy (Rathus, 2003). The physical changes of puberty are the most obvious signs of adolescence. During puberty the reproductive system matures. Within a few years, a child's body is transformed into an adult body. The boy's testes release large quantities of testosterone, which result in facial and body hair, voice deepening, muscle development, and overall growth in height and weight. The female ovaries release large quantities of estrogen and the adrenal gland releases the adrenal hormone, resulting in breast development, menstruation, body shape changes, and growth in height. Both sexes undergo a growth spurt, a rapid gain in height; however, girls encounter their growth spurt before boys. Eventually, however, boys catch up to girls and tend to be taller and ultimately heavier. Testosterone and estrogen are released in both boys and girls, but each sex receives a larger amount of one.

Sexual maturation is one of the most important aspects of puberty. From middle childhood, the body changes into a reproductive system. The average age of menarche (first menstruation) for girls is 12.5, and the average age for spermarche (first ejaculation) is 13 for males. Although the signs of puberty seem quite sudden, the hormonal changes that underlie puberty begin much earlier. By the time the results of the hormonal changes are evident, they have been under way for some time. In addition to sexual maturation, there are skeletal system changes so that adolescents increase in height; their joints develop further, allowing better coordination. The muscular system continues to develop so that adolescents become stronger and have a high level of physical performance.

One of the ways scientists have searched for the causes of mental illness is by studying the development of the brain from birth to adulthood. New technologies have enabled them to track the growth of the brain and to study the connections between brain function, development, and behavior. This research has turned up some surprises, among them the discovery of striking changes taking place during the teen years (National Institute of Mental Health, 2012).

Contrary to earlier thoughts, the adolescent brain continues to grow and develop (Johnson, Blum, & Giedd, 2009). Recent research by Johnson and colleagues reveals the development of the frontal lobes during adolescence and indicates that they may not be fully developed until age 25. The frontal lobes direct the executive functions of planning, memory, and impulse control. One interpretation of these findings is that, in teens, the parts of the brain involved in keeping emotional, impulsive responses in check are still reaching maturity. This may help to explain adolescents' appetite for novelty and tendency to act on impulse without regard for risk.

Although much is being learned about the adolescent brain, it is not yet possible to know to what extent a particular behavior or ability is the result of a feature of brain structure. Changes in the brain take place in the context of many other factors, such as genetics, childhood experiences, family, friends, community, and culture.

Cognitive Development
Adolescence is marked by changes in thinking. Piaget named the time period from age 11 or 12 to adulthood the *formal operational stage* of cognitive development, which is the final stage of his developmental theory. The formal operational stage of cognitive development is characterized by increased cognition in many areas. Adolescents can think about possibilities rather than only about concrete events, as in the previous stage (concrete operational stage), and they can think abstractly. They can mentally solve hypothetical problems, which is a marked difference from the previous stage. One consequence of this new thinking, however, is that teens may think they know the answers to complex and multidimensional problems. Sometimes they become critical of their parents and their parents' choices. For example, a teen may think that she knows how to have a good marriage and criticize her mother for what she did wrong to ruin her own marriage. It is noteworthy that not all individuals reach the formal operational stage or all of the cognitive gains in it; even those who go to college do not pass all formal operational tests.

Adolescents are able to think about how things could be rather than merely how they are. Adolescent thinking is characterized by hypothetical thought. The teenager may think hypothetically about what life will be like if she or he stays close to home for college or goes far away. Sometimes this new capacity for thinking frustrates parents because teens are constantly trying out their new ideas of politics, education, and relationships, for example. They may make judgments about morality, and they often challenge traditional ideas.

Adolescents are also capable of deductive reasoning, and this is one of the primary reasons why courses such as geometry are taught in high school rather than earlier. Teens are able to reason about if-then statements. They can systematically solve problems by starting with a premise and testing hypotheses. Adolescent science projects often reflect their deductive thinking capabilities.

Adolescent thinking is characterized by egocentric thoughts. Teens tend to overestimate their significance among friends and groups and feel that other people are keenly interested in them. They may feel that they have an imaginary audience, that everyone is watching them. This helps explain why they will spend a large amount of time getting ready, choosing an outfit, or fixing their hair. Alternatively, a teen may not want to go to a particular store for fear that someone might see her there, even though the person seeing her would also be in the store. With this elevated sense of importance, teens may imagine their own lives as ultimately being magical and heroic. For example, a teen may feel that all violence is wrong regardless of the reason because all individuals are created equal and deserve respect. She may feel that, if she could only tell the US attorney general about this, he would understand this wrongdoing and change policies regarding violence in our country.

Adolescents become more aware during adolescence—they become more aware of themselves, others, and their place in the world. This combination of egocentrism and thinking about possibilities rather than realities makes adolescence a time when teens feel that they have explored all rational solutions to a problem, but they rarely have done so. The egocentrism in their thinking influences their ability to consistently make well-informed decisions.

Social Development

In addition to Erickson's psychosocial crises, many other developmental activities affect social development in adolescence. Even though the adolescent years can be trying for parents who are struggling to understand the changes in their child, children with strong attachments to their parents are able to weather the tasks of adolescence better than those with poor attachments, and these attachments will remain strong during adolescence despite the influence of peers. Strong attachments to parents are predictive of high academic achievement and good peer relationships (Black & McCartney, 1997). Similarly, teens who have good relationships with their parents are less likely to use drugs in both adolescence and adulthood. However, teens and parents tend to bicker and argue more at home during adolescence. They fight about petty things such as hair, clothing, and cleaning. Teens often try to obtain adult privileges during adolescence and seek privacy. Although this can be a trying time, it is developmentally appropriate as teens try to embrace tasks of adulthood with new cognitive skills and access to social functions.

One of the primary tasks of adolescence is the discovery of self. Self-esteem often changes in adolescence. Adolescents have generally high levels of self-esteem, but this varies from individual to individual. Some factors associated with a decline in self-esteem include school transition, late physical development, poor academic performance, and drug use. Children whose parents use an authoritative style of parenting have generally higher levels of self-esteem. Research also shows that both boys and girls who have an androgynous or masculine self-concept/identity have higher self-esteem (Burnett, Anderson, & Heppner, 1995) although cross-cultural research suggests that this may not be true for all cultures (Lobel, Slone, & Winch, 1997).

Peer relationships become important during middle childhood, but they become even more so during adolescence. Friendships take on new functions. Intimacy and loyalty become important. Adolescents search for psychological closeness to their friends; they tend to feel that nobody understands them (Rathus, 2003), and their friends provide a forum in which to feel understood. Adolescent friendships are also characterized by loyalty: sticking up for one another becomes important in the cohesion of friendships.

Another component of friendships is self-disclosure, in which teens tell each other personal things about themselves to be held in confidence among friends. Such intimacy among friends is not seen in middle school children but is an important part of adolescent friendships. Friends also provide social support to one another, and this helps ease coping with physical and emotional challenges. Adolescents get to know their friends better as people, including their dreams and goals, rather than just as playmates. They try to preserve friendships because of their shared intimacy and loyalty, and they try to resolve conflicts with their close friends as opposed to just ending the friendship.

Peer groups and cliques also form among teen friends with similar characteristics. Peer groups become more prevalent in adolescence. Teens gather in groups with shared liking of activities and often thoughts. The peer group is structured, often around shared family background, socioeconomic status, and attitudes. Peer pressure frequently has a negative connotation, but it is not always bad. Peer groups often pressure friends to abstain from drugs or smoking and can serve many positive functions. Special peer groups, often referred to as *cliques*, such as the brains, jocks, druggies, and popular kids, form during school. Cliques frequently have a shared language (also seen in middle childhood), dress, and behaviors or activities. Association with peer groups and cliques changes over time, however. Toward late adolescence teens are less concerned with cliques because, if they have attained identity achievement, they have less need for crowd or peer influence with their identity. At any rate, peer groups help shape adolescent thinking and exploration of identities.

One of the challenges of adolescent relationships is the development of romantic relationships. Friendships in middle childhood are primarily among same-sex friends, but adolescent friendships change to include members of the opposite sex. Not all different-sex friendships evolve into romantic relationships, but most teens have a conceptual understanding of being in love with another. As in same-sex friendships, girls tend to seek psychological closeness with members of the opposite sex through self-disclosure, whereas boys seek this less. Romantic relationships tend to be intense but short-lived. Adolescence is a time of sexual exploration, although the degree of this is influenced by peers, family structure, and religious upbringing.

Although romantic relationship development is important in adolescence, so is the decision about one's individual sexual development. By the time they complete high school, the majority of males and females are likely to have engaged in sexual intercourse (Miller, Levin, Whitaker, & Xu, 1998). Social factors are good predictors of the likelihood of sexual activity, including low socioeconomic status, lack of adult supervision, and familial acceptance of dating and sex, as well as child sexual abuse (Herrenkohl, Herrenkohl, Egolf, & Russo, 1998).

Much of our developmental theories focus on heterosexual sexual development, but recent research has also looked at the unique challenges of gay and lesbian adolescents. Gay and lesbian adolescents face unique challenges compared to their heterosexual counterparts, including whether or not to disclose their sexual orientation and how to handle the response from peers and family. Furthermore, gay and lesbian teens have a smaller dating pool because many teens are still discovering their sexuality. Many teens do not label themselves as gay or lesbian, but rather remain undecided in adolescence as they are discovering their sexual and personal identities. At any rate, both heterosexual and gay and lesbian teens face many of the same insecurities and challenges. Males in both groups are more likely to drink alcohol, females in both groups are more likely to diet, and both groups are likely to fear rejection from their partners. However, many adolescent lesbians and gays feel different from their heterosexual peers (Wormer, Wells, & Boes, 2000).

The Brain

Throughout this book, brain research targeted to each mental health disorder or problem will be discussed. Knowledge gained through research examining brain development and changes that occur related to mental health disorders and trauma helps us understand what the child is experiencing biologically and its impact on development. In social work practice with children, it is important to be aware of the changes in brain function that occur with all mental health disorders. The size of a child's brain is 80 percent the size of an adult brain by age 2 and 90 percent by age 5. It is extremely important for social workers and others working with children who are experiencing social, emotional, and behavioral problems to conduct thorough bio-socio-ecological assessments prior to treatment.

To understand the role of the brain in mental illness, it is important to have a basic understanding of how the brain works. The brain is made up of three basic units: the forebrain, consisting of the cerebrum and hidden structures of the inner brain; midbrain, consisting of the uppermost part of the brainstem; and hindbrain, consisting of the spinal cord, brainstem, and cerebellum (National Institutes of Health, 2014). Within these units are specialized areas working together to mediate different functions of the body.

The regions of the brain consist of gray and white matter. Gray matter consists mostly of the cell bodies of nerve cells, called neurons. These neurons communicate with billions of synapses and stimulate sacs that release the chemicals known as *neurotransmitters* into the synapses. Neurotransmitters attach to the receptors of other cells and can either change the properties of the new cells or transmit to another cell if the cell is also a neuron. These neurotransmitters seem to play significant roles in mental illnesses.

Gray matter is associated with intelligence. It is responsible for gathering information from sensory organs and passing the information to where it needs to go. White matter, which consists of axons of nerve cells and myelin, makes up other parts of the brain and is responsible for helping gray matter communicate to the rest of the body. Gray and white matter continue to transform through early adulthood.

The brain develops from less complex structures, such as the brain-stem (lower part of the brain that connects the spinal cord to the cerebral hemispheres), to the more complex structures of the reticular activating system (RAS) located within the brainstem and one of the most important structures in the brain. The RAS is made up of billions of neurons and glial cells organized into systems with the purpose of sensing, processing, storing, perceiving, and acting on both the internal and external environments. Neurons are the raw material of the brain, and glial cells are supportive cells located in the brain and spinal cord, also known as the *central nervous system*.

The RAS is involved in arousal, anxiety, and modulation of limbic and cortical processing. The limbic system, located in the cerebrum part of the brain, has been found to be responsible for regulating emotions and forming memories. It is also responsible for affect regulation and the development of attachment. It consists of key structures such as the hypothalamus, hippocampus, amygdala, and locus coeruleus. The hypothalamus regulates our ability to control anger and aggressive behavior. It also regulates things such as hunger, ability to feel pleasure, sexual satisfaction, and the autonomic nervous system that controls our arousal responses and the physical aspects connected to our arousal responses such as breathing, pulse rate, and blood pressure.

The cognitive aspects of memory are stored in the hippocampus. The hippocampus plays a major role in memory and learning and in activities of the autonomic nervous system and the neuroendocrine system. It is located near the cortex and lower diencephalic (back of the forebrain) areas of the brain. It is believed to play a significant role in the pathophysiology of anxiety and panic attacks due to excess noradrenergic influences from the locus coeruleus. It is further believed that the hippocampus plays a role in the behavioral inhibitory system that acts to stop socially inappropriate behavior. Repeated stress inhibits development of neurons (specialized cells that conduct electrochemical impulses) and causes atrophy of dendrites (short branched fibers where nerve impulses are generated). This results in functional problems with memory and learning.

The amygdala is located in the cerebral hemispheres of the brain. The emotional aspects of memory are stored in the amygdala. The amygdala is the most sensitive brain structure for the emergence of *kindling*, which causes spontaneous electric discharges. Kindling results in long-term alterations in neuronal excitability, which can affect behavior. The amygdala plays a key role in emotional memory processing, interpreting and integrating emotional functions. It also plays a role in fear conditioning and control of aggressive oral and sexual behavior. Key to orchestrating a response to areas of the brain, the amygdala is involved in motor, autonomic nervous system, and neuroendocrine areas of the central nervous system.

The locus coeruleus, part of the catecholamine system, functions as a general regulator for noradrenergic tone and activity. The ventral tegmental nucleus is also part of the catecholamine system. The catecholamine system plays a critical role in regulating arousal; vigilance; affect; and stress, behavioral irritability, locomotion, attention, sleep, and startle responses. The locus coeruleus is a bilateral nucleus of norepinephrine-containing neurons that regulates the sympathetic nervous system and activities of the autonomic system and hypothalamic-pituitary-adrenal axis. If incoming sensory information is threatening, the locus coeruleus increases its activity and releases norepinephrine (a neurotransmitter) into key areas of the brain and body. When norepinephrine is released, changes occur in heart rate, blood pressure, respiratory rate, muscle tone, and glucose mobilization, resulting in the release of the potentially brain-damaging hormones adrenocorticotropin and cortisol. The ventral tegmental nucleus also releases norepinephrine when activated by acute stress.

When subjected to extreme stress, the body responds by releasing hormones such as cortisol or adrenaline, which have been shown to damage brain cells, disrupt homeostasis, impair memory, and affect the sympathetic nervous and endocrine systems. The changes in these systems thus effect changes in other body systems, such as the cardiovascular, respiratory, and muscular systems. Acute stress resulting in neurophysiologic activation is reversible; however, these changes can be irreversible in cases of stress at high levels of frequency, duration, or intensity. Brain research on mental health disorders focuses on the amygdala, hippocampus, and prefrontal cortex regions of the brain.

Sound Techniques for Intervention with Youth

Three overarching practice orientations have been identified as beneficial for working with youth. These include relationship-oriented practice, empowerment-oriented practice, and collaboration-oriented practice (Almqvist & Lassinantti, 2017). The next section will provide details about each of these techniques.

The first orientation that we will discuss is *relationship-oriented practices.* Good relationship quality between the social worker and youth is essential. Youth are more engaged in and satisfied with services as well as have more favorable treatment outcomes when there is a good-quality relationship between the youth and the helping professional (Iachini, Hock, Thomas, & Clone, 2015; Ungar, Liebenberg, & Ikeda, 2014; Ungar, Liebenberg, Landry, & Ikeda, 2012).

One of the first ways to build a relationship or therapeutic alliance with youth is to develop rapport with them. Authenticity, empathy, and trust are crucial to the development of rapport with youth (Almqvist & Lassinantti, 2017). Establishing trust is especially crucial when working with children who have experienced trauma (Almqvist & Lassinantti, 2017; Lanktree et al., 2012; Purvis, McKenzie, Razuri, Cross, & Buckwalter, 2014). Listening to youth and their family's perspectives, viewing them as experts in their own lives and experiences, and being nonjudgmental and respectful are other ways that practitioners can build rapport (Iachini et al., 2015; Munford & Sanders, 2017).

Youth report they prefer relationships where the professional is authentic, nonjudgmental, and genuinely cares about them (Cahill, Holt, & Kirwan, 2015; Ungar et al., 2012, 2014; Zlotowitz, Barker, Moloney, & Howard, 2016). Youth tend to respond better when the practitioner adopts a more informal approach (Greeson, Richard, Barth, Hurley, & Sisson, 2009). Additionally, youth tend be more responsive when the services are based on outreach rather than in formal office settings (Greeson et al., 2009). Youth also report that it is important to them that the helping professional does not give up on them when the youth try to push them away (Munford & Sanders, 2017).

Once rapport is established, continuity is crucial to maintaining a good relationship and therapeutic alliance between the youth and the professional (Cahill et al., 2015; Greeson et al., 2009; Ådanes & Steihaug, 2016). This is important because there is evidence of a positive correlation between the continuity of a therapeutic relationship and positive therapeutic outcomes as well as client satisfaction (Ungar, Liebenberg, Dudding, Armstrong, & van de Vijver, 2013; Ungar et al., 2014). Moreover, continuity of the relationship can mitigate the fragmentation of care (Ådanes & Streihaug, 2016).

At times, youth's behavior may make it difficult to establish a good relationship (Malvaso, Delfabbro, Hackett, & Mills, 2016). However, by engaging in interpersonal skills such as warmth and a nonauthoritarian style, this may be overcome (Malvaso et al., 2016). Professionals need to understand the nature and purpose of *resistance* as a first step in delivering interventions with youth (Munford & Sanders, 2017). Resistance is a way for youth to manage and make sense of their circumstances (Severinsson & Markström, 2015). Practitioners should strive to understand the context of youth's lives and experiences as well as realize what the youth contributes to the relationship (Forrester, Westlake, & Glynn, 2012).

Effective practitioners acknowledge that although the youth may have faced numerous adversities, they have negotiated and navigated resources as well as developed coping strategies to manage their circumstances (Munford & Sanders, 2017). It is imperative that practitioners nurture the self-efficacy of the youth in the helping relationship, and, in that sense, resistance is the youth engaging in his or her self-efficacy (Watson, 2011). Furthermore, when professionals refrain from labeling the client as "bad" and instead reframe them as youth trying to manage difficult issues and circumstances, youth are more likely to engage with them (Munford & Sanders, 2017). Utilizing the motivational interviewing technique of "rolling with the resistance" to help reflect on their actions and emotions is one way that practitioners can work with resistance rather than against it (Watson, 2011, p. 468).

The second type of orientation is *empowerment-oriented practices* with youth. One of the best ways to empower youth is to involve them in the decision-making process (Almqvist & Lassinantti, 2017). Youth respond well when they are involved in the decision-making process (Almqvist & Lassinantti, 2017) because it increases their sense of agency (Almqvist & Lassinantti, 2017). One of the best predictors of treatment success is whether the provider has engaged the client's personal agency (Ungar et al., 2013).

Additionally, providers should strive to empower youth by focusing on their strengths, giving them the opportunities to share their views, and providing information about different treatment options, as well as providing them time to make the choice (Malvaso et al., 2016). This is not to say that youth should be left on their own to make a decision; instead, professionals should discuss decisions with youth if they feel that the youth is making a less than wise decision (Malvaso et al., 2016). Providing flexible and accessible services, such as walk-in services, is another way to empower youth (Malvaso et al., 2016). However, walk-in services may not be the best option for all client populations and thus should be provided as a complement to rather than a replacement for treatment as usual (Barwick et al., 2013).

Families can also be empowered when providers involve them in discussions about their child's treatment, as appropriate. Empowering families requires that providers are open to and respect the family's priorities (Ungar et al., 2012). Families often experience their involvement in treatment as a way to be protective of the youth as well as to enhance family communication (Ungar et al., 2012).

The third type of orientation is *collaboration-oriented practices*. In addition to collaborating directly with youth and their families, helping professionals must also collaborate with other professionals, agencies, and systems. Youth with mental health needs and their families are frequently involved with various systems and services. Service fragmentation often occurs when the youth is involved with several agencies and there is a lack of care coordination (Almqvist & Lassinantti, 2017). The lack of coordination of care can result in youth receiving care that does not address their overall needs (Almqvist & Lassinantti, 2017).

Collaboration between providers may occur in three different ways (Bunger, 2010). Collaboration efforts can be orchestrated in a pooled, sequential, or reciprocal manner (Bunger, 2010). *Pooled efforts* require the least interaction. In this case each service provider works independently, but the combination of the work impacts the outcome. *Sequential collaboration* occurs when one provider screens for a problem and another professional provides the treatment. Finally, *reciprocal collaboration* is characterized by providers' willingness to adjust their services based on the other services that the client receives. Providing client case management is one way to help with service coordination when a client is receiving care from multiple disciplines or setting. Case management serves as a "bridge" to connect clients to various services (Bunger, 2010, p. 213). Case management is an example of pooled collaboration. *Wraparound service,* on the other hand, is an example of reciprocal collaboration as it integrates assessment and planning and neatly ties services together to address the needs of the youth and their family.

References

Ådnanes, M., & Steihaug, S. (2016). You never know what happens next: Young adult service users' experience with mental health care and treatment through one year. International. *Journal of Integrated Care, 16*(3), 1–11.

Almqvist, A., & Lassinantti, K. (2017). Social work practices for young people with complex needs: An integrative review. *Child & Adolescent Social Work Journal, 35*(3), 207–219. doi:10.1007/s10560-017-0522-4

Barwick, M., Urajnik, D., Sumner, L., Cohen, S., Reid, G., Engel, K., & Moore, J. E. (2013). Profiles and service utilization for children accessing a mental health walk-in clinic versus usual care. *Journal of Evidence-Based Social Work, 10*(4), 338–352.

Black, K., & McCartney, K. (1997). Adolescent females' security with parents predicts the quality of peer interactions. *Social Development, 6,* 91–110.

Bunger, A. C. (2010). Defining service coordination: A social work perspective. *Journal of Social Service Research, 36*(5), 385–401

Burnett, J., Anderson, W., & Heppner, P. (1995). Gender roles and self-esteem: A consideration of environmental factors. *Journal of Counseling and Development, 73,* 323–326.

Cahill, O., Holt, S., & Kirwan, G. (2015). Key working in residential child care: Lessons from research. *Children and Youth Services Review, 65,* 216–223.

Forrester, D., Westlake, D., & Glynn, G. (2012). Parental resistance and social worker skills: towards a theory of motivational social work. *Child & Family Social Work, 17*(2), 118–129.

Greeson, J., Richard, K. P., Barth, P., Hurley, S., & Sisson, J. (2009). Contributions of therapist characteristics and stability to intensive in-home therapy youth outcomes. *Research on Social Work Practice, 19*(2), 239–250

Grotevant, H. D. (1998). Adolescent development in family contexts. In N. Eisenberg (Vol. Ed.) & W. Damon (Series Ed.), *Handbook of child psychology: Social, emotional, and personality development, Vol. 3* (pp. 1097–1149). New York: Wiley.

Herrenkohl, E., Herrenkohl, R., Egolf, B., & Russo, M. (1998). The relationship between early maltreatment and teenage parenthood. *Journal of Adolescence, 21,* 291–303.

Hutchison, E. D. (2018). *Dimensions of human behavior: The changing life course* (6th ed.).Thousand Oaks, CA: Sage Publications.

Hutchison, E. D. (2019). *Dimensions of human behavior: Person in environment life course* (6th ed.) Thousand Oaks, CA: Sage.

Iachini, A. L., Hock, R. M., Thomas, M., & Clone, S. (2015). Exploring the youth and parent perspective on practitioner behaviors that promote treatment engagement. *Journal of Family Social Work, 18*(1), 57–73. doi:10.1080/10522158.2014.974293

Johnson, S., Blum, R., & Giedd, J. (2009). Adolescent maturity and the brain: The promise and pitfalls of neuroscience research in adolescent health policy. *Journal of Adolescent Health, 45,* 216–221.

Lanktree, C. B., Briere, J., Godbout, N., Hodges, M., Chen, K., Trimm, L., & Freed, W. (2012). Treating multi-traumatized, socially marginalized children: Results of a naturalistic treatment outcome study. *Journal of Aggression, Maltreatment & Trauma, 21*(8), 813–828.

Lobel, T., Slone, M., & Winch, G. (1997). Masculinity, popularity, and self-esteem among Israeli preadolescent girls. *Sex Roles, 36,* 385–408.

Malvaso, C., Delfabbro, P., Hackett, L., & Mills, H. (2016). Service approaches to young people with complex needs leaving out-of home care. *Child Care in Practice, 22*(2), 128–147.

Marcia, J. E. (1966). Development and validation of ego-identity status. *Journal of Personality and Social Psychology, 3,* 551–558.

Miller, K. S., Levin, M. L., Whitaker, D. J., & Xu, X. (1998). Patterns of condom use among adolescents: The impact of mother-adolescent communication. *American Journal of Public Health, 88,* 1542–1544.

Munford, R., & Sanders, J. (2017). Harnessing resistance in interventions with young people. *Journal of Social Work Practice, 31*(1), 79–93. doi:10.1080/02650533.2016.1164127

National Institute of Mental Health. (2012). *The teen brain: Still under construction* (NIH Publication No. 11–4929). Retrieved from http://www.nimh.nih.gov/health/publications/the-teen-brain-still-under-construction/index.shtml

National Institutes of Health. (2014). *Brain basics: Know your brain* (NIH Publication No. 11–3440a). Bethesda, MD: Author. Retrieved from http://www.ninds.nih.gov/disorders/brain_basics/know_your_brain.htm

Purvis, K. B., Mc Kenzie, L. B., Razuri, E. B., Cross, D. R., & Buckwalter, K. (2014). A trust-based intervention for complex developmental trauma: A case study from a residential treatment center. *Child & Adolescent Social Work Journal, 31*(4), 355–368.

Rathus, S. A. (2003). *Voyages in childhood*. Belmont, CA: Wadsworth, Thompson Learning.

Scannapieco, M., & Connell-Carrick, K. (2005). *Understanding child maltreatment: An ecological and developmental perspective*. New York: Oxford University Press.

Severinsson, S., & Markström, A. (2015). Resistance as a means of creating accountability in child welfare institutions. *Child & Family Social Work, 20*(1), 1–9.

Sokol, J. T. (2009). Identity development throughout the lifetime: An examination of Eriksonian theory. *Graduate Journal of Counseling Psychology, 1*, article 14. Retrieved from http://epublications.marquette.edu/gjcp/vol1/iss2/14

Ungar, M., Liebenberg, L., Dudding, P., Armstrong, M., & van de Vijver, F. J. R. (2013). Patterns of service use, individual and contextual risk factors, and resilience among adolescents using multiple psychosocial services. *Child Abuse & Neglect, 37*(2–3), 150–159.

Ungar, M., Liebenberg, L., & Ikeda, J. (2014). Young people with complex needs: Designing coordinated interventions to promote resilience across child welfare, juvenile corrections, mental health and education services. *British Journal of Social Work, 44*(3), 675–693.

Ungar, M., Liebenberg, L., Landry, N., & Ikeda, J. (2012). Caregivers, young people with complex needs, and multiple service providers: A study of triangulated relationships. *Family Process, 51*(2),193–206.

Watson, J. (2011). Resistance is futile? Exploring the potential of motivational Interviewing. *Journal of Social Work Practice, 25*(4), 465–479.

Wormer, K., Wells, J., & Boes, M. (2000). *Social work with lesbians, gays, and bisexuals: A strengths perspective*. Boston: Allyn Bacon.

Zlotowitz, S., Barker, C., Moloney, O., & Howard, C. (2016). Service users as the key to service change? The development of an innovative intervention for excluded young people. *Child and Adolescent Mental Health, 21*(2), 102–108.

4

Childhood Trauma

Types and Incidence of Trauma

Social work has spent a long time trying to better understand how childhood trauma might affect children's well-being, their development, and their futures. Studies over the past 5 years have attempted to expand this knowledge base by strengthening earlier findings and providing new ones. These studies will be discussed and analyzed throughout this chapter, but first we must engage in a brief discussion about the different types of trauma that a child may experience and the prevalence of that trauma within the United States. This analysis will set up the lens under which we will look at, analyze, and interpret the findings in the literature.

Academics have measured types of trauma in different ways and with different labels; however, there is a clear consensus in the literature that there are five main types of trauma that a child may experience. These include physical abuse, sexual abuse, emotional abuse, physical neglect, and emotional neglect (Ballard et al., 2015; Berenz et al., 2018; Bernstein et al., 2003; De Venter et al., 2017; Ferrer et al., 2017; Hornor, 2015). There are slight variations in the way these are described and labeled in the literature, but, overall, researchers seem to agree that these are the main five trauma types. This is further confirmed by the fact that most researchers utilize the Childhood Trauma Questionnaire (CTQ), developed by Bernstein et al. (2003), which categorizes trauma in a similar way (Kilian et al., 2017; Kim, Jin, Jung, Hahn, & Lee, 2017; Lazary, Eszlari, Juhasz, & Bagdy, 2016; Monteleone et al., 2015; Müller, Bertsch, Bülau, Herpertz, & Buchheim, 2018). By using these five subtypes we can better assess the prevalence of each type of trauma in our communities.

Understanding the Mental Health Problems of Children and Adolescents. Kirstin Painter and Maria Scannapieco, Oxford University Press (2021). © Oxford University Press. DOI: 10.1093/oso/9780190927844.003.0004

One way to monitor the prevalence of childhood trauma or adverse childhood experiences (ACE) is through the Behavioral Risk Factor Surveillance System (BRFSS). The BRFSS is a system that randomly surveys adults regarding their health conditions and risk factors (including ACE). Data have been collected from 32 states and the District of Columbia between 2009 and 2014. The following tables show participant demographics and prevalence statistics for the 2010 BRFSS (Centers for Disease Control and Prevention, 2015).

Demographic Information	Percent (N = 53,784)
Gender	
Female	51.2%
Male	48.8%
Race/Ethnicity	
White	85.1%
Hispanic/Latino	3.7%
Asian/Pacific Islander	3.2%
African-American	4.6%
Other	3.4%
Age (years)	
18–29	13.6%
30–39	20.8%
40–49	21.4%
50–59	18.6%
60 and over	25.6%
Education	
Not High School Graduate	5.6%
High School Graduate	30.5%
Some College	26.8%
College Graduate or Higher	37.1%

ACE Category	Women Percent (N = 32,539)	Men Percent (N = 21,245)	Total Percent (N = 53,784)
ABUSE			
Emotional Abuse	34.1%	35.9%	35.0%
Physical Abuse	15.8%	15.9%	15.9%

ACE Category	Women Percent (N = 32,539)	Men Percent (N = 21,245)	Total Percent (N = 53,784)
Sexual Abuse	15.2%	6.4%	10.9%
HOUSEHOLD CHALLENGES			
Intimate Partner Violence	15.6%	14.2%	14.9%
Household Substance Abuse	27.2%	22.9%	25.1%
Household Mental Illness	19.3%	13.3%	16.3%
Parental Separation or Divorce	23.1%	22.5%	22.8%
Incarcerated Household Member	5.2%	6.2%	5.7%

Number of Adverse Childhood Experiences (ACE Score)	Women Percent (N = 32,539)	Men Percent (N = 21,245)	Total Percent (N = 53,784)
0	40.0%	41.4%	40.7%
1	22.4%	24.9%	23.6%
2	13.4%	13.2%	13.3%
3	8.0%	8.1%	8.1%
4 or more	16.2%	12.4%	14.3%

These findings can help social workers, policymakers, and other professionals gain a better understanding of the unique needs of different individuals and the types of trauma that they may experience. Overall, it seems like ACE prevalence between men and women is about the same in each category. However, there is a significant difference in sexual abuse experiences, with the prevalence in women being almost three times that of men. The existence of these differences is why categorization of trauma and prevalence research is so important. Understanding the prevalence and types of childhood trauma that people experience can help social workers develop interventions that not only address the negative manifestations of trauma but also help prevent long-term developmental or neurological effects.

How Is Trauma Manifested?

The literature shows that childhood trauma can manifest itself in three major ways. Trauma can manifest itself through mental health conditions, risky behaviors, and negative developmental outcomes (Carliner, 2016; Imperatori et al., 2017; Jansen et al., 2016; Lazary et al., 2016; Levenson & Grady, 2016). Gaining a better understanding of these trauma manifestations can help social workers develop interventions that can be preventative in nature and not just treatment strategies that are implemented after the symptoms are manifested.

Childhood Trauma and Mental Health

Childhood trauma can affect an individual's mental health by causing, exacerbating, and/or influencing the way they experience or cope with mental illness. Studies have found that childhood trauma can influence the symptomatology and experience of depression and anxiety (Berenz et al., 2018; De Venter at al., 2017; Lazary et al., 2016; Shevlin, McElroy, & Murphy, 2015; Vares et al., 2016). Different types of trauma have been associated with varying degrees of distress tolerance (Berenz et al., 2018). These findings are significant because they can help determine a child's risk for developing mental illness based on their ability to cope and tolerate distress. Those who have experienced childhood trauma have increased rates of anxiety disorders and a greater chronicity of symptoms (De Venter et al., 2017). Similarly, studies have found childhood trauma to be associated with higher rates of major depressive disorder, increased vulnerability for developing depression, and increased depression severity (Gamache, Martin, Van Ryzin, & Dishion, 2016; Kim et al., 2017; Lazary et al., 2016; Vares et al., 2016). These findings show strong empirical evidence that childhood trauma can lead to increased rates and severity of generalized anxiety and major depressive disorder.

Similarly, childhood trauma has also been found to be associated with other mental disorders including schizophrenia, mood disorders, and post-traumatic stress disorder (PTSD) (Dale et al., 2018; Hyland et al., 2017; Jansen et al., 2016; Noto et al., 2015; Ruby, Rothman, Corcoran, Goetz, & Malaspina, 2017; Utzinger et al., 2016). For schizophrenia, individuals with childhood trauma may experience poorer functioning during early psychosis, an increase in positive symptoms, dysthymic symptoms, and changes in amygdala-to-whole-brain volume ratios (Alameda et al., 2017; Ruby et al., 2017). In addition, these individuals may experience a decrease in negative symptoms and whole-brain volumes. For mood disorders (such as bipolar disorder and borderline personality disorder), individuals with childhood trauma may have a lower response to lithium during treatment, increased rates of bipolar or borderline personality disorders, an increase in prodromal symptoms (social withdrawal, decreased functioning, and anhedonia), and increased clinical severity (Etain et al., 2017; Ferrer et al., 2017; Jansen et al., 2016; Noto et al., 2015). Finally, for PTSD (for a more robust discussion of PTSD please refer to Chapter 7), individuals who experience childhood trauma may experience higher rates of PTSD, greater psychological distress, greater symptom severity, lower levels of respiratory sinus arrhythmia, higher heart rate, atypical physiological regulations of stress, higher externalizing symptoms, increased sleep disturbances, and increased risk for developing complex PTSD (Dale et al., 2018; Darnell et al., 2018; Gamache et al., 2016; Hyland et al., 2017; Thordardottir et al., 2016). Something important to consider is that some of the mediating and moderating effects described in this section can vary based on other factors such as gender and type of trauma. Social workers must be mindful of these when interpreting findings and utilizing them in the implementation of new strategies that aim to prevent or address the mental health needs of individuals who have experienced childhood trauma.

Childhood Trauma and Risky Behaviors

The negative biopsychosocial outcomes of childhood trauma can leave an individual at increased risk for engaging in risky behaviors later in life. Early childhood trauma can increase the risk of engaging in addictive behaviors such as drug and alcohol use and gambling, as well as for developing substance abuse disorders (Carliner et al., 2016; Imperatori et al., 2017; Jester, Steinber, Heitzeg, & Zucker, 2015; Nierop et al., 2016). Some of these effects have been attributed to an increase in craving reactivity and pathological dissociations associated with individuals who experienced childhood trauma (Imperaroti et al., 2017; Trautmann, Kräplin, Dieterich, Richter, & Muehlhan, 2018). Childhood trauma may also increase an individual's propensity to engage in criminogenic behaviors and sexual deviance, and it may lead to criminogenic effects in adulthood (Halsey, 2018; Levenson & Grady,

2016; Martin, Eljdupovic, McKenzie, & Colman, 2015). Understanding how childhood trauma may predict an individual's involvement in risky behaviors later in life can help social workers address these individuals' mental health needs early and provide them with healthy coping strategies that can keep them away from substance abuse, gambling, and crime.

Childhood Trauma and Development

The effects of childhood trauma can also be seen in a child's biopsychosocial development. Although the studies mentioned earlier point to developmental deficits that may lead to risky behaviors and mental illness, other studies expand on this literature and shed light on the ways in which childhood trauma may significantly affect a child's development. The literature shows developmental deficits from childhood to adulthood, such as academic premorbid adjustment (precursor to schizophrenia), cardiovascular disease symptoms (mediated by early pubertal maturation), insecure/avoidant attachment styles, delayed development of worthiness, and a decreased use of adaptive coping skills (Cristobal, Santelices, & Fuenzalida, 2017; Kilian et al., 2017; Lei, Beach, & Simmons, 2018; McCormack & Thomson, 2017; Perlman, Dawson, Dardis, Egan, & Anderson, 2016). These findings inform our understanding of how childhood trauma may lead to negative developmental outcomes.

One of the main development areas negatively impacted by childhood trauma is attachment. Maladaptive attachment styles can become a major factor that can not only affect a child's development, but can also affect their parenting style, attachment to their own children as adults, and ability to create a therapeutic alliance and may become a risk factor for sexual disorders (Cristobal et al., 2017; Lafrenaye-Dugas, Godbout, & Hébert, 2018). Insecure attachment styles resulting from childhood trauma can lead to deficits in an adult's reflective functioning and mentalization (Cristobal et al., 2017). In addition, avoidant attachment patterns have been identified as the mediator between childhood trauma and the decreased use of adaptive coping skills (Perlman et al., 2016). Research also shows that adults who experienced childhood trauma may struggle in their ability to understand their own identify and to learn how to separate their "adult identity" from their "traumatized child" identity due to the delayed development of worthiness resulting from childhood trauma (McCormack & Thomson, 2017). These findings further support the proposition that childhood trauma may lead to significant developmental deficits that can affect a child throughout his or her life. Future research and social work practice must continue this line of inquiry and look for better interventions that might help address the needs of children and ameliorate the developmental deficits resulting from childhood trauma.

Trauma-Informed Care

The manifestations of trauma just discussed demonstrate the need for social workers to implement trauma-informed care (TIC) into their practice. Understanding how childhood trauma can affect a child's relationships, future, and overall well-being can help in the design and implementation of TIC practices. In the literature we find programs and interventions that have attempted to address these needs and reduce the effects of childhood trauma.

Trauma and Attachment Group Program

The CASA Trauma and Attachment Group (TAG) Program is one of many that aim to provide services for children who have experienced trauma. Its goal is to help children struggling with attachment issues (a major developmental area impacted by childhood trauma) (Ashton, O'Brien-Langer, & Silverstone, 2016). Children who participated in TAG showed significant improvements in attachment and communication as well as a decrease in the number of discipline practices and relational frustration. Parents also benefitted from this intervention by demonstrating improved reflective functioning and a reduction of symptoms associated with PTSD. Those who administered and participated in the program report three major themes that they believe accounted for the program's success (Ashton, O'Brien-Langer, Olson, & Silverstone, 2017). The first was the importance given to the relationship between the caregiver and the child as well as the involvement of the caregiver in the healing process. The second was the group process and the benefits of participating in a therapeutic group setting. The third was the psychoeducation-based content and the knowledge acquired about the effects of trauma. Understanding what makes TAG successful can help future programs design and implement effective strategies that can help children and their families with trauma. The positive outcomes of TAG show what an effective trauma-informed model can look like, and they highlight the importance of involving parents in the healing process

Head Start Trauma Smart Program

The Head Start Trauma Smart (HSTS) program is another example of how social workers can implement TIC into their practice (Holmes, Levy, Smith, Pinne, & Neese, 2015). This program aimed to decrease chronic stress from early trauma, foster social/cognitive development, and create a trauma-informed culture for children, parents, and staff in a school setting. The program was designed to integrate different treatment modalities (training, classroom consultation, intensive therapy, and peer mentoring) and provide support and skills training to all caregivers (e.g., parent, teacher, therapist, etc.). The hope was that early intervention could help reduce the negative developmental outcomes of childhood trauma. An evaluation of the program found significant improvements in a child's externalizing and internalizing behaviors after participating in the program, as well as an overall satisfaction with the program expressed by all caregivers (e.g., parents, teachers, administrators) (Holmes et al., 2015). These findings demonstrate that early interventions do work and may help significantly reduce the long-lasting negative effects that trauma can have on a child's life and their relationships.

Practitioner Workshop Program

Other TIC programs indirectly help children who have experienced trauma, and they do this by improving the training of practitioners who work with them. Palfrey et al. (2018) evaluated a workshop that provided TIC training for professionals in hospital and community settings (included nursing, medical, and allied health professionals). Participating in the program improved practitioners' ability to incorporate TIC into their practice, increased the number of trauma assessments they used, and increased their emphasis on establishing a therapeutic alliance. In addition, professionals who participated in the program reported increased confidence and awareness and a better attitude toward treatment of and work with individuals who have experienced trauma, which also increased the practitioners' willingness to include trauma histories in a patient's file. Reductions were also found in the barriers that previously prevented the incorporation of trauma into treatment, such as the fear of increasing distress by asking about trauma and the feelings of being ill-equipped or not properly trained to address trauma. These findings are significant because they demonstrate the need to develop interventions that not only address the needs of trauma victims but also the need to train and prepare the medical professionals that work with them.

Other TIC Programs

There are a wide variety of TIC programs across the nation, but, for the purposes of this chapter, we will only mention a few more that are noteworthy. As mentioned earlier, well-trained health professionals can provide better services for individuals who have experienced trauma. Therefore, strategies have been implemented that aim to incorporate TIC (e.g., behavioral health, case management, and care coordination) into primary care settings (Freed & SmithBattle, 2016; Machtinger, Cuca, Khanna, Dawson Rose, & Kimberg, 2015). These changes have proved to be beneficial not only for the patients who experienced the trauma but also for their relatives, friends, and communities. These changes can also be beneficial for providers and staff by improving their relationships with their patients and, in turn, improving the healing process (Machtinger et al., 2015). Other TIC programs have focused on providing better access to health care, TIC for the homeless, and TIC in kinship care settings (Foli, Woodcox, Kersey, & Zange, 2018; Randhawa et al., 2018; Williams, 2016). The list goes on, but it is evident that TIC is an integral part of every social service organization in our nation. Any professional who works with trauma victims, regardless of the setting, must understand TIC, the challenges associated with it, and the needs of these traumatized individuals. Organizations must look for ways to incorporate TIC into their practice by addressing the needs of trauma victims and training their staff on how to best address these needs.

Neuroscience and Trauma

Childhood trauma has been found to be associated with neurobiological deficits that can lead to negative life outcomes. Research shows that early trauma experiences can lead to lower levels of gray matter in the brain, a decrease in functioning of the medial prefrontal cortex and the amygdala, changes in executive function, and deficits in emotion regulation (Bachi et al., 2018; Cisler, 2017; Cross, Fani, Powers, & Bradley, 2017). These deficits can lead to an increased risk for cocaine use disorder, dissociation, and trauma-related disorders (Bachi et al., 2016; Cross et al., 2017). Some of these negative outcomes and increased risk factors have also been attributed to reactions and dysregulations between the hypothalamic-pituitary-adrenal (HPA) axis, genes, and the epigenetic process, causing areas of the brain to be vulnerable during early periods of development (Cross et al., 2017; Vangeel et al., 2018). Childhood trauma may also lead to negative changes in the structure, function, and connectivity of different areas of the brain (e.g., hippocampus, prefrontal cortex, and amygdala) (Cisler, 2017; Cross et al., 2017; Janiri et al., 2017; Martin-Blanco et al., 2016). Connections have also been found between childhood trauma and immune system development (Danese & Lewis, 2017). Researchers found that childhood trauma may have a similar biological response to physical trauma in triggering an activation of the innate immune system, which can affect brain functioning and development and in turn affect an individual's response to life stressors (Danese & Lewis, 2017). These effects and neurobiological outcomes from childhood trauma may help explain this population's high risk for psychopathology.

Neuroscience and Mental Illness

Changes in the response systems (hippocampus and amygdala) to stress and emotion regulation resulting from childhood trauma can impact the risk for and manifestation of mental illness. Experiences of childhood trauma also can increase the risk of and manifestation of trauma-related disorders (e.g., PTSD, depression, etc.), bipolar disorders, eating disorders, and schizophrenia (Cross et al., 2017; Janiri et al., 2017; Martin-Blanco et al., 2016; Monteleone et al., 2015; Ruby et al., 2017). Childhood trauma has been found to modulate the effects of bipolar disorder on gray matter volumes: healthy individuals who experienced childhood trauma were characterized by decreased bilateral gray matter volumes, while individuals who had bipolar disorder and childhood trauma were characterized by increased deep gray matter volumes (Janiri et al., 2017). Other studies have found that childhood trauma can lead to a blunted cortisol awakening response for individuals with eating disorders, which might be due to the dysregulation of the HPA axis resulting from the trauma. The literature also shows effects on the manifestation of schizophrenia (Ruby et al., 2017). Childhood trauma has been associated with an increase in positive symptoms, an increase in dysthymic symptoms, a decrease in negative symptoms, a decrease in whole-brain volumes, and an increase in amygdala-to-whole-brain volume ratios (Ruby et al., 2017), once again highlighting the significant role that trauma can play in the development and manifestation of mental illness. These findings demonstrate how childhood trauma can have different neurobiological effects depending on an individual's mental health and neurological resilience.

Neuroscience and TIC

Earlier in this chapter we discussed the importance of implementing TIC in our practice. Now we'd like to show an example of how neuroscience can be utilized as a tool to enhance our TIC programs. Ryan, Lane, and Powers (2017) evaluated and examined a program whose goal was to provide a multidisciplinary model for treating complex trauma in early childhood. Its emphasis was on the healing power of safe relationships and on the actions that activate specific areas of the brain. The components of the program included trauma-informed play therapy, strengths-based trauma-informed childhood education, occupational therapy, and caregiver therapy. The program provided healing for both the child and caregiver while simultaneously providing the child with adaptive self-regulation and socioemotional tools. This program is an example of how TIC can integrate our knowledge of neurobiology with empirically supported therapeutic interventions. This area might benefit from further study as we learn more about the brain and the ways in which new technological advances can be applied in a therapeutic setting.

References

Alameda, L., Golay, P., Baumann, P. S., Progin, P., Mebdouhi, N., Elowe, J., & Conus, P. (2017). Mild depressive symptoms mediate the impact of childhood trauma on long-term functional outcome in early psychosis patients. *Schizophrenia Bulletin, 43*(5), 1027–1035.

Ashton, C. K., O'Brien-Langer, A., Olson, K., & Silverstone, P. H. (2017). Qualitative reflections: CASA's Trauma and Attachment Group (TAG) program for youth who have experienced early developmental trauma. *Journal of the Canadian Academy of Child and Adolescent Psychiatry, 26*(1), 12–20.

Ashton, C., O'Brien-Langer, A., & Silverstone, P. (2016). The CASA Trauma and Attachment Group (TAG) program for children who have attachment issues following early developmental trauma. *Journal of the Canadian Academy of Child and Adolescent Psychiatry, 25*(1), 35-42.

Bachi, K., Parvaz, M. A., Moeller, S. J., Gan, G., Zilverstand, A., Goldstein, R. Z., & Alia-Klein, N. (2018). Reduced orbitofrontal gray matter concentration as a marker of premorbid childhood trauma in cocaine use disorder. *Frontiers in Human Neuroscience, 12.* Retrieved from https://doi.org/10.3389/fnhum.2018.00051

Ballard, E. D., Van Eck, K., Musci, R. J., Hart, S. R., Storr, C. L., Breslau, N., & Wilcox, H. C. (2015). Latent classes of childhood trauma exposure predict the development of behavioral health outcomes in adolescence and young adulthood. *Psychological Medicine, 45*(15), 3305–3316. Retrieved from https://doi.org/10.1017/S0033291715001300

Berenz, E. C., Vujanovic, A. A., Rappaport, L., Kevorkian, S., Gonzalez, R. E., Chowdhury, N., . . . Amstadter, A. B. (2018). Childhood trauma and distress tolerance in a trauma-exposed acute-care psychiatric inpatient sample. *Psychological Trauma, 10*(3), 368–375. Retrieved from https://doi.org/10.1037/tra0000300

Bernstein, D. P., Stein, J. A., Newcomb, M. D., Walker, E., Pogge, D., Ahluvalia, T., . . . Zule, W. (2003). Development and validation of a brief screening version of the childhood trauma questionnaire. *Child Abuse Neglect. 27*, 169–190. doi:10.1016/S0145-2134(02)00541-0

Carliner, H., Keyes, K. M., McLaughlin, K. A., Meyers, J. L., Dunn, E. C., & Martins, S. S. (2016). Childhood trauma and illicit drug use in adolescence: A population-based national comorbidity survey replication–adolescent supplement study. *Journal of the American Academy of Child & Adolescent Psychiatry, 55*(8), 701–708. Retrieved from https://doi.org/10.1016/j.jaac.2016.05.010

Centers for Disease Control and Prevention. (2015). Behavioral risk factor surveillance system survey ACE data, 2009–2014. Department of Health and Human Services, Centers for Disease Control and Prevention.

Cisler, J. M. (2017). Childhood trauma and functional connectivity between amygdala and medial prefrontal cortex: A dynamic functional connectivity and large-scale network perspective. *Frontiers in Systems Neuroscience, 11.* Retrieved from http://search.ebscohost.com/login.aspx?direct=true&db=psyh&AN=2017-24278-001&site=ehost-live

Cristobal, P. S., Santelices, M. P., & Fuenzalida, D. A. M. (2017). Manifestation of trauma: The effect of early traumatic experiences and adult attachment on parental reflective functioning. *Frontiers in Psychology, 8.* Retrieved from http://search.ebscohost.com/login.aspx?direct=true&db=psyh&AN=2017-14924-001&site=ehost-live

Cross, D., Fani, N., Powers, A., & Bradley, B. (2017). Neurobiological development in the context of childhood trauma. *Clinical Psychology, 24*(2), 111–124. Retrieved from https://doi.org/10.1111/cpsp.12198

Dale, L. P., Shaikh, S. K., Fasciano, L. C., Watorek, V. D., Heilman, K. J., & Porges, S. W. (2018). College females with maltreatment histories have atypical autonomic regulation and poor psychological wellbeing. *Psychological Trauma, 10*(4), 427–434. Retrieved from https://doi.org/10.1037/tra0000342

Danese, A., & Lewis, S. J. (2017). Psychoneuroimmunology of early-life stress: The hidden wounds of childhood trauma? *Neuropsychopharmacology, 42*(1), 99–114. Retrieved from https://doi.org/10.1038/npp.2016.198

Darnell, D., Flaster, A., Hendricks, K., Kerbrat, A., & Comtois, K. A. (2018). Adolescent clinical populations and associations between trauma and behavioral and emotional problems. *Psychological Trauma.* Retrieved from https://doi.org/10.1037/tra0000371

De Venter, M., Van Den Eede, F., Pattyn, T., Wouters, K., Veltman, D. J., Penninx, B. W. J. H., & Sabbe, B. G. (2017). Impact of childhood trauma on course of panic disorder: Contribution of clinical and personality characteristics. *Acta Psychiatrica Scandinavica, 135*(6), 554–563. Retrieved from https://doi.org/10.1111/acps.12726

Etain, B., Lajnef, M., Brichant, P. C., Geoffroy, P. A., Henry, C., Gard, S., . . . Bellivier, F. (2017). Childhood trauma and mixed episodes are associated with poor response to lithium in bipolar disorders. *Acta Psychiatrica Scandinavica*, *135*(4), 319–327. Retrieved from https://doi.org/10.1111/acps.12684

Ferrer, M., Andión, Ó., Calvo, N., Ramos-Quiroga, J., Prat, M., Corrales, M., & Casas, M. (2017). Differences in the association between childhood trauma history and borderline personality disorder or attention deficit/hyperactivity disorder diagnoses in adulthood. *European Archives of Psychiatry & Clinical Neuroscience*, *267*(6), 541–549. Retrieved from https://doi.org/10.1007/s00406-016-0733-2

Foli, K. J., Woodcox, S., Kersey, S., & Zhang, L. (2018). Addressing the wicked problem of childhood trauma through a nursing and cooperative extension system collaboration. *Public Health Nursing*, *35*(1), 56–63. Retrieved from https://doi.org/10.1111/phn.12375

Freed, P., & SmithBattle, L. (2016). Promoting teen mothers' mental health. *American Journal of Maternal/Child Nursing*, *41*(2), 84–89. Retrieved from http://search.ebscohost.com/login.aspx?direct=true&db=psyh&AN=2016-13540-002&site=ehost-live

Gamche Martin, C., Van Ryzin, M. J., & Dishion, T. J. (2016). Profiles of childhood trauma: Betrayal, frequency, and psychological distress in late adolescence. *Psychological Trauma*, *8*(2), 206–213. Retrieved from https://doi.org/10.1037/tra0000095.supp (Supplemental)

Halsey, M. (2018). Child victims as adult offenders: Foregrounding the criminogenic effects of (unresolved) trauma and loss. *British Journal of Criminology*, *58*(1), 17–36. Retrieved from https://doi.org/10.1093/bjc/azw097

Holmes, C., Levy, M., Smith, A., Pinne, S., & Neese, P. (2015). A model for creating a supportive trauma-informed culture for children in preschool settings. *Journal of Child & Family Studies*, *24*(6), 1650–1659. Retrieved from https://doi.org/10.1007/s10826-014-9968-6

Hornor, G. (2015). Childhood trauma exposure and toxic stress: What the PNP needs to know. *Journal of Pediatric Health Care*, *29*(2), 191–198. Retrieved from https://doi.org/10.1016/j.pedhc.2014.09.006

Hyland, P., Murphy, J., Shevlin, M., Vallières, F., McElroy, E., Elklit, A., . . . Cloitre, M. (2017). Variation in post-traumatic response: The role of trauma type in predicting ICD-11 PTSD and CPTSD symptoms. *Social Psychiatry & Psychiatric Epidemiology*, *52*(6), 727–736. Retrieved from https://doi.org/10.1007/s00127-017-1350-8

Imperatori, C., Innamorati, M., Bersani, F. S., Imbimbo, F., Pompili, M., Contardi, A., & Farina, B. (2017). The association among childhood trauma, pathological dissociation and gambling severity in casino gamblers. *Clinical Psychology & Psychotherapy*, *24*(1), 203–211. Retrieved from https://doi.org/10.1002/cpp.1997

Janiri, D., Sani, G., Rossi, P. D., Piras, F., Iorio, M., Banaj, N., . . . Spalletta, G. (2017). Amygdala and hippocampus volumes are differently affected by childhood trauma in patients with bipolar disorders and healthy controls. *Bipolar Disorders*, *19*(5), 353–362. Retrieved from https://doi.org/10.1111/bdi.12516

Jansen, K., Cardoso, T. A., Fries, G. R., Branco, J. C., Silva, R. A., Kauer-Sant'Anna, M., . . . Magalhaes, P. V. S. (2016). Childhood trauma, family history, and their association with mood disorders in early adulthood. *Acta Psychiatrica Scandinavica*, *134*(4), 281–286. Retrieved from https://doi.org/10.1111/acps.12551

Jester, J. M., Steinberg, D. B., Heitzeg, M. M., & Zucker, R. A. (2015). Coping expectancies, not enhancement expectancies, mediate trauma experience effects on problem alcohol use: A prospective study from early childhood to adolescence. *Journal of Studies on Alcohol and Drugs*, *76*(5), 781–789. Retrieved from https://doi.org/10.15288/jsad.2015.76.781

Kilian, S., Burns, J. K., Seedat, S., Asmal, L., Chiliza, B., Plessis, S. D., . . . Emsley, R. (2017). Factors moderating the relationship between childhood trauma and premorbid adjustment in first-episode schizophrenia. *Plos One*, *12*(1). Retrieved from http://search.ebscohost.com/login.aspx?direct=true&db=psyh&AN=2017-04052-001&site=ehost-live

Kim, J. S., Jin, M. J., Jung, W., Hahn, S. W., & Lee, S.-H. (2017). Rumination as a mediator between childhood trauma and adulthood depression/anxiety in non-clinical participants. *Frontiers in Psychology*, *8*. Retrieved from https://doi.org/10.3389/fpsyg.2017.01597

Lafrenaye-Dugas, A.-J., Godbout, N., & Hébert, M. (2018). Cumulative childhood trauma and therapeutic alliance: The moderator role of attachment in adult patients consulting in sex therapy. *Journal of Sex & Marital Therapy*, *44*(7), 1–12. Retrieved from https://doi.org/10.1080/0092623X.2018.1447057

Lazary, J., Eszlari, N., Juhasz, G., & Bagdy, G. (2016). Genetically reduced faah activity may be a risk for the development of anxiety and depression in persons with repetitive childhood trauma. *European Neuropsychopharmacology*, *26*(6), 1020–1028. Retrieved from https://doi.org/10.1016/j.euroneuro.2016.03.003

Lei, M.-K., Beach, S. R. H., & Simons, R. L. (2018). Childhood trauma, pubertal timing, and cardiovascular risk in adulthood. *Health Psychology*, *37*(7), 613–617. Retrieved from https://doi.org/10.1037/hea0000609

Levenson, J. S., & Grady, M. D. (2016). The influence of childhood trauma on sexual violence and sexual deviance in adulthood. *Traumatology*, *22*(2), 94–103. Retrieved from https://doi.org/10.1037/trm0000067

Machtinger, E. L., Cuca, Y. P., Khanna, N., Rose, C. D., & Kimberg, L. S. (2015). From treatment to healing: The promise of trauma-informed primary care. *Women's Health Issues*, *25*(3), 193–197. Retrieved from https://doi.org/10.1016/j.whi.2015.03.008

Martin, M. S., Eljdupovic, G., McKenzie, K., & Colman, I. (2015). Risk of violence by inmates with childhood trauma and mental health needs. *Law and Human Behavior*, *39*(6), 614–623. Retrieved from https://doi.org/10.1037/lhb0000149.supp

Martín-Blanco, A., Ferrer, M., Soler, J., Arranz, M., Vega, D., Calvo, N., . . . Pascual, J. (2016). The role of hypothalamus-pituitary-adrenal genes and childhood trauma in borderline personality disorder. *European Archives of Psychiatry & Clinical Neuroscience*, *266*(4), 307–316. Retrieved from https://doi.org/10.1007/s00406-015-0612-2

McCormack, L., & Thomson, S. (2017). Complex trauma in childhood, a psychiatric diagnosis in adulthood: Making meaning of a double-edged phenomenon. *Psychological Trauma*, *9*(2), 156–165. Retrieved from https://doi.org/10.1037/tra0000193

Monteleone, A. M., Monteleone, P., Serino, I., Scognamiglio, P., Genio, M., & Maj, M. (2015). Childhood trauma and cortisol awakening response in symptomatic patients with anorexia nervosa and bulimia nervosa. *International Journal of Eating Disorders*, *48*(6), 615–621. Retrieved from https://doi.org/10.1002/eat.22375

Müller, L. E., Bertsch, K., Bülau, K., Herpertz, S. C., & Buchheim, A. (2018). Emotional neglect in childhood shapes social dysfunctioning in adults by influencing the oxytocin and the attachment system: Results from a population-based study. *International Journal of Psychophysiology*. Retrieved from https://doi.org/10.1016/j.ijpsycho.2018.05.011

Nierop, M., Bak, M., Graaf, R., Have, M., Dorsselaer, S., & Winkel, R. (2016). The functional and clinical relevance of childhood trauma-related admixture of affective, anxious and psychosis symptoms. *Acta Psychiatrica Scandinavica*, *133*(2), 91–101. Retrieved from https://doi.org/10.1111/acps.12437

Noto, M. N., Noto, C., Caribé, A. C., Miranda-Scippa, Â., Nunes, S. O., Chaves, A. C., . . . Brietzke, E. (2015). Clinical characteristics and influence of childhood trauma on the prodrome of bipolar disorder. *Revista Brasileira de Psiquiatria, 37*(4), 280–288. Retrieved from https://doi.org/10.1590/1516-4446-2014-1641

Palfrey, N., Reay, R. E., Aplin, V., Cubis, J. C., McAndrew, V., Riordan, D. M., & Raphael, B. (2018). Achieving service change through the implementation of a trauma-informed care training program within a mental health service. *Community Mental Health Journal*. Retrieved from https://doi.org/10.1007/s10597-018-0272-6

Perlman, M. R., Dawson, A. E., Dardis, C. M., Egan, T., & Anderson, T. (2016). The association between childhood maltreatment and coping strategies: The indirect effect through attachment. *Journal of Genetic Psychology, 177*(5), 156–171. Retrieved from https://doi.org/10.1080/00221325.2016.1220912

Randhawa, G., Azarbar, A., Dong, H., Milloy, M., Kerr, T., & Hayashi, K. (2018). Childhood trauma and the inability to access hospital care among people who inject drugs. *Journal of Traumatic Stress. 31*, 383–390. Retrieved from https://doi.org/10.1002/jts.22286

Ruby, E., Rothman, K., Corcoran, C., Goetz, R. R., & Malaspina, D. (2017). Influence of early trauma on features of schizophrenia. *Early Intervention in Psychiatry, 11*(4), 322–333. Retrieved from https://doi.org/10.1111/eip.12239

Ryan, K., Lane, S. J., & Powers, D. (2017). A multidisciplinary model for treating complex trauma in early childhood. *International Journal of Play Therapy, 26*(2), 111–123. Retrieved from https://doi.org/10.1037/pla0000044

Shevlin, M., McElroy, E., & Murphy, J. (2015). Loneliness mediates the relationship between childhood trauma and adult psychopathology: Evidence from the adult psychiatric morbidity survey. *Social Psychiatry and Psychiatric Epidemiology, 50*(4), 591–601. Retrieved from https://doi.org/10.1007/s00127-014-0951-8

Thordardottir, E. B., Hansdottir, I., Valdimarsdottir, U. A., Shipherd, J. C., Resnick, H., & Gudmundsdottir, B. (2016). The manifestations of sleep disturbances 16 years posttrauma. *Sleep, 39*(8), 1551–1554. Retrieved from https://doi.org/10.5665/sleep.6018

Trautmann, S., Kräplin, A., Dieterich, R., Richter, J., & Muehlhan, M. (2018). The role of childhood trauma and stress reactivity for increased alcohol craving after induced psychological trauma: An experimental analogue study. *Psychopharmacology*. Retrieved from https://doi.org/10.1007/s00213-018-4979-4

Utzinger, L. M., Haukebo, J. E., Simonich, H., Wonderlich, S. A., Cao, L., Lavender, J. M., . . . Crosby, R. D. (2016). A latent profile analysis of childhood trauma in women with bulimia nervosa: Associations with borderline personality disorder psychopathology. *International Journal of Eating Disorders, 49*(7), 689–694.

Vangeel, E. B., Kempke, S., Bakusic, J., Godderis, L., Luyten, P., Van Heddegem, L., . . . Claes, S. (2018). Glucocorticoid receptor DNA methylation and childhood trauma in chronic fatigue syndrome patients. *Journal of Psychosomatic Research, 104*, 55–60. Retrieved from https://doi.org/10.1016/j.jpsychores.2017.11.011

Vares, E. A., Salum, G. A., Spanemberg, L., Caldieraro, M. A., Souza, L. H. de, Borges, R. de P., & Fleck, M. P. (2016). Childhood trauma and dimensions of depression: A specific association with the cognitive domain. *Revista Brasileira de Psiquiatria, 38*(2), 127–134. Retrieved from https://doi.org/10.1590/1516-4446-2015-1764

Williams, M. E. (2016). Integrating early childhood mental health and trauma-informed care for homeless families with young children. *Pragmatic Case Studies in Psychotherapy, 12*(2), 113–123. Retrieved from https://doi.org/10.14713/pcsp.v12i2.1968

5

Depressive Disorders

Feeling sad or down is common for all children and teens. Situational depression due to a best friend moving away, loss of a pet, or making a bad grade is expected. *Clinical depression*, however, also known as *depressive disorder*, goes beyond situational depression. Persistent feelings of sadness and changes in behavior such as decreased interest in favorite activities, isolation, changes in sleeping or eating habits, and decreased grades can be an indication of a more serious problem (American Psychiatric Association, 2013). When feelings of sadness persist and a child or teenager has difficulty functioning in daily life, the situation needs to be taken seriously and not ignored.

Children do experience serious depression. The reality is that as many as 1 in 33 children experience clinical depression, meaning a serious depression that significantly interferes with their lives (Merikangas et al., 2010). Merikangas and colleagues reported that, as youth reach adolescence, these numbers change to as many as 1 in 8 experiencing serious depression. A nationally representative survey on health risk behaviors, the Youth Risk Behavior Survey (YRBS), is conducted with high school students every 2 years by the Centers for Disease Control and Prevention (CDC). The YRBS asks questions about high-risk substance use, sexual behavior, violence victimization, and mental health and suicide. One of the questions asks students if, in the past 12 months, they *ever felt so sad or hopeless almost every day for 2 weeks or more in a row that you stopped doing some usual activities*. From 2007 through 2017, the percent of students that reported they experienced feelings of persistent sadness or hopelessness increased significantly (28.5 percent in 2007; 31.5 percent in 2017). A comparison based on race and gender found that females (41.1 percent) were significantly more likely than males (21.4 percent) to have experienced these persistent feelings, and Hispanic youth (33.7 percent) experienced these feelings at significantly different rates than white youth (30.2 percent) or black youth (29.2 percent). When depression is ignored, it can lead to academic underachievement, social isolation, difficult relationships with family and friends, increased risk of

Understanding the Mental Health Problems of Children and Adolescents. Kirstin Painter and Maria Scannapieco,
Oxford University Press (2021). © Oxford University Press. DOI: 10.1093/oso/9780190927844.003.0005

drug and alcohol abuse, and increased risk for suicide (National Institute of Mental Health, n.d.-a, n.d.-b).

Causes of Depression

The causes of depression in children and teenagers are similar to the causes of depression in adults. It is believed that depression is caused by a combination of risk factors such as genetic vulnerability, biochemical disturbances in the brain, environment, poor coping or problem-solving skills, and family history (National Institute of Mental Health, n.d.-a). Children with a family history of depression are two to three times more likely to experience depression are than children without such a family history (National Research Council and Institute of Medicine, 2009; Tsuang, Bar, Stone, & Farone, 2004; Tsuang & Faraone, 1990).

Stressful life events such as the death of a caregiver, divorce, or a chaotic living environment can be triggers of serious depression. Other triggers may include moving to a new school, failing a grade, or being bullied. Children and teenagers who have experienced abuse, neglect, a chronic illness, or other traumatic event are at a higher risk of developing serious depression. Youth in the child welfare and juvenile justice systems have been found to experience higher rates of serious depression than other youth.

Depression and the Brain

Research suggests that mood disorders such as depression are a result, at least to some extent, of disruption in the emotional centers of the brain. Brain research on the biology of depression has focused on the limbic system, hypothalamus, and three neurotransmitters: serotonin, norepinephrine, and dopamine (Krishnan et al., 2004). The limbic system is made up of many structures that regulate functions in the body (Kandel, Schwartz, & Jessell, 2000). The amygdala and hippocampus, two structures of the limbic system, are involved in regulating emotion. The hypothalamus regulates anger, aggression, hunger, the ability to feel pleasure, sexual arousal, and stress response.

When we think, feel, or react, neurotransmitters send messages through the limbic system. Serotonin, norepinephrine, and dopamine are the neurotransmitters that transmit messages in the limbic system and hypothalamus. Researchers have found a connection between these three neurotransmitters and clinical depression, but just how they are connected is not quite known (National Institute of Mental Health, n.d.-a). What is known is that levels of these neurotransmitters are altered in persons with depression. Researchers are not sure which comes first. Either a person becomes depressed, resulting in changes in the levels of the serotonin, norepinephrine, or dopamine, or changes in the levels of the neurotransmitters cause depression. Researchers continue to study the underlying causes of depression in an effort to better understand them and to develop more effective treatments. For example, the hormone cortisol has been found to be elevated in depressed persons (Tsuang & Faraone, 1990).

Researchers are also studying genes that they believe make some people susceptible to depression. One study funded through National Institute of Mental Health (NIMH) (Hyde et al., 2016) found 17 genetic variations at 15 genomes linked to depression and found evidence of a genetic overlap between depression and other mental illnesses. The researchers used data collected through a prior genome study and combined it with data collected from people who purchased their own genetic profiles through a company that offers direct-to-customer DNA testing and consented for use of their DNA in research studies. This research has the potential to lead to new and better treatments for depression.

Signs and Symptoms of Depression

There are many signs suggesting that a child or adolescent is experiencing depression and is in need of an evaluation by a mental health professional. Changes in sleeping and eating patterns can be a sign of depression. The youth may begin sleeping too much or have difficulty falling or staying asleep and/or experience significant weight gain or loss. One may notice changes in cognitions, behavior, and personality. Irrational beliefs can lead a once confident youth to become highly sensitive to rejection or failure. These feelings are often not based in the reality of the situation. A once happy youth may exhibit frequent tearfulness or sadness. Both children and adolescents experiencing depression may exhibit self-destructive behaviors or overreact emotionally to what may seem to be small things to those around them. A decrease in self-esteem is usually evident. It is common for youth experiencing depression to begin talking about themselves in self-deprecating or negative ways. When these youth look in the mirror, they may see a distorted version of themselves. They may perceive themselves to be ugly or fat.

Changes in motivation and energy level are also very common. The youth may seem to move more slowly, talk more slowly, or not seem interested in anything. A classic sign of depression in youth is a decreased interest in things once enjoyed and a decreased interest in hanging out with friends, such as when the youth who once enjoyed playing basketball after school or going to the mall to hang out with friends stops engaging in these social activities and begins spending more and more time isolated in his or her room. It is common for depressed teenagers to begin listening to music about death or aggressive subjects or to draw pictures or write about subjects that include death, suicide, or morbid subjects. In children, signs of depression can often be seen in their play. Their play may involve aggression that is directed toward themselves or others, or it may persistently involve themes that are sad.

Significant change in school attendance or decrease in grades is also very common. The youth no longer seems to care about completing homework or worry about grades. He or she may have trouble focusing in class or be found to sleep during class. Many depressed youth begin refusing to go to school due to somatic complaints such as headaches or stomachaches. There are several general categories of depression in the *Diagnostic and Statistical Manual of Mental Disorders* (DSM), each distinguished by the severity, duration, and cause of symptoms. This book will address major depressive disorder (MDD), persistent depressive disorder (PDD or dysthymia), and a newly added diagnosis to the DSM that is specific to children, *disruptive mood dysregulation disorder* (DMDD; American Psychiatric Association, 2013).

Major Depressive Disorder

MDD is considered the most serious form of depression. MDD can significantly interfere in a youth's ability to function and with their mental and physical well-being. As specified in the DSM-5, a person meets the criteria for major depressive disorder if he or she has experienced at least five symptoms, one of which is either a depressed mood or a loss of interest or pleasure most of the day, almost every day, during the same 2-week period. Other symptoms include significant changes in weight loss when not dieting or weight gain (for children this can include failure to reach an expected weight), too much or too little sleep, restlessness (psychomotor agitation) or slowed psychomotor functioning (psychomotor retardation), fatigue or loss of energy, feelings of worthlessness or excessive or inappropriate guilt, trouble thinking or concentrating, indecisiveness, and thoughts of death or suicidal ideation (thinking about suicide). In addition, the symptoms must cause clinically significant distress or impairment in the youth's level of daily functioning, representing a significant decrease from prior functioning. The episode must not be attributable to the physiological effects of a substance, a physical medical condition, or another mental illness. When criteria are met for major depression, the current clinical status or features of the depression are identified with specifiers. The specifiers for depression are mild, moderate, and with psychotic features.

Persistent Depressive Disorder

PDD is a chronic form of depression characterized by onset in childhood, adolescence, or early adulthood (APA, 2013). PDD is a combination of the previous diagnoses of dysthymia and chronic MDD. The symptoms are not as severe as those of major depression, but they linger for long periods, often 2 or more years. To be diagnosed with PDD, a person must experience a depressed mood for most of every day, most days of the week, for at least 2 years (1 year for children). He or she must also experience two or more depressive symptoms but not have met the criteria for a major depressive episode. Studies have found that somewhere in the range of 10–25 percent of persons with PDD will go on to develop major depression.

Disruptive Mood Dysregulation Disorder

The DSM-5 includes for the first time a relatively new depressive disorder specific to children: DMDD is characterized by recurrent severe temper outbursts that are disproportionate to the situation or cause, incongruous with a youth's developmental level, and occur in at least two settings (home, school, or with peers) for at least 1 year and must be without interruption for more than 3 months (APA, 2013). The youth's mood between outbursts is characterized by chronic irritability. The extreme irritability and anger must be present almost every day for most of the day. The age of onset must be by the age of 10 and cannot be diagnosed for the first time before the age of 6 or after the age of 18. The outbursts may present as verbal and/or behavioral and occur three or more times a week for at least 1 year without having three or more consecutive months without the outbursts. DMDD was added to the DSM due to a concern in the field that some children and adolescents are inappropriately diagnosed with bipolar disorder because the frequency of children and adolescents being given this diagnosis has significantly increased over the past 25 years (Copeland et al., 2013). Pediatric visits with a diagnosis of bipolar disorder in the US have increased significantly. In 1994–1995, it was estimated to be 25 per 100,000; in 2002–2003, it increased to 1,003 per 100,000 (Moreno et al., 2007). The major concern in misdiagnosing youth as having bipolar disorder is due to increases in the prescribing of atypical antipsychotics to youth, which can result in serious physical health problems (Kealy et al., 2014). What differentiates youth with DMDD from those with bipolar disorder is that those with DMDD do not experience the episodic depression, mania, or hypomania characteristics of bipolar disorder (see Chapter 13). DMDD is differentiated by another diagnosis, intermittent explosive disorder (IED), based on the frequency of outburst requirement (two per week for IED and three per week for DMDD). Furthermore, although youth with IED can experience persistent irritability, there is not a requirement for persistent irritability in IED.

DMDD and oppositional defiant disorder (ODD) both include the criteria for irritability and temper outbursts; however, the requirement for DMDD is more severe than ODD (three outbursts per week compared to two per week). DMDD also has a longer duration requirement (12 compared to 6 months) and must result in profound impairment across two settings. ODD does not have this requirement. Due to the relative newness of the DMDD diagnosis, there are gaps in knowledge of the disorder. The prevalence of DMDD is not yet known, but it is estimated to be somewhere from 2 percent to 5 percent (APA, 2013).

Depression in Children and Adolescents

Depression occurs equally among younger male and female children. However, after puberty, females are twice as likely as males to experience major depression. Once any young person has experienced a depressive episode, he or she is at a high risk of developing another depressive episode.

In general, 60 percent of persons who have experienced a major depressive episode will go on to have a second one. A person who experiences major depression as a child is five times more likely to experience major depression as an adult (Cyranowski, Frank, Young, & Shear, 2000; Weissman et al., 1990).

When a young person is assessed for depression, it is important to consider whether the information he or she provides is factual. Some youth may not be open to treatment and therefore may deny having problems. Other youth may lack self-awareness or the ability to communicate their thoughts and feelings, thus making it difficult to determine if there is a problem. It is always important to interview others involved in the youth's life, including a primary caregiver and if possible a teacher or other closely connected persons to get a clear picture of the problems.

Self-Harming Behaviors

Self-harm, intentionally causing bodily harm to oneself, has become a major concern. Self-harm is used as a way to cope with anger, frustration, or emotional pain or to relieve tension. The literature refers to this as *nonsuicidal self-injury* (NSSI). NSSI is strongly linked to child sexual abuse, eating disorders, substance abuse, posttraumatic stress disorder, borderline personality disorder, depression, and anxiety disorders (Gluck, 2012; Yates, 2004). Self-injury refers to a broad range of behaviors, the most common being cutting. *Cutting* is intentionally scratching or cutting one's body with an object sharp enough to break the skin and make it bleed. People may cut themselves on their legs, belly, arms, or wrists, usually in places where they can hide the injury with clothing. Other self-injuring behaviors (not exhaustive) include

- Severe pinching with fingernails or other objects to the point of bleeding;
- Banging or punching objects or oneself to the point of bruising or bleeding;
- Biting to the point that bleeding occurs or marks remain on the skin;
- Pulling out hair, eyelashes, or eyebrows;
- Burning the skin;
- Embedding objects into the skin.

Teenage girls seem to be at most risk of self-injuring behaviors; however, boys engage in this behavior as well (Cyranowski et al., 2000). An estimated

1 in 5 females engage in self-injurious behaviors each year compared to 1 in 7 of their male peers (Gluck, 2012). Sexual orientation is also linked to self-injury, with bisexual and questioning youth at a higher risk than their heterosexual peers.

Self-injuring behaviors generally take place in private and are hidden by the person, making it difficult to identify prevalence rates. It is a myth that people self-injure purely to seek attention. Research studies have found that self-injury is more common than once thought, with a lifetime prevalence of 12–37.2 percent in secondary school populations (Swannell et al., 2014). Self-injuring behaviors can last well into adulthood. They can be an indication of depression or other psychiatric illnesses. Although the intent of self-harm is not to commit suicide, this behavior may be a sign of suicidal ideation.

Teenagers cut themselves for various reasons. Most self-injury experts agree that cutting shows some addictive qualities and may serve as a form of self-medication. For some people cutting is a way to cope with the pain of strong emotions, intense pressure, or relationship problems. Often individuals who cut do not know how to talk about their feelings; they cut to express strong feelings of rage, sorrow, rejection, desperation, and loneliness. They engage in self-injuring behavior sometimes as a way to avoid suicide and as a means of relieving pain and/or feeling something. The purpose of self-injury is often the opposite of suicide; the objective is generally to feel better, not to end life. People who self-injure are not doing it for pure attention-seeking. Although 60 percent of individuals with a history of self-injury report not considering suicide, NSSI may best be understood as a symptom of distress that, if it does not relieve the pain, may lead to suicidal behavior (Whitlock & Knox, 2007). It is important to emphasize that individuals with a history of self-injury are at a higher risk for suicidal ideation and need to be assessed for suicide risk.

Suicide

Suicide is a serious public health problem. It is the second leading cause of death for youth aged 10–24 (Centers for Disease Control [CDC], 2019). The CDC (2019) estimates that approximately 16 percent of high school students seriously consider suicide each year, 13 percent have a suicide plan, and 8 percent attempt suicide. Suicide is a complex issue resulting from a combination of individual, environmental, social, cultural, and economic factors

(US Department of Health and Human Services [DHHS], 2012). Depression increases the risk of suicide in children and adolescents; however, depression is not the only mental health problem associated with suicidal behavior. Other mental health problems such as eating disorders, anxiety, psychosis, substance abuse, and behavioral disorders can also be contributing factors.

In 2001, David Satcher, the then Surgeon General issued the first national strategy for suicide prevention that set forth a national agenda that consisted of 11 goals and 68 objectives (US DHHS, 2001). This strategy led to the creation of the National Suicide Prevention Lifeline (800–273–TALK/8255) and the establishment of the Suicide Prevention Resource Center (SPRC). Building from the work of the 2001 national agenda for suicide prevention, the Surgeon General and the National Strategy for Suicide Prevention Task Force released an updated prevention strategy (DHHS, 2012). The report provides the following multilevel approach to the prevention of suicide, a program in which we can all play an important role (DHHS, 2012, pp. 12–13).

A Comprehensive Approach to Suicide Prevention

This description highlights some of the many clinical and community services and supports that should be available to a person who struggles with depression and thoughts of suicide.

In the community, when the person interacts with family members, friends, physicians, and others:

- Reduced prejudice about mental disorders and suicide makes it more likely that the person will let others know about symptoms and seek help;
- Responsible media reporting of mental illness and suicide reduces prejudice and prevents contagion;
- A well-implemented public awareness campaign raises cognizance of the signs and symptoms of mental disorders and risks for suicide and of where help is available locally;
- Training of community service providers makes it easier to identify the person at risk and increases appropriate referrals;
- Systems are in place to ensure that the person is referred to and safely transported to the appropriate facility for evaluation; and
- Reducing access to lethal means makes it less likely that the person will engage in suicidal behaviors.

At the primary care provider or emergency department:

- Screening improves the likelihood that the person will receive appropriate evaluation and treatment;

- Training on recognition of risk and quality of care increases the likelihood of a good outcome;
- The care provider accurately diagnoses and records the problems and ensures that the appropriate public health surveillance systems are notified or made aware of the diagnoses;
- The implementation of trauma-informed policies and practices ensures that the person is treated with respect and in a way that promotes healing and recovery;
- Easy access to mental health care referrals for individuals with suicide risk increases the likelihood of a better outcome;
- Education efforts by health care providers increase knowledge of the warning signs of suicide risk among the individual and his or her family and/or support network; and
- Continuous care and improved aftercare leads to better monitoring and follow-up of the at-risk individual over time.

In the community, while receiving care:
- Reduced prejudice regarding mental health issues and suicide leads to greater acceptance by family members and friends;
- The availability of high-quality mental health services that are linguistically and culturally appropriate makes it less likely that depression or related problems will recur;
- Sharing information, with the person's permission, among care providers allows treatment to be better coordinated and collaborative; and
- Resources are available to offer social support, resiliency training, problem-solving skills, and other protective factors to the person and his or her family members and/or support network.

In the community, after the person recovers:
Education efforts help the person and his or her family members and/or support network maintain physical, mental, emotional, and spiritual health and well-being; and

Systems are in place to evaluate the effectiveness and efficiency of the interventions provided

Unfortunately, despite increased efforts and available evidence-based interventions aimed at the prevention of suicide, suicide rates in the US continue to rise. According to the National Vital Statistics System of the CDC, for youth aged 10–14, suicide is the third leading cause of death, and it is the second leading cause of death for those 15–24 years old (CDC, 2019). Significant increases in suicide deaths have occurred in youth aged 10 through 19 from 2008 through 2017 (see Figure 5.1). Most disturbingly, there has been a significant increase in suicides for 10- to 12-year-olds in the United States (CDC, 2019).

As addressed in the section on cognitive development in Chapter 3, teenagers have the capacity for new thinking during adolescence. They can imagine a perfect world; cognitively, they explore solutions to problems and imagine an array of possibilities before them. Although this increase in cognitive sophistication is tremendous, for some teens it also opens the door to thinking about various possibilities, including death. Teens face many stressors. They have access to drugs and alcohol as well as guns, which are readily available in today's society, and they may have fewer social supports than before. With many parents working and time spent alone at home watching TV or playing video games, teens can easily isolate themselves. Adolescents who are depressed may experience family problems, have emotional problems, and may contemplate suicide. They may exhibit warning signs including changes in sleeping and eating, and they may become agitated easily and neglect their personal appearance. They may see death as one of many options to escape circumstances they consider unbearable. Suicidal

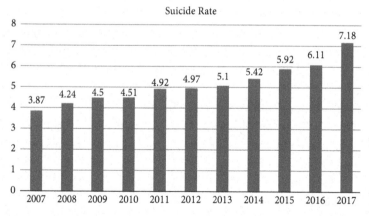

Figure 5.1 2007–2017, United States suicide injury deaths and rates per 100,000 all races, both sexes, age 10–19

Taken from https://webappa.cdc.gov/cgi-bin/broker.exe

ideation becomes a major threat when the person (1) has a plan for death, (2) has the means to accomplish the plan, and (3) lacks supervision so that time for actualizing the plan is available.

Suicidal ideation in youth should always be taken seriously and assessed properly. The most obvious consequence of suicide is death, but there are also the consequences experienced by the friends and family left behind. Suicide affects entire communities. It often leaves people feeling shame or guilt and questioning why they missed or ignored the signs or cries for help. They may also experience anger and/or depression. When there is a failed suicide, it can leave the person with a serious injury such as a traumatic brain injury or paralysis. Failed suicides can also have the unintentional consequence of economic burden as a result of lost productivity and increased health care costs related to injury. A study conducted at the NIMH on youth suicide risk screening in emergency rooms (Lanzillo et al., 2019) found that 7 percent of youth aged 10–12 seeking help for physical concerns screened positive for suicide risk. The US Surgeon General (US DHHS, 2012) estimates that more than 90 percent of children and adolescents who take their lives have a mental health disorder such as depression. Sadly, most youth do not get needed mental health treatment. Less than half of teens who attempt suicide received mental health services in the year prior to their attempt. Those who did receive mental health treatment appeared to have terminated treatment prematurely. This suggests a need to understand the reasons for early termination and to develop strategies to improve treatment completion. It is important to note that not everyone with suicidal ideation has a diagnosable mental illness.

Risk and Protective Factors

Risk factors are characteristics associated with suicide. They are not necessarily the direct cause of suicide, but they are contributors to the increased risk for suicide. Protective factors are characteristics that buffer against suicide. When suicidal ideation is assessed, these factors should be considered. For instance, a higher risk of suicide exists for youth who have previously attempted suicide or have a family member who committed suicide. Drug and alcohol use or abuse increases the risk of suicide. Gender and race/ethnicity are factors. Males are more likely to die from a suicide attempt than females (83 percent compared to 17 percent). Hispanic and Native American/

Box 5.1 Risk and protective factors associated with suicide

Risk factors
- Family history of suicide
- Family history of child maltreatment
- Previous suicide attempt(s)
- History of mental disorders, particularly clinical depression
- History of alcohol and substance abuse
- Feelings of hopelessness
- Impulsive or aggressive tendencies
- Cultural and religious beliefs about suicide (e.g., belief that suicide is a noble resolution of a personal dilemma)
- Local epidemics of suicide
- Isolation, or a feeling of being cut off from other people
- Barriers to accessing mental health treatment
- Loss (relational, social, work, or financial)
- Physical illness
- Easy access to lethal methods
- Unwillingness to seek help

Protective factors
- Effective clinical care for mental, physical, and substance abuse disorders
- Easy access to a variety of clinical interventions and support for help seeking
- Family and community support (connectedness)
- Support from ongoing medical and mental health care relationships
- Skills in problem solving, conflict resolution, and nonviolent ways of handling disputes
- Cultural and religious beliefs that discourage suicide and support instincts for self-preservation

---

Alaskan Native youth have higher rates of suicide than white non-Hispanic or black youth. According to the CDC (Eaton et al., 2012), risk and protective factors associated with suicide include those listed in Box 5.1.

Warning Signs

Most often (4 out of 5 times), suicidal teens exhibit clear warning signs. Clear warning signs include an obsession with death that is evidenced through a youth's conversations, writings, music, or artwork. Youth may stop participating in things they once enjoyed. Often suicidal youth will experience extreme changes in their personality and behaviors, including irrational or bizarre behavior. Making direct or indirect suicidal threats and giving away belongings are also common. The US Department of Health and Human Services offers the mnemonic *IS PATH WARM?* as a tool to identify red flags indicating suicidal ideation.

- Ideation: Threatened or communicated
- Substance abuse: Excessive or increased
- Purposeless: No reasons for living
- Anxiety: Agitation/insomnia
- Trapped: Feeling there is no way out
- Hopelessness
- Withdrawing: From friends, family, society
- Anger (uncontrolled): Rage, seeking revenge
- Recklessness: Risky acts, unthinking
- Mood changes (dramatic)

Addressing Suicidal Ideation

Too often, warning signs go ignored because we believe that the person is just trying to get attention. It is common for people to refuse to believe that a young person would follow through with taking his or her own life. There is also a mistaken belief that a discussion of suicide may increase someone's suicidal ideation. Both of these are myths. Young people do commit suicide, and discussing and questioning a youth about suicidal ideation will not put the idea of suicide into his or her head or result in increased suicidality. Ignoring the warning signs can result in serious consequences. If you identify or suspect suicidal ideation, it is important to address the issue head on. Question the youth as to whether he or she is having thoughts about harming him- or herself. If you find that the young person is having suicidal ideation, determine if he or she has a determined time-frame and a plan for committing suicide. A youth with imminent suicidal ideation, meaning that he or she has a plan and the means to carry it out, should never be left alone. In the helping profession, we have a duty to protect. This is a time when we have to consider whether or not to break confidentiality. It is important that someone, usually the primary caregiver, knows about the situation and promises to watch the youth and ensure that he or she gets professional care. If the threat or attempt of suicide is serious, psychiatric hospitalization may be indicated as a means of monitoring the youth to ensure safety and offer intensive treatment.

Suicide contracts are a controversial preventative intervention that many counselors, therapists, and sometimes even family members try to implement. In such a contract, the suicidal person is asked to sign a document agreeing not to harm him- or herself. The document, which is not legally binding, sets out a plan and a promise to call someone rather than hurting him- or herself. The controversy with this intervention is that a person may appear to agree with the contract and sign it but then not follow through with the agreement. Sometimes people with suicidal intent will suddenly say that they feel better and no longer plan to commit suicide as a way to be left alone so that they can kill themselves. Whether or not someone will follow through with attempting suicide is unpredictable. Understanding the level of psychological distress the youth is experiencing can be a guide. Evidence supporting interventions for suicidal ideation will be addressed in Chapter 6.

Eating Disorders

Eating disorders are complex medical and psychiatric conditions characterized by severe disturbances in how a person views food intake. They are a serious public health problem due to the negative physical, emotional, and mortality consequences. While they are not depressive disorders, people with eating disorders commonly have co-occurring mood and/or anxiety disorders (Grilo, White, & Masheb, 2009). Due to the high occurrence of depressive disorders, high suicide rates, and serious health complications that accompany eating disorders, we decided to include a brief discussion of the three most common eating disorders: binge eating disorder, bulimia nervosa, and anorexia nervosa.

Onset of eating disorders commonly occurs during the teen years and early adulthood but can occur anytime across the lifespan, even in early childhood. Though they are more common in females, they also affect males and nonbinary individuals (Diemer et al., 2015). They affect an estimated 2.7 percent of adolescents aged 13–18. Youth with eating disorders often have to contend with teasing and bullying by both peers and family members.

Like other disorders, the causes of eating disorders are multifaceted. There are genetic, environmental (e.g., physical illness, life stressors, being bullied), and societal (e.g., media) contributors. Researcher have found that youth who engage in dieting are five times more likely to have an eating disorder. Alarmingly, a study on body image found that 25 percent of elementary girls diet on a regular basis (Smolak, 2011). Youth who restrict their diet to extreme levels are 18 times more likely to develop an eating disorder than other youth (Golden, Schneider, & Wood, 2016). Eating disorders can result in serious physical health problems. They can negatively affect the cardiovascular, gastrointestinal, neurological, and endocrine systems. Death rates related to eating disorders range from approximately 3.9 percent to 5.2 percent. They have the highest mortality rate of any mental health disorder, second only to opioid overdoses (Chesney, Goodwin, & Fazel, 2014). The mortality rate is based both on death related to suicide and to medical complications such as heart attacks or kidney failure. Signs that a child or adolescent has an eating disorder or is at high risk of developing an eating disorder include eating in secret, calorie counting, binging and/or purging, preoccupation with food, and a fear of becoming fat.

Binge Eating Disorder (BED)

Binge eating disorder (BED) is a new diagnosis first appearing in the DSM 5. In the DSM-IV (1994), it was listed in the appendix to be used as a specifier when diagnosing Eating Disorder Not Otherwise Specified. It was added to the DSM 5 due to extensive research studies published in peer reviewed journals supporting BED as a stand-alone diagnosis. The DSM 5 diagnostic criteria for binge eating disorder include:

- Recurrent episodes of binge eating. An episode of binge eating is characterized by both of the following:
  o Eating, in a discrete period of time (e.g., within any two-hour period), an amount of food that is definitely larger than most people would eat in a similar period of time under similar circumstances
  o A sense of lack of control over eating during the episode (e.g., a feeling that one cannot stop eating or control what or how much one is eating)
- The binge-eating episodes are associated with three (or more) of the following:
  o Eating much more rapidly than normal
  o Eating until feeling uncomfortably full

o Eating large amounts of food when not feeling physically hungry
o Eating alone because of feeling embarrassed by how much one
  is eating
o Feeling disgusted with oneself, depressed, or very guilty afterward
- Marked distress regarding binge eating is present.
- The binge eating occurs, on average, at least once a week for 3 months.
- The binge eating is not associated with the recurrent use of inappropriate compensatory behavior (e.g., purging) and does not occur exclusively during the course of anorexia nervosa, bulimia nervosa, or avoidant/restrictive food intake disorder.

An estimated 33 percent of people with binge eating disorder have co-occurring depression (Hudson, Hiripi, Pope, & Kessler, 2007; Milos, Spindler, Buddeberg, & Crameri, 2003; US National Library of Medicine, 2017). Binging behavior can result in people feeling a loss of control and extreme feelings of guilt, depression, disgust, and/or low self-esteem. People with a binge eating disorder do not purge, fast, or exercise excessively. Most often people who binge eat are overweight or obese.

Bulimia Nervosa

Bulimia nervosa is similar to binge eating disorder but differs in that it includes behaviors to prevent weight gain. Co-occurring depression affects approximately 36–50 percent of people with bulimia (Hudson et al., 2007; Milos et al., 2003; US National Library of Medicine, 2017). The DSM diagnostic criteria include:

- Recurrent episodes of binge eating. An episode of binge eating is characterized by both of the following:
  o Eating, in a discrete period of time (e.g., within a 2-hour period), an amount of food that is definitely larger than what most people would eat during a similar period of time and under similar circumstances.
  o Lack of control over eating during the episode (e.g., a feeling that you cannot stop eating, or control what or how much you are eating).

- Recurrent inappropriate compensatory behavior to prevent weight gain, such as self-induced vomiting, misuse of laxatives, diuretics, or other medications, fasting, or excessive exercise.
- The binge eating and inappropriate compensatory behaviors both occur, on average, at least once a week for 3 months.
- Self-evaluation is unduly influenced by body shape and weight.
- Binging or purging does not occur exclusively during episodes of behavior that would be common in those with anorexia nervosa.

Anorexia Nervosa

Anorexia nervosa is the characterized by self-starvation, excessive weight loss, and negative body image. For children this can be a lack of weight gain appropriate to their height, body type, and age. Of those with anorexia, it is estimate that from 32 percent to 39 percent have a co-occurring depressive disorder. People with anorexia restrict their calorie intake through means such as restricting high-calorie food, compulsive exercising, vomiting, and taking laxatives. The onset of anorexia can occur at any age, but it most commonly occurs during adolescence. Anorexia is more common in females, making up approximately 85–90 percent of people with the disorder.

The symptoms of anorexia can be life-threatening due to the significant toll it takes on the cardiovascular, gastrointestinal, neurological, and endocrine systems. The mortality rate for anorexia is estimated to be 10 percent (Arcelus, Mitchell, Wales, & Nielsen, 2011). Because the body does not get the nutrients it needs to function, it slows down. When this happens, it can result in the following problems:

- Abnormally slow heart rate and low blood pressure
- Damage to the structure and function of the heart; increased risk of heart failure
- Reduction of bone density
- Muscle loss and weakness
- Severe dehydration, which can result in kidney failure
- Edema
- Fainting, fatigue, lethargy, and overall weakness
- Dry skin and hair, brittle hair and nails, hair thinning and hair loss

- Anemia (can lead to fatigue, shortness of breath, increased infections, and heart palpitations)
- Severe constipation
- Arrested sexual maturity and growth failure
- Drop in internal body temperature, growth of a soft layer of hair to keep the body warm
- Loss of menstrual cycle
- Infertility and other fetal complications

To receive a diagnosis of anorexia nervosa, the following criteria must be met (APA, 2013):

- Restriction of energy intake relative to requirements leading to a significantly low body weight in the context of age, sex, developmental trajectory, and physical health.
- Intense fear of gaining weight or becoming fat, even though underweight.
- Disturbance in the way in which one's body weight or shape is experienced, undue influence of body weight or shape on self-evaluation, or denial of the seriousness of the current low body weight.

Screening Tools

Eating Disorders

SCOFF

The SCOFF is a valid and reliable screening tool for eating disorders. It was developed as an alternative to the existing tools which were cumbersome to complete and most often required a specialist to interpret (Morgan, Reid, & Lacey, 2000). SCOFF stands for sick, control, one, fat, food. The SCOFF consists of five yes/no questions focused on eating behavior and feelings. If a person answers "yes" to two or more of the questions, referral to an eating disorder professional for further evaluation is warranted. More information on the SCOFF can be found at: http://www.aafp.org/afp/2003/0115/p297.html

Eating Disorder Examination Questionnaire

The Eating Disorder Examination Questionnaire (EDE-Q) is a 22-item questionnaire designed to screen for eating disorders in a primary care setting

(Mond, Hay, Rodgers, Owen, & Beumont, 2004). A version of the EDE-Q was developed for adolescents aged 14–18 (EDE-A) (Fairburn, Cooper, & O'Connor, 2014). The version for adults 18 years and older asks how many days in the past 28 days (4 weeks) the person experienced things such as feeling faint, fear over losing control over eating, and limiting the amount of food. It also asks how many times they engaged in behaviors such as binging, vomiting, and taking laxatives. The EDE-A is similar to the adult version in terms of the questions, but it asks about the past 2 weeks rather than 4 weeks. The EDE-A can be accessed at https://www.corc.uk.net/outcome-experience-measures/eating-disorder-examination/.

Depression

There are many valid and reliable rating scales that can be used to screen children for depression. Many of these tools can be administered by a pediatrician, school social worker, child welfare workers, counselors, or other professionals working with children. Some of these tools are available free. Others are subject to copyright and require permission for use or purchase. The following are a few examples of measurement tools for assessing depression.

Children's Depression Rating Scale-Revised
The Children's Depression Rating Scale-Revised (CDRS-R), developed by Poznanski and Mokros (1996), was designed for assessing depressive symptoms in 6- to 12-year-olds. It is also a useful tool for measuring response to treatment across time. The CDRS-R is administered through a semi-structured interview conducted with either the youth or an adult who knows the child well. It takes approximately 15–20 minutes to administer. It was designed to rate across 17 symptom areas, including the DSM criteria for depression. The CDRS-R can be purchased online from Western Psychological Services.

Children's Depression Inventory 2nd Edition
The Children's Depression Inventory 2nd Edition (CDI 2) assesses for cognitive, affective, and behavioral signs of depression in youth aged 7–17 (Kovacs, 2010). The CDI consists of a youth self-report and parent and teacher questionnaires. The youth tool includes 29 items that focus on emotional problems and functional impairment. It takes approximately 10–15

minutes to complete. A shorter version of the CDI 2 that takes approximately 5 minutes to complete is available. The CDI 2 toolkit can be purchased online from Pearson Assessments.

Center for Epidemiological Studies Depression Scale Modified for Children
The Center for Epidemiological Studies Depression Scale Modified for Children (CES-DC) is a self-report tool designed to assess depression in youth aged 6–17 (Faulstich, Carey, Ruggiero, Enyart, & Gresham, 1986; Radloff, 1977). The CES-DC is a self-administered 20-item scale. Youth are asked to rate the level to which they have experienced certain feelings. This scale takes about 5 minutes to complete and can be downloaded free from Bright Futures (http://www.brightfutures.org).

The Beck Depression Inventory for Youth and the Beck Depression Inventory-II Student
The Beck Depression Inventory for Youth (BDI-Y) for ages 7–14 and the Beck Depression Inventory-II (BDI-II) Student for ages 13 and older are commonly used tools for the early identification and screening of depressive symptoms (Beck, Ward, & Mendelson, 1961). The BDI-Y consists of 20 self-report items that are written at a second-grade level. The BDI-II consists of 21 self-report items. Both tools take between 5 and 10 minutes to complete and can be purchased from Pearson (http://www.pearsonclinical.com).

Case Studies

The following are case studies that relate to depression. In the next chapter, we will explore evidence-based treatments and practices for depression. We will return to the case studies presented here to learn about the actual types of interventions that were provided to the youth in these studies and learn to determine which interventions are most appropriate.

Mary
Mary is a 16-year-old in the ninth grade. Her family is considered a very loving upper-class family. Mary made straight A's and rarely missed a day of school through elementary and middle school. She took piano lessons and played the trumpet in the school band. She was very involved in the youth group at her church. About midway through the ninth grade, Mary

started complaining of stomachaches and refused to go to school. She did this two to three times a week. When she stayed at home, she stayed in bed and slept. She ate very little at meals. Mary's mother took her to see her primary care physician. Her doctor ran all sorts of medical tests to determine the cause of her stomach problems. No medical cause could be found. Mary continued to complain and miss school. She got to the point where she refused to go to school altogether. She did not pick up her trumpet, play her piano, or hang out with her church youth group. She missed so much school that her grades went from A's to F's and she was at risk of having to repeat the ninth grade.

Here are some questions about Mary's case:

1. What symptoms was Mary experiencing?
2. Does she meet the criteria for a diagnosis of any of the types of depression? Explain. If she does, which one?
3. Based on your current knowledge, what interventions would you suggest? Do you believe that the appropriate intervention or treatment was provided?
4. Who should be included in the treatment planning and interventions?
5. What barriers might get in the way of effectively intervening?
6. What suggestions, thoughts, or ideas do you have for the other members of her family?

David

David was 9 years old when his father died. After the death of his father, David's behavior changed. He started to exhibit aggressive behavior. He tormented and hit his younger brother for no obvious reason. He began to sit in his tree house by himself for hours on end drawing bloody and gruesome pictures of monsters killing people. In school, he had difficulty focusing on and completing his work. When his teacher tried to redirect him, he started yelling that he sucked and could not do the assignment because he was stupid. Sometimes when he was asked to do the simplest of tasks at home, he would bang his head on the floor or hit walls. After approximately 6 weeks of this new behavior, his mother decided to take him to see a mental health professional.

Consider the following questions:

1. What symptoms was David experiencing?
2. Does he meet the criteria for a diagnosis of any of the types of depression? Explain. If he does, which one?
3. Based on your current knowledge, what interventions would you suggest? Do you believe that the appropriate intervention or treatment was provided?
4. Who should be included in the treatment planning and interventions?
5. What barriers might get in the way of effectively intervening?
6. What suggestions, thoughts, or ideas do you have for the other members of his family?

References

American Psychiatric Association. (1994). *Diagnostic and statistical manual of mental disorders* (4th ed.). Washington, DC: Author.

American Psychiatric Association. (2013). *Diagnostic and statistical manual of mental disorders* (5th ed.). Washington, DC: Author.

Arcelus, J., Mitchell, A. J., Wales, J., & Nielsen, S. (2011). Mortality rates in patients with anorexia nervosa and other eating disorders: A meta-analysis of 36 studies. *Archives of General Psychiatry*, 68(7), 724–731.

Beck, A. T., Ward, C., & Mendelson, M. (1961). Beck depression inventory (BDI). *Archives of General Psychiatry*, 4, 561–571.

Centers for Disease Control and Prevention (CDC). (2019). Suicide among youth. Retrieved from https://www.cdc.gov/healthcommunication/toolstemplates/entertainmented/tips/SuicideYouth.html

Centers for Disease Control and Prevention (CDC), National Center for Health Statistics (NCHS), National Vital Statistics System (n.d.). 10 leading causes of death, United States. Retrieved April 8, 2019, from https://webappa.cdc.gov/cgi-bin/broker.exe

Chesney, E., Goodwin, G. M., & Fazel, S. (2014). Risks of all-cause and suicide mortality in mental disorders: a meta-review. *World Psychiatry*, 13(2), 153–160.

Copeland, W. E., Angold, A., Costello, E. J., Egger, H. - (2013). Prevalence, comorbidity, and correlates of DSM-5 proposed disruptive mood dysregulation disorder. *American Journal of Psychiatry*, 170, 173–179.

Cyranowski, J. M., Frank, E., Young, E., & Shear, M. K. (2000). Adolescent onset of the gender difference in lifetime rates of major depression. *Archives of General Psychiatry*, 57, 21–27.

Diemer, E. W., Grant, J. D., Munn-Chernoff, M. A., Patterson D. A., Duncan, A. E. (2015). Gender identity, sexual orientation, and eating-related pathology in a national sample of college students. *Journal of Adolescent Health*, 57(2), 144–149.

Eaton, D. K., Kann, L., Kinchen, S., Shanklin, S., Flint, K. H., Hawkins, J., . . . Wechsler, H. (2012). Youth risk behavior surveillance—United States, 2011. *Morbidity and Mortality Weekly Report*, 61(4). Retrieved from http://www.cdc.gov/mmwr/pdf/ss/ss6104.pdf

Fairburn, C., Cooper, Z., & O'Connor, M. (2014). *Eating Disorder Examination* (Edition 17.0D; April, 2014). New York: Guilford Press.

Faulstich, M. E., Carey, M. P., Ruggiero, L., Enyart, P., & Gresham, F. (1986). Assessment of depression in childhood and adolescence. An evaluation of the Center for Epidemiological Studies Depression Scale for Children (CES-DC). *American Journal of Psychiatry, 143,* 1024–1027.

Gluck, S. (2012). Self injury, self harm statistics and facts, healthy place. Retrieved May 8, 2019, from https://www.healthyplace.com/abuse/self-injury/self-injury-self-harm-statistics-and-facts

Golden, N. H., Schneider, M., & Wood, C. (2016). Preventing obesity and eating disorders in adolescents. *Pediatrics, 138*(3). doi:10.1542/peds.2016-1649

Grilo, C. M., White, M. A., & Masheb, R. M. (2009). DSM-IV psychiatric disorder co-morbidity and its correlates in binge eating disorder. *International Journal of Eating Disorders, 42,* 228–234. doi:10.1002/eat.20599

Hudson, J. I., Hiripi, E., Pope, H. G. Jr, & Kessler, R. C. (2007). The prevalence and correlates of eating disorders in the National Comorbidity Survey Replication. *Biological Psychiatry, 61*(3), 348–358.

Hyde, C. L., Nagle, M. W., Tian, C., Chen, X., Paciga, S. A., Wendland, J. R., . . . Winslow, A. R. (2016). Identification of 15 genetic loci associated with risk of major depression in individuals of European descent. *Nature Genetics.* doi:10.1038/ng.3623

Kandel, E. R., Schwartz, J. H., & Jessell, T. M. (2000). *Principles of neural science* (4th ed.). New York: McGraw-Hill.

Kealey, E., Hudson Scholle, S., Byron, S. C., Hoagwood, K., Leckman-Westin, E., Kelleher, K., & Finnerty, M. (2014). Quality concerns in antipsychotic prescribing for youth: A review of treatment guidelines. *Academic Pediatrics, 14*(5), 68–75.

Kovacs. (2010). *The Children's Depression Inventory* (2nd ed.) (CDI 2).

Krishnan, K., Taylor, W. D., McQuoid, D. R., MacFall, J. R., Payne, M. E., Provenzale, J. M., & Steffens, D. C. (2004). Clinical characteristics of magnetic resonance imaging-defined subcortical ischemic depression. *Biological Psychiatry, 55,* 390–397.

Lanzillo, E. C., Horowitz, L. M., Wharff, E. A., Sheftall, A. H., Pao, M., & Bridge, J. A. (2019). The importance of screening preteens for suicide risk in the emergency department. *Hospital Pediatrics, 9*(4), 305–307.

Merikangas, K. R., He, J., Burstein, M., Swanson, S. A., Avenevoli, S., Cui, L., . . . Swendsen, J. (2010). Lifetime prevalence of mental disorders in US adolescents: Results from the National Comorbidity Study-Adolescent Supplement (NCS-A). *Journal of the American Academy of Child & Adolescent Psychiatry, 49,* 980–989.

Milos, G., Spindler, A., Buddeberg, C., & Crameri, A. (2003). Axes I and II comorbidity and treatment experiences in eating disorder subjects. *Psychotherapy and Psychosomatics, 72*(5), 276–285.

Mond, J. M., Hay, P. J., Rodgers, B., Owen, C., & Beumont, P. J. (2004). Validity of the Eating Disorder Examination Questionnaire (EDE-Q) in screening for eating disorders in community samples. *Behaviour, Research and Therapy, 42*(5), 551–567.

Moreno, C., Laje, G., Blanco, C., Jiang, H., Schmidt, A. B., & Olfson, M. (2007). National trends in the outpatient diagnosis and treatment of bipolar disorder in youth. *Archives of General Psychiatry, 64,* 1032–1039.

Morgan, J. F., Reid, F., & Lacey, J. J. (2000). The SCOFF questionnaire: A new screening tool for eating disorders. *Western Journal of Medicine, 172*(3), 164–165.

National Institute of Mental Health. (n.d.-a). Depression in children and adolescents. Retrieved from http://www.nimh.nih.gov/health/topics/depression/depression-in-children-and-adolescents.shtml

National Institute of Mental Health. (n.d.-b). Suicide: A major, preventable mental health problem: Facts about suicide and suicide prevention among teens and young adults. Retrieved from http://www.nimh.nih.gov/health/publications/suicide-a-major-preventable-mental-health-problem-fact-sheet/teen-suicide.pdf

National Research Council and Institute of Medicine. (2009). *Depression in Parents, Parenting, and Children: Opportunities to Improve Identification, Treatment, and Prevention. Committee on Depression, Parenting Practices, and the Healthy Development of Children. Board on Children, Youth, and Families.* Division of Behavioral and Social Sciences and Education. Washington, DC: The National Academies Press.

Poznanski, M. D., & Mokros, H. B. (1996). *Children's depression rating scale-Revised (CDRS-R).* Los Angeles: Western Psychological Services.

Radloff, L. S. (1977). The CES-D scale: A self-report depression scale for research in the general population. *Applied Psychological Measurement, 1,* 385–401.

Smolak, L. (2011). Body image development in childhood. In T. Cash & L. Smolak (Eds.), *Body image: A handbook of science, practice, and prevention* (2nd ed., pp. 67–75). New York: Guilford.

Swannell, S. V., Martin, G. E., Page, A., Hasking, P., & St. John, N. J. (2014). Prevalence of non-suicidal self-injury in nonclinical samples: systematic review, metal-analysis and meta regression. *Suicide and Life-Threatening Behavior, 44*(3), 273–303.

Tsuang, M. T., Bar, J. L., Stone, W. S., & Faraone, S. V. (2004). Gene-environment interactions in mental disorders. *World Psychiatry, 3*(2), 73–83.

Tsuang, M. T., & Faraone, S. V. (1990). *The genetics of mood disorders.* Baltimore, MD: Johns Hopkins University Press.

US Department of Health and Human Services (DHHS). (2001). *National strategy for suicide prevention: Goals and objectives for action.* Rockville, MD: HHS.

US Department of Health and Human Services (DHHS) Office of the Surgeon General and National Action Alliance for Suicide Prevention. (2012, September). *National Strategy for Suicide Prevention: Goals and objectives for action.* Washington, DC: HHS.

US National Library of Medicine. (2017, July 3). *NIH Categorical Spending -NIH Research Portfolio Online Reporting Tools (RePORT).* Washington, DC: US National Library of Medicine.

Weissman, M. M., Wolk, S., Goldstein, R. B., Moreau, D., Adams, P., Greenwald, S., . . . Wichramaratne, P. (1990). Depressed adolescents grown up. *Journal of the American Medical Association, 281,* 1701–1713.

Whitlock, J. L., & Knox, K. (2007). The relationship between suicide and self-injury in a young adult population. *Archives of Pediatrics and Adolescent Medicine, 161,* 634–640. Retrieved from http://www.selfinjury.bctr.cornell.edu/publications/a3.pdf

Yates, T. M. (2004). The developmental psychopathology of self-injurious behavior: Compensatory regulation in posttraumatic adaptation. *Clinical Psychological Review, 24,* 35–74.

6

Treatment of Depressive Disorders

Medication and psychotherapy are the two most common treatments for depression. Eighty percent of persons who receive treatment experience improvement in their depression (National Institute of Mental Health, 2005). The type of treatment prescribed by a doctor depends on the type and level of depression. Medication is indicated mostly for persons with major depression, although it can be used to treat less severe forms of depression as well. Medication does not provide a cure, but it can help the body regulate its own chemistry to control the symptoms of depression. The amount of control varies from person to person. Psychotherapy helps a person change faulty thinking and poor coping into positive thinking and coping. Research has found that a combination of medication and psychotherapy has the best results in reducing levels of depression.

Antidepressant Medication

There are currently approximately 25 different antidepressant medications that help the body regulate the neurotransmitters dopamine, serotonin, and/or norepinephrine in the brain. These neurotransmitters are essential for normal brain activity. There are four main classes of antidepressants, each acting on different neurotransmitters: serotonin reuptake inhibitors (SSRIs), serotonin norepinephrine reuptake inhibitors (SNRIs), monoamine oxidase inhibitors (MOAIs), and tricyclic antidepressants (TCAs). Different people will respond to these medications differently (Trivedi et al., 2006). It is not easy to determine in advance which medication a person will respond to best. Antidepressants take up to 4 weeks to work, so it is important for patients to give the medication enough time before determining that it does not work.

The most popularly prescribed antidepressants are fluoxetine (Prozac), paroxetine (Paxil), escitalopram (Lexapro), citalopram (Celexa), and sertraline (Zoloft). These medications are in the SSRI class, meaning that they affect the concentration and activity of one specific neurotransmitter

Understanding the Mental Health Problems of Children and Adolescents. Kirstin Painter and Maria Scannapieco,
Oxford University Press (2021). © Oxford University Press. DOI: 10.1093/oso/9780190927844.003.0006

Table 6.1 Selective serotonin reuptake inhibitors

Brand name	Generic name
Celexa	Citalopram
Lexapro	Escitalopram
Luvox	Fluvoxamine
Luvox CR	Fluvoxamine CR
Paxil	Paroxetine
Prozac	Fluoxetine
Zoloft	Sertraline

in the brain known as serotonin. The SSRIs are popular due to their high level of effectiveness in reducing symptoms and their low risk of side effects and overdoses. This class of medication is the most popular for treating children and adolescents. Table 6.1 lists selective SSRI medications by brand and generic names.

The SNRIs form a newer class of medications. This class has been found to be effective in alleviating symptoms of depression and anxiety. The SNRIs target both the serotonin and norepinephrine receptors in the brain. As shown in Table 6.2, examples of SNRI medications include desvenlafaxine (Pristiq), duloxetine (Cymbalta), and venlafaxine (Effexor). The SSRIs and SNRIs have been found to have relatively equal response rates.

There are also atypical antidepressants that have been approved by the US Food and Drug Administration (FDA) for treating depression. Each of these medications works differently from other atypical antidepressants and from the other classes of antidepressants. What they have in common

Table 6.2 Serotonin norepinephrine reuptake inhibitors

Brand name	Generic name
Cymbalta	Duloxetine
Effexor (XR)	Venlafaxine (XR)
Pristiq	Desvenlafaxine
Savella	Milnacipran
Fetzima	Levomilnacipran

Table 6.3 Atypical medications

Brand name	Generic name
Wellbutrin	Bupropion
Remeron	Mirtazapine
Nefazodone (discontinued)	Dutonin, nefadar, serzone
Oleptro	Trazodone

with each other and with other antidepressants is that they affect dopamine, serotonin, and/or norepinephrine in some way that changes the balance of these neurotransmitters to affect mood. The exact way in which they affect the neurotransmitters is unknown. These medications share common side effects: dry mouth, constipation, and dizziness. In addition, each one causes side effects that are different from those caused by the others. Table 6.3 lists atypical medications.

TCAs and MAOIs are older classes of antidepressants. Both tricyclics and MAOIs are far less expensive than the other two classes of medications and come in generic forms; however, there is a high risk of side effects. Tricyclics affect serotonin and norephinephrine, and MAOIs block the effect of an enzyme in the brain that prevents the breakdown of serotonin and norephinephrine. Tricyclic overdose is a serious issue because it does not take much more than a normal dosage to cause an overdose. Overdose is also a serious issue for MAOIs. In addition to the long list of side effects for MAOIs, there is a risk of experiencing a severe spike in blood pressure. Although these medications are not in the first line of antidepressants prescribed, they are still prescribed to people who do not respond to the newer medications. Brand names and generic names of tricyclic antidepressants and monoamine oxidase inhibitors are listed in Tables 6.4 and 6.5, respectively.

Antidepressant Medication Use in Children and Adolescents

Unfortunately, there have been few studies on the effectiveness of antidepressant medications in treating children or adolescents, although antidepressants are commonly prescribed for children and can be effective. Currently, there are two antidepressants approved by the FDA for treating major depressive disorder. Prozac is approved for treating depression in

Table 6.4 Tricyclic antidepressants

Brand name	Generic name
Adapin	Doxepin
Anafranil	Clomiprimine
Aventyl	Nortriptyline
Elavil	Amitriptyline
Ludiomil	Maprotiline
Norpramin	Desipramine
Pamelor	Nortriptyline
Sinequan	Doxepin
Surmontil	Trimipramine
Tofranil	Imipramine
Vivactil	Protriptyline

children aged 8 and older; Lexapro is approved for youth 12 and older. When a medication has not been studied and approved by the FDA to treat certain conditions or certain age groups, it is prescribed *off-label*. Although SSRI antidepressants are the most frequently prescribed for young people, research studies have found a link between SSRI and SNRI medications and increased suicidal thoughts and behaviors. A review of data from 24 clinical trials evaluating the effectiveness of antidepressants on children and adolescents revealed an increased risk for suicidality in the youths taking antidepressants compared to the control group who received a placebo (Bridge et al., 2007). Due to the findings of this review, the FDA gave SSRI and SNRI medications *black box warnings*, the most serious medication warning given by the FDA, about the possible increased risk of suicide they can cause in young people. These warnings appear on the labels of prescription medications to alert

Table 6.5 Monoamine oxidase inhibitors

Brand name	Generic name
Marplan	Isocarboxid
Nardil	Phenelzine
Parnate	Tranylcypromine

consumers of any serious safety concerns (i.e., serious side effects or life-threatening risks).

When a youth is prescribed an antidepressant, it is important to monitor him or her for unusual changes in behavior and suicidal ideation. When prescribing an antidepressant, the doctor must weigh the increased risk of suicide against the potential benefit of the medication. Untreated persons who are depressed are at an increased risk of attempting or committing suicide as well.

Cognitive-Behavioral Therapy

Cognitive-behavioral therapy (CBT) is the most extensively tested psychosocial treatment for depression. It has been found to be effective in treating both children and adolescents experiencing depression (Burns & Hoagwood, 2002; Burns, Hoagwood, & Mrazek, 1999; Jensen, Weersing, Hoagwood, & Goldman, 2005; Kazdin & Weisz, 1998). Developed in the 1960s by Aaron T. Beck, CBT focuses on changing how one thinks and acts as a means of improving depression. This is based on the theory that depression is both caused and maintained by negative or irrational beliefs that affect behavior (Beck, 1967, 1970; Clark, Beck, & Alford, 1999). When people learn to recognize and evaluate the rationality of these negative, irrational beliefs, they can replace them with healthier thoughts and change their negative behaviors to healthier ones. This in effect will improve their mood. Because CBT has been extensively tested and found effective in treating depression, it is often a cornerstone in evidence-based treatments for depression.

CBT is structured and time-limited, lasting from 14 to 16 weeks. Treatment is goal-oriented and focuses on the *what* and *how* of specific problems occurring in the immediate present. CBT does not focus on the *why* of a person's thinking. The first goal of CBT is to help youth realize that they can control their own behaviors and therefore can change their depression. This technique is known as *cognitive restructuring*. The therapist works with the youth to change irrational and negative thought patterns by teaching strategies to stop, confront, and change these thought patterns.

The client takes an active role in treatment. Mood diaries or emotions charts are common tools used to assist the young person in monitoring thoughts, actions, physiological sensations, emotions, and events and in becoming aware of how these factors affect depression. The therapist also teaches the youth problem-solving, coping, self-monitoring, relaxation, and social skills. Learning ways to relax in stressful situations helps the youth feel more competent and opens the door to trying out other skills. Homework is used as a strategy for increasing learning and integrating the skills being developed.

Penn Resiliency Program

The Penn Resiliency Program (PRP) is a curriculum-based intervention aimed at promoting resilience and prevention of depressive symptoms in youth from ages 10 to 14. It was developed by Karen Reivich and Jane Gillham at the University of Pennsylvania. This program has been highly researched and found to be effective in youth across ethnic and culturally diverse populations (Brunwasser, Gillham, & Kim, 2009; Cardemil, Reivich, Beevers, Seligman, & James, 2007). It uses a small-group format that can be applied in schools or clinical settings. The curriculum can be used by teachers, counselors, or therapists.

The first five sessions of PRP utilize cognitive-behavioral techniques aimed at helping youth identify their self-talk and faulty thinking and learn to adapt their thinking to be more flexible. Youth learn about the link between thoughts and feelings and different thinking styles, thereby challenging their thinking. The remainder of the sessions (6–12) focus on teaching the youth coping, problem-solving, assertiveness and negotiating, decision-making, and social skills aimed at helping them manage day-to-day stressors. In all of the sessions, youth practice their new skills through games and activities. More information on PRP can be found at https://ppc.sas.upenn.edu/services/penn-resilience-training

Adolescents Coping with Depression

Adolescents Coping with Depression (CWD-A) was designed for adolescents from ages 12 to 18 (Lewinsohn, Clarke, Hops, & Andrews, 1990). It is a cognitive-behavioral intervention conducted in small groups of 4–10 youths. The curriculum consists of 16 2-hour sessions. The focus of CWD-A is on helping youth monitor their mood, change unrealistic thinking, increase participation in pleasant activities, and decrease anxiety. As with the other interventions using a CBT approach, adolescents are taught new skills such as social skills, communication skills, and conflict resolution. The manual for CWD-A is accompanied by a workbook for group participants. The workbook includes parallel exercises for each session as well as homework exercises.

CWD-A also includes materials for a caregiver group to accompany the youth group. The caregiver group focuses on teaching caregivers about adolescent depression and describing the skills being taught to the youth. In addition, caregivers are taught how to better communicate with and support children as they work through their depression. Caregivers also have a workbook and complete homework assignments. For more information, visit http://www.kpchr.org/research/public/acwd/acwd.html.

Interpersonal Psychotherapy

Interpersonal psychotherapy (IPT) was originally developed to treat adults experiencing depression (Mufson, Pollack Dorta, Moreau, & Weissman, 2004). It has since been found to be effective in treating adolescents experiencing depression. It is a very didactic therapy with overarching goals to decrease depressive symptoms and improve interpersonal relationships. The underlying basis of IPT is that depression can be caused, maintained, or buffered by the quality of relationships with others.

Interpersonal Psychotherapy for Depressed Adolescents

IPT for Depressed Adolescents (IPT-A) is a manualized version of IPT (Mufson et al., 1994) targeted to treating adolescents 12 through 18 years old who experience an acute onset of major depression. The treatment consists of 12–16 sessions conducted individually or in a group format. Therapists may choose to also include up to three sessions with parents. This program was developed to address relationship problems specific to adolescence, such as interpersonal relationships with the opposite sex, problems with parental authority, and peer pressure. It is meant to be implemented by master's- or doctoral-level clinicians.

The first focus of IPT is to provide education on the causes, correlates, and etiology of depression; to explore the youth's interpersonal relationships with others; and to identify a specific problem area that will be targeted during treatment. Once the problem area has been identified, the therapist educates the youth on the connection between relationship problems and depression. The next strategy of IPT is to help the youth clarify their expectations of relationships and teach them new skills aimed at improving significant relationships. During sessions, the youth practices the new skills with the therapist through role-playing. Once a certain level of mastery is achieved, the youth uses the techniques outside of therapy sessions. Through this process, the therapist helps link improvement in mood to the new ways of communicating with others and solving problems. ITP-A has been evaluated in both individual and group treatment formats and with an ethnically/racially diverse population. Studies have reported that youth receiving IPT-A experienced significant improvement in symptoms of depression, anxiety, and overall functioning (e.g., Gunlicks-Stoessel et al., 2010; Gunlicks-Stoessel & Mufson, 2011; O'Shea, Spence, & Donovan, 2015). More information is available at https://iptinstitute.com/.

Dialectical Behavior Therapy for Adolescents

Dialectical Behavior Therapy (DBT) is a CBT approach developed to treat chronically suicidal adults, in particular, people with borderline personality disorder (BPD) (Linehan, 1993). DBT combines behavior therapy and mindfulness. *Mindfulness* is a state of being aware of the present moment and observing your thoughts and body sensations (Brown & Ryan, 2003). Several randomized controlled studies have found it to be significantly more effective in reducing suicidal and nonsuicidal self-harm behaviors (e.g., Carter, Willcox, Lewin, Conrad, & Bendit, 2010; Linehan, Armstrong, Suarez, Allmon, & Heard, 1991; Verheul et al., 2003). DBT was adapted for treating adolescents (DBT-A) with repeated suicidal and nonsuicidal self-harm behavior (Miller, Muehlenkamp, & Jacobson, 2008). DBT-A is a manualized therapy lasting 16 weeks. The youth participates in weekly individual therapy sessions for 1 hour per week. Concurrently, caregivers participate in weekly skills training groups with other caregivers. Family therapy is added as needed. It also includes a module aimed at training adolescents new skills designed to modulate their emotional dysregulation, which is a trait found in people who frequently self-harm. DBT-A has been found to be significantly more effective in treating youth with repeated suicidal and nonsuicidal self-harm behavior than treatment as usual (i.e., counseling) (e.g., Katz, Cox, Gunasekara, & Miller, 2004; Goldstein, Axelson, Birmaher, & Brent, 2007).

Case Studies

Mary

Mary is the 16-year-old from a loving upper-class family introduced in Chapter 5. She did very well in school, making straight A's and having near perfect attendance through elementary and middle school. She was actively involved in many extracurricular activities.

About midway through the ninth grade, Mary began having somatic complaints and missed 2–3 days of school each week. She slept more than usual and ate much less than usual. She went from being a straight-A student to being an F student. No medical cause could be found for these changes. Her primary care doctor suggested that she see a counselor.

Her mother spoke with friends to find a counselor. She was referred to a counselor who was trained in CBT. Mary's mood improved somewhat after 3 weeks of counseling, but she was still experiencing depressive symptoms. Her counselor referred Mary to a psychiatrist. The psychiatrist started Mary on a low dose of Paxil. After 2 weeks on the medication, her mood improved significantly. She continued with counseling for the full 12 sessions of CBT.

Each week while she was on the medication and receiving counseling, Mary continued to improve. By the end of CBT, she was feeling like her old self. Her mother set an appointment for Mary and her to meet with the school counselor and all Mary's teachers. As a group, they came up with a plan to help Mary get her grades up. She was allowed to retake tests that she had failed and redo major assignments. She was able to complete these things while keeping up with her other school work.

David

David is the 9-year-old introduced in Chapter 5 whose father had passed away. After the death of his father, his behavior changed drastically. He became very aggressive toward others. He began to isolate himself and to draw death-themed pictures. At school, he had difficulty focusing on and completing his work. When asked to do the simplest of tasks at home or school, he would bang his head on the floor or hit walls. After approximately 6 weeks of this behavior, his mother took him to see a therapist.

The therapist helped David talk about the loss of his father. She worked with him to express his feelings, either verbally or through art. She taught him relaxation techniques to use when he felt stressed. David maintained a diary, in which he wrote down the activities of his day and his feelings about the activities. The therapist used the diary to help David change his negative thoughts into active coping strategies.

For the last 15 minutes of each session, David's mother joined in the session. The therapist modeled and taught her how to respond in supportive ways to David's emotions. After eight sessions, David was expressing his feelings better and experiencing a significant decrease in aggressive behavior.

Study Questions

1. What do these real-life scenarios have in common?
2. What are the differences?
3. After you learned what happened to each of the youths, do you have any different thoughts on how you would have handled the situation if you were the families' social worker?

References

Beck, A. T. (1967). *The diagnosis and management of depression*. Philadelphia: University of Pennsylvania Press.

Beck, A. T. (1970). *Depression: Causes and treatment*. Philadelphia: University of Pennsylvania Press.

Bridge, J. A., Iyengar, S., Salary, C. B., Barbe, R. P., Birmaher, B., Pincus, H. A., ... Brent, D. A. (2007). Clinical response and risk for reported suicidal ideation and suicide attempts in pediatric antidepressant treatment, a meta-analysis of randomized controlled trials. *Journal of the American Medical Association, 297,* 1683–1696.

Brown, K. W., & Ryan, R. M. (2003). The benefits of being present: mindfulness and its role in psychological well-being. *Journal of Personality and Social Psychology, 84*(4), 822–848.

Brunwasser, S. M., Gillham, J. E., & Kim, E. S. (2009). A meta-analytic review of the Penn Resiliency Program's effect on depressive symptoms. *Journal of Consulting and Clinical Psychology, 77*, 1042–1054.

Burns, B. J., & Hoagwood, K. (Eds.). (2002). *Community treatment for youth: Evidence-based interventions for severe emotional and behavioral disorders.* New York: Oxford University Press.

Burns, B. J., Hoagwood, K., & Mrazek, P. J. (1999). Effective treatment for mental disorders in children and adolescents. *Clinical Child and Family Psychology Review, 2*, 199–254.

Cardemil, E. V., Reivich, K. J., Beevers, C. G., Seligman, M. E. P., & James, J. (2007). The prevention of depressive symptoms in low-income, minority children: Two-year follow-up. *Behaviour Research and Therapy, 45*, 313–327.

Carter, G. L., Willcox, C. H., Lewin, T. J., Conrad, A. M., & Bendit, N. (2010). Hunter DBT project: Randomized controlled trial of dialectical behavior therapy in women with borderline personality disorder. *Australia and New Zealand Journal of Psychiatry, 44*, 162–173.

Clark, D. A., Beck, A. T., & Alford, B. A. (1999). *Scientific foundations of cognitive theory and therapy of depression.* New York: John Wiley.

Goldstein, T. R., Axelson, D. A., Birmaher, B., & Brent, D.A. (2007). Dialectical behavior therapy for adolescents with bipolar disorder: A 1-year open trial. *Journal of the American Academy of Child and Adolescent Psychiatry, 46*, 820–830.

Gunlicks-Stoessel, M., & Mufson, L. (2011). Early patterns of symptom change signal remission with interpersonal psychotherapy for depressed adolescents. *Depress Anxiety, 28*(7), 525–531.

Gunlicks-Stoessel, M., Mufson, L., Jekal, A., & Turner, J. (2010). The impact of perceived interpersonal functioning on treatment for adolescent depression: IPT-A versus treatment as usual in school-based health clinics. *Journal of Counseling and Clinical Psychology, 78*(2), 260–267.

Jensen, P. S., Weersing, R., Hoagwood, K. E., & Goldman, E. (2005). What is the evidence for evidence-based treatments? A hard look at our soft underbelly. *Mental Health Services Research, 7*, 53–74.

Katz, L. Y., Cox, B. J., Gunasekara, S., & Miller, A. L. (2004). Feasibility of dialectical behavior therapy for suicidal adolescent inpatients. *Journal of the American Academy of Child and Adolescent Psychiatry, 43*, 276–282.

Kazdin, A. E., & Weisz, J. R. (1998). Identifying and developing empirically supported child and adolescent treatments. *Journal of Counseling and Clinical Psychology, 66*, 19–36.

Lewinsohn, P. M., Clarke, G. N., Hops, H., & Andrews, J. (1990). Cognitive-behavioral group treatment of depression in adolescents. *Behavior Therapy, 21*, 385–401.

Linehan, M. M. (1993). *Cognitive-behavioral treatment of borderline personality disorder.* New York: Guilford Press.

Linehan, M. M., Armstrong, H. E., Suarez, A., Allmon, D., & Heard, H. L. (1991). Cognitive-behavioral treatment of chronically parasuicidal borderline patients. *Archives of General Psychiatry, 48*, 1060–1064.

Miller, A. L., Muehlenkamp, J. J., & Jacobson, C. M. (2008). Fact or fiction: Diagnosing borderline personality disorder in adolescents. *Clinical Psychology Review, 28*, 969–981.

Mufson, L., Moreau, D., Weissman, M. M., Wickramaratne, P., Martin, J., & Samoilov, A. (1994). Modification of interpersonal psychotherapy with depressed adolescents

(IPT-A): Phase I and phase II studies. *Journal of the American Academy of Child and Adolescent Psychiatry, 33*, 695–705.

Mufson, L., Pollack Dorta, K., Moreau, D., & Weissman, M. (2004). *Interpersonal psychotherapy for depressed adolescents*. New York: Guilford Press.

National Institute of Mental Health. (2005). Antidepressant medications for children and adolescents: Information for parents and caregivers. Retrieved from http://www.nimh.nih.gov/about/updates/2005/antidepressant-medications-for-children-and-adolescents-information-for-parents-and-caregivers.shtml

O'Shea, G., Spence, S. H., & Donovan, C. L. (2015). Group versus individual interpersonal psychotherapy for depressed adolescents. *Behavioural and Cognitive Psychotherapy, 43*(1), 1–19.

Trivedi, M. H., Fava, M., Wisniewski, S. R., Thase, M. E., Quitkin, F., Warden, D., . . . Rush, J. A. (2006). Medication augmentation after the failure of SSRIs for depression. *New England Journal of Medicine, 354*, 1243–1252.

Verheul, R., Van Den Bosch, L. M., Koeter, M. W., De Ridder, M. A., Stijnen, T., & Van Den Brink, W. (2003). Dialectical behaviour therapy for women with borderline personality disorder: 12-month, randomized clinical trial in the Netherlands. *British Journal of Psychiatry, 182*, 135–140.

7

Anxiety Disorders

Of all the mental health problems experienced by children and adolescents, anxiety disorders are the most common, affecting as many of 31.9 percent of youth by the age of 18, with approximately 8 percent experiencing a serious anxiety problem (Kessler, Petukhova, Sampson, Zaslavsky, & Wittchen, 2012; Merikangas et al., 2010). All youth experience anxiety at different points in their lives. Moderate levels of anxiety, stress, fear, and worry are normal feelings until they severely interfere with daily life. Normal anxiety will usually extinguish when the situation causing the anxiety is resolved or as the youth is able to use coping skills to manage the anxiety. However, when anxiety reaches a level at which it is interrupting daily life for an extended period of time, intervention is needed. Youth experiencing an anxiety disorder are more likely to have difficulty with school, friendships, and family. As with other mental disorders, untreated anxiety disorders can last into adulthood and can lead to drug and alcohol misuse.

Signs and Symptoms

Anxiety disorders share features of excessive stress, anxiety, and fear. The anxiety experienced is the anticipation that something unpleasant is going to happen, and, in response, a person experiences physical and biological reactions that are not due to a medical problem (American Psychiatric Association, 2013). The responses may include an increase in heart rate, profuse sweating, heartburn, headaches or other body aches, gastrointestinal problems, or nausea, for example. Types of anxiety disorders include generalized anxiety disorder, social phobia, panic disorder, separation anxiety disorder, panic disorder, and specific phobias. Obsessive-compulsive disorder (OCD) and posttraumatic stress disorder (PTSD), though not included in the *Diagnostic and Statistical Manual of Mental Disorders* (DSM) as anxiety disorders, are included in this chapter since they share many similarities with anxiety disorders. Each anxiety disorder has distinct characteristics,

Understanding the Mental Health Problems of Children and Adolescents. Kirstin Painter and Maria Scannapieco, Oxford University Press (2021). © Oxford University Press. DOI: 10.1093/oso/9780190927844.003.0007

but the symptoms overlap those of other anxiety disorders. Along with anxiety disorders, children or adolescents may experience *panic attacks* or *agoraphobia*. Both panic attacks and agoraphobia can occur as part of almost any anxiety disorder, although not all persons with an anxiety disorder experience them.

Anxiety disorders begin earlier in development than other mental health disorders. The median age of onset for anxiety disorders is 12 years; however, different types of anxiety disorders develop at different stages of development (Merikangas et al., 2010). Young children are more likely to experience phobias and anxiety separation while adolescents tend to experience social anxiety. In childhood, anxiety disorders are equally prevalent in males and females; however, during adolescence females have two times the frequency of any diagnosable anxiety disorder (Merikangas et al., 2010).

Causes of Anxiety Disorders

Anxiety disorders are the result of a combination of genetics and environmental risks (National Institute of Mental Health [NIMH], n.d.). Causes and correlates of anxiety vary based on the specific disorder, but all anxiety disorders include both genetic and environmental factors (NIMH, n.d.). Environmental factors that increase the risk of developing an anxiety disorder include a person's personality, experiencing or witnessing a traumatic event, stressful life events, relationship problems, and health problems, to name a few. Research studies of families and twins have found that anxiety disorders can be heritable (Hettema, Neale, & Kendler, 2001; Hettema, Prescott, Myers, Neale, & Kendler, 2005; Kaabi et al., 2006; Maron, Hettema, & Shlik, 2010).

Anxiety and the Brain

There are many unknowns about the role the brain plays in anxiety disorders, specifically the role of neuroendocrine influence (the relationship between the nervous and endocrine systems), neurotransmitters (chemicals in the nervous system that transmit information between nerve cells), and disruptions in the nervous system. Most of what is known about the brain and its relationship to the development of anxiety disorders comes from neuroimaging studies of adults; however, findings of studies with children and adolescents are consistent with findings of studies conducted with adults (Blackford & Pine, 2012; Wehry et al., 2015). Studies suggest that dysfunction of the amygdala (responsible for memory, emotions, fear responses, and survival instincts) and the prefrontal cortex (responsible for complex cognitive behavior, personality expression, decision making, and moderating social behavior) regions of the brain are critical to fear behaviors (Davis, 1992). In normal development of fear, the prefrontal cortex modulates amygdala reactions. Research suggests that youth with anxiety disorders exhibit overactivity in the amygdala (Martin, Ressler, Binder, & Nemeroff, 2009).

Panic Disorder

Although the DSM includes panic disorder, in which a person experiences recurrent, unexpected attacks of intense fear or discomfort during times when there is no real danger or threat, panic attacks often occur along with other mental health disorders. When this is the case, the panic attack is coded as a *specifier* to the other disorder. The symptoms experienced during a panic attack are very intense and scary for the person experiencing them. They can also be scary for an observer. During a panic attack, a person may feel as if he or she is going crazy or may die. The symptoms of panic attacks are much more intense than the symptoms experienced due strictly to anxiety, and they can occur in the context of any anxiety disorder and sometimes in conjunction with other disorders. Panic attacks last for a discrete period of time, with the symptoms of the panic peaking within 10 minutes. According to the DSM, during a true panic attack, four or more of the following symptoms will be experienced:

- Palpitations, pounding heartbeats, or accelerated heart rate
- Sweating, trembling, or shaking
- Sensations of shortness of breath or smothering
- Feelings of choking, chest pain, or discomfort
- Nausea or abdominal distress
- Dizziness, unsteadiness, lightheadedness, or faintness
- Feelings of being outside of reality (called derealization) or detached from oneself (called depersonalization)
- Fear of losing control or going crazy

- Fear of dying
- Feelings of numbness or tingling sensations (called paresthesias)
- Chills or hot flushes

Agoraphobia

Agoraphobia is characterized by extreme fear of being in a place or a situation from which there is no escape as, for example, in a large crowd, on a train, or in an elevator. The person may be fearful of losing control in public or experiencing a panic attack in front of others and being embarrassed or not having the help he or she needs. Persons with agoraphobia begin avoiding places or situations in which they feel unsafe or unable to maintain control. As time goes on, they find fewer places where they can go without fear. Many become prisoners in their own homes.

Panic Disorder with or without Agoraphobia

When a person experiences recurrent, unexpected panic attacks that are not associated with any specific trigger and cannot be attributed to another mental health disorder, substance abuse, or general medical condition, he or she may meet the criteria for panic disorder. For at least 1 month following an unexpected panic attack, the person must experience ongoing fear of having another attack, excessive worry about the causes or consequences of attacks, and/or a significant change in behavior resulting from the attacks. Panic disorder usually begins during late adolescence or early adulthood. It can begin in childhood, although this is rare. A child or teenager who has a biological parent, sibling, or other first-degree relative with a panic disorder is up to eight times more likely to develop a panic disorder (American Psychiatric Association, 2013).

Separation Anxiety Disorder

Separation anxiety disorder (SAD) usually begins in childhood. All children experience separation anxiety as part of normal childhood development, beginning around 7 months and subsiding by 3 years of age (American

Psychiatric Association, 2013). Approximately 4–5 percent of children and 1–2 percent of adolescents experience separation anxiety disorder. The average age of onset is 7½ years old, and it is more common in girls than boys. With SAD, a youth experiences extreme levels of fear and anxiety that are out of proportion to the situation and to their developmental age. This fear and anxiety significantly affect daily functioning and can prevent youth from participating in independent activities, particularly those occurring away from home. They may refuse to go to school or to play with friends for fear of being separated from their family. Older youth may experience excessive worry that something bad will happen to them or their family, such as a serious car wreck or the sudden death of a parent. When onset is acute, it can often be traced to a precipitating factor such as loss of a parent or other loved one, changing schools, or traumatic experience.

Diagnosing Separation Anxiety

For a youth to be diagnosed with separation anxiety, he or she must be experiencing a level of anxiety that is inappropriate for his or her developmental stage and excessive when he or she is threatened with being separated from home or from an individual with whom he or she is attached, usually a parent. The anxiety must be so severe that it significantly interferes with daily functioning or relationships. According to the DSM-5 (American Psychiatric Association, 2013), to be diagnosed with separation anxiety, the youth must exhibit three or more of the following symptoms over a time span of at least 4 weeks:

- Recurrent excessive distress when separation from home or major attachment figures occurs or is anticipated
- Persistent and excessive worry about losing or having harm befall major attachment figures
- Persistent and excessive worry that an untoward event will lead to separation from a major attachment figure (e.g., getting lost or kidnapped)
- Reluctance or refusal to go to school or elsewhere because of fear of separation
- Persistent and excessive fear of or reluctance to be alone or without major attachment figures at home or without significant adults in other settings

- Persistent reluctance or refusal to go to sleep without being near a major attachment figure or to sleep away from home
- Repeated nightmares involving the theme of separation
- Repeated complaints of physical symptoms (such as headaches, stomachaches, nausea, or vomiting) when separation from major attachment figures occurs or is anticipated

Social Phobia

Social phobia is considered one of the most common mental health disorders, affecting nearly 13 percent of people across their lifespans. Someone who experiences social phobia has excessive fear about being in certain social situations. We all experience some level of nervousness in situations in which we have to give a speech or presentation or perform in front of others. Although we are nervous, we are able to give the speech or perform. People with social phobia experience extreme fear of and anxiety about being judged or evaluated by other people. The fear experienced is unreasonable for the situation and severely interferes with a person's functioning. A person who is exposed to the feared situation experiences severe anxiety symptoms such as panic attacks.

Persons with social phobia are often characterized as being quiet, shy, aloof, nervous, or unfriendly. Their fear can interfere with their ability to be social or make friends. It is not the case that they do not want to be part of a social group or develop friendships; it is the extreme fear that paralyzes them and prevents them from engaging in such interactions.

Diagnosing Social Phobia

To be diagnosed with social phobia, a person must meet the criteria specified in the DSM. First is a persistent fear of social situations in which a person perceives that others may scrutinize him or her or in which he or she may act in a way that is embarrassing or humiliating. The fear of these social situations results in significant levels of anxiety. The person either avoids these situations or endures them with intense anxiety or distress. Second, adults must recognize that their anxiety is excessive or out of proportion for the situation. The response to the anxiety may take the form of a panic attack or other extreme responses. The level of anxiety or distress must interfere with daily living. The symptoms must not be attributable to a medical condition or another mental health problem.

Children and Social Phobia

For someone younger than 18 to be diagnosed with social phobia, the symptoms must last at least 6 months. The youth must be capable of having age-appropriate social relationships. The anxiety-provoking situations must be experienced in settings with peers and not only with adults.

Unlike adults, children do not have to have insight that their fear is unreasonable for the situation. When they do realize that their fear is not normal, they may try to conceal the problem. Children may also express their anxiety differently from the way adults express it. Children may express their anxiety through crying or temper tantrums. They may avoid social situations in which they will be with unfamiliar people.

Generalized Anxiety Disorder

Generalized anxiety disorder (GAD) is characterized by excessive worry about everyday life. The types of worry differ from person to person and may focus on things from the past, present, or future. As with other disorders discussed here, the worry causes significant interference with daily functioning. GAD is often accompanied by somatic problems such as rapid heart rate, shortness of breath, chronic physical health problems, and gastric problems including nausea or diarrhea. People with GAD may also experience trembling, being easily startled, and substance abuse.

Diagnosing Generalized Anxiety Disorder

The DSM criteria for GAD include excessive anxiety and worry almost every day for at least 6 months that affects multiple different events or activities, as well as difficulty controlling the worry. Adults must meet both criteria, whereas children are required to meet only one. Three of the following symptoms (one for children) must also be present:

- Restlessness or feeling on edge
- Being easily fatigued
- Difficulty concentrating/mind going blank
- Irritability
- Muscle tension
- Sleep disturbance

Children and Generalized Anxiety Disorder

As stated earlier, children do not need to have as many of the symptoms of GAD as do adults in order to meet criteria for the diagnosis. Common worries experienced by children often focus on the health of their family or themselves, their level of competence in school or athletics, their past actions, and future events. The fears experienced are not realistic and are excessive for the child's developmental level. It is important for the mental health professional to evaluate whether the fears are based in reality. For example, a child about to have surgery may experience fear of dying. Once the surgery has passed, the fear will dissipate. In meeting the criteria for GAD, the child must have difficulty controlling worry, and daily functioning must be significantly impaired.

Obsessive-Compulsive Disorder

Obsessive-compulsive disorder (OCD) is a very disruptive disorder prevalent in approximately 1–2 percent of the population, with 25 percent of those experiencing onset by age 14. OCD causes significant distress and frustration. It can be triggered by environmental or stressful factors, including normal developmental transitions such as starting school. When we think of OCD, we tend to think of people who have to wash their hands repeatedly before they can leave the bathroom or those who turn the light switch on and off over and over. Youth with OCD experience excessive worry about bad things happening to themselves or someone they care about or become excessively preoccupied with something. The level of worry is far beyond a normal child's level of worry and is not usually related to anything realistic. These excessive intrusive thoughts or worries are called *obsessions*. Although obsessions can present around many different issues, some of the more common obsessions experienced by children and adolescents include the following:

- Constant worry that something is going to harm family or self
- Fear of germs or contamination
- Intrusive sounds or words
- Religious preoccupation
- Preoccupation with body wastes
- Intrusive thoughts related to sex or aggression

Trying to ignore or suppress an obsession only increases its intensity and the associated discomfort, which often leads to the development of compulsions. *Compulsions* are repetitive behaviors or mental acts that are performed to reduce the stress or prevent something bad from happening. They are excessive and usually not related to the situation to be avoided. They interfere with a person's functioning. The following compulsions are the most common among children and teens:

- Repeated hand washing, showering, or teeth brushing
- Repeated rituals such as turning a light on and off a certain number of times before leaving a room
- Repeatedly rechecking something, such as seeing if a door is locked
- Having to touch an object over and over
- Rituals to prevent harming self or others
- Rituals of ordering or arranging things, such as ensuring that all the books on a bookshelf are perfectly aligned
- Counting rituals such as counting to 100 before starting some task
- Hoarding and collecting things
- Cleaning rituals related to the house or other items

The conduct of these rituals can take lots of patience on the part of families, caregivers, teachers, and others spending time with a youth. Trying to stop the youth from completing the ritual can result in serious behavior problems such as severe tantrums. A caregiver's failure to recognize the child's need to conduct rituals can also result in serious problems.

There are common signs that youth may be experiencing an obsession or compulsion. A youth's hands may be raw from constant washing, or he or she may use a large amount of paper towels or soap. A caregiver may notice that a child's homework has holes in the paper due to excessive erasing or that a child is spending hours on homework but not completing it. Normal daily activities may take an exceptionally long time to complete, such as showers that take 2 hours each morning. Youth may voice fear of being contaminated and respond by refusing to eat a meal if someone touches their plate or food, for example. Children may refuse to leave the house for fear that something really bad will happen to their parent.

Obsessions and/or compulsions in a child or adolescent often result in isolation from others. They can become so intrusive that the youth does not have time to participate in life. Furthermore, he or she will become isolated from friends and family due to the actual obsession or compulsion or the need to hide these symptoms from others and avoid the associated stigma.

Diagnosing Obsessive-Compulsive Disorder

To be diagnosed with OCD, a person must experience obsessions and/or compulsions that are time-consuming and cause marked distress. These thoughts or rituals often interfere with daily functioning, resulting in a person missing work or being late to work, school, or appointments. To be diagnosed with OCD, adults must recognize that their obsessions or compulsions are excessive and not normal. The need to recognize the irrationality of thoughts and/or behaviors does not apply to children. Children do not have to recognize that their obsessions or compulsions are not normal; however, those who do recognize the irrationality may try to hide it from others.

Posttraumatic Stress Disorder

Posttraumatic stress disorder (PTSD) is a mental health disorder resulting from a traumatic event in the environment that changes a person's brain chemistry. It is often associated with veterans returning from war, and it is one of the most common mental health problems experienced by maltreated children. Children who have experienced severe physical abuse or domestic violence are at a high risk for developing PTSD. Because of the prevalence of PTSD in maltreated children, more attention will be focused on this disorder.

PTSD is a form of *hyperarousal response*, meaning that it is a state of increased mental and physiological tension. The response is the result of the brain's inability to process and store the memories of a traumatic event. Persons who develop PTSD have either experienced or witnessed some tragic event involving actual or threatened death or serious injury to themselves or someone else. They respond to the event with feelings of complete helplessness or intense fear and re-experience it in one of several ways. Reliving of the experience often occurs in flashbacks of the event. People may experience recurrent nightmares of the event or intrusive images or thoughts of the event. They may experience a sound, smell, sight, or feeling that reminds them of the event and causes a physiological response or intense distress psychologically.

Along with flashbacks or dreams of the event, other symptoms may include diminished interest or participation in significant activities, feelings of detachment or estrangement from others, restricted range of affect, difficulty falling or staying asleep, irritability or outbursts of anger, difficulty concentrating, hypervigilance, and exaggerated startle response (American Psychiatric Association, 2013).

Posttraumatic Stress Disorder and the Brain

Research studies on PTSD have found that persons with PTSD experience changes in their brain chemistry and functioning (Kandel, Schwartz, & Jessell, 2000; Perry, 2006; Solomon & Heide, 2005; Teicher et al., 2003; Van der Kolk, 1987). It has been found that adults with PTSD have increased heart rates and higher blood pressure than adults without PTSD. They also experience conditioned anxiety, agitation, and panic states. The majority of studies in the literature have been conducted with adults rather than with children. Psychophysiological studies on adults with PTSD have reported heightened baseline autonomic activation as evidenced by increased heart rate, systolic blood pressure, and forehead electromyography. Other psychophysiological studies have found that adult PTSD patients have a more marked conditioned autonomic hyperactivity as well as conditioned anxiety, agitation, and panic states. High levels of catecholamines, neurotransmitters in the central and peripheral nervous systems (i.e., dopamine, noreprinephrine, and adrenaline), and their metabolites in plasma and urine suggest evidence of central and/or peripheral noradrenergic system dysfunction. In other words, there is evidence that highened levels of catecholamines and metabolites may be an indication of PTSD.

PTSD is considered a developmental disorder for children in that, as neurons are being developed and differentiated, damaging changes are occurring in the child's brain due to the changes and quantity of neurotransmitters resulting from trauma. These altered neurotransmitters thus alter the development of catecholamine receptor/effector systems and the functions mediated by them. Children who develop PTSD have alterations in their central and autonomic nervous systems, higher than normal levels of endogenous opiates in the brain, and an elevation of thyroid functioning. They have been found to excrete high levels of norepinephrine in urine, thus signifying a high level of circulating catecholamine. Evidence suggests that childhood trauma interferes with central nervous system maturation and causes lasting neurological changes. It is believed that some biochemical, functional, and structural changes in the brain are related to early and more chronic abuse and neglect that affect the process of brain development. Researchers have found that higher levels of exposure to violence result in more serious changes in the brains of children. Two studies of childhood PTSD both found abnormal functioning of the autonomic nervous system mediated by the main catecholamines which are adrenaline (epinephrine), noradrenaline (norepinephrine), and dopamine (Perry, 1994). When a person gets stressed, the adgrenal glands make large amounts of these catecholamines which help the body respond to stress. The first study examined dysregulation of the brain stem catecholamines and the second study examined heart rate changes for children diagnosed with PTSD. The combination of the findings of these two studies suggests poorly integrated brainstem function, increased sympathetic tone, and overreactive and poorly regulated brainstem catecholamine systems, meaning that brain development is significantly affected in children with PTSD.

Diagnosing Posttraumatic Stress Disorder

In the DSM-5 (American Psychiatric Association, 2013), PTSD is in a new chapter on trauma- and stressor-related disorders along with reactive attachment disorder, disinhibited social engagement disorder, acute stress disorder, and adjustment disorders. The disorders in this group are all characterized by exposure of a person to a catastrophic or aversive event followed by the expression of a clinical level of distress that may present itself in an internalized manner (anxiety or fear) or an externalized manner (anger or aggression).

To be diagnosed with PTSD, a child must experience symptoms associated with PTSD for a month or longer, and these symptoms must cause significant problems in the ability to function in normal activities and relationships. Following the traumatic event, the child must experience at least three symptoms related to persistently avoiding anything that may be associated with the trauma and have a general lack of responsiveness. In other words, as specified in the DSM, the child must present with at least three of the following symptoms:

- Avoidance of thoughts, feelings, or conversations associated with the trauma
- Avoidance of activities, places, or people that arouse recollections of the trauma
- Inability to recall an important aspect of the trauma
- Markedly diminished interest or participation in significant activities
- Feeling of detachment or estrangement from others
- Restricted range of affect (e.g., does not expect to have a career, marriage, children, or a normal lifespan)

He or she must also experience persistent symptoms of increased arousal (not present before the trauma) as indicated by two (or more) of the following:

- Difficulty falling or staying asleep
- Irritability or outbursts of anger
- Difficulty concentrating
- Hypervigilance
- Exaggerated startle response

Children and Posttraumatic Stress Disorder

It can be difficult to diagnose PTSD in children due to the presentation of the symptoms. A child's symptoms may present similarly to those of another mental illness such as attention deficit hyperactivity disorder, conduct disorder, or bipolar disorder. The presentation of symptoms can also be different for children than for adults. For example, rather than having nightmares of the event, children commonly experience nightmares that are unrecognizable. Younger children may repetitively act out themes of the trauma in their play.

Assessment of PTSD in children necessitates a full psycho-social-emotional-biological evaluation across all areas of a child's life. The evaluation must include information from multiple persons involved in the child's life such as teachers, family members, coaches, or any others intimately involved with the child. Structured assessment instruments specific to the symptoms of PTSD in youth are also important to include in making the diagnosis.

The specific symptoms or disorders a child develops from maltreatment are based on the age of the child; the duration, extent, and level of abuse; the child's adaptive style; and other factors in the child's life such as emotional support received. Research on child maltreatment in PTSD has found that family history can affect the presentation of symptoms in childhood PTSD (Terr, 1991). For example, a child with a family history of schizophrenia has a higher likelihood of developing psychotic symptoms whereby the child loses touch with reality in response to maltreatment. The child may experience an inability to think clearly or understand reality, difficulty communicating effectively, or inability to behave appropriately, or he or she may respond to situations with exaggerated behaviors or with complete numbness.

A child whose family history includes anxiety disorders is more likely to develop symptoms of anxiety or an anxiety disorder, and a child with a family history of sociopathy and substance abuse is more likely to develop symptoms similar to conduct disorder. High rates of mental health problems and histories of trauma exposure and abuse have been found in adjudicated female youth. The variance in the presentation of symptoms makes identifying and treating PTSD in children very challenging. It is even more challenging in infants and children under the age of 4 because DSM 5 criteria are not sensitive enough to pick up PTSD in these younger children and infants. These young children often do not experience the hallmark features of adult PTSD, such as flashbacks and avoidance behaviors. Instead, symptoms of PTSD can be observed in a child's repetitive play, in which he or she reenacts a traumatic theme. When reminders of the trauma occur, children often experience intense distress that can manifest itself as difficulty concentrating, disturbed sleep, irritability, or anger outbursts. Although less is known about children responding to maltreatment with dissociation, some children with PTSD will develop symptoms such as diminished interest in regular activities, blunted affect, listlessness, and/or detachment. Lack of under-standing or recall of the trauma by the child adds to the difficulty.

Screening Tools for Anxiety

There are many tools for screening or assessing for symptoms of anxiety. The instruments discussed here are just examples of existing tools. Although there are many others, these three have been tested and found to be valid and reliable for assessing anxiety in children. Some of these tools are com-pleted by a clinician. Others are self-reports completed by the youth or care-giver reports completed by the caregiver about the child. None of these tools should be used as the sole criterion for diagnosing an anxiety disorder; how-ever, they can be useful in screening for anxiety or for monitoring treatment effectiveness.

The Spence Children's Anxiety Scale

The Spence Children's Anxiety Scale (SCAS; Spence, Barrett, & Turner, 2003) is a tool used to assess the severity of anxiety symptoms across six anx-iety domains (generalized anxiety, panic/agoraphobia, social phobia, separa-tion anxiety, OCD, and physical injury fears). The SCAS is available in three forms: youth self-report, caregiver report, and a caregiver preschool report. Each version of the scale takes about 5–10 minutes to complete. Youth or the caregivers rate the frequency with which the youth experiences symptoms (*never, sometimes, often,* and *always*). The SCAS is sensitive to changes in symptoms; therefore, it is useful for monitoring the effectiveness of treat-ment. It has been translated into multiple languages. All versions of the scale are available free at http://www.scaswebsite.com.

Beck Anxiety Inventory for Youth

The Beck Anxiety Inventory for Youth (BYI) (Beck, Beck, & Jolly, 2005) is a 20-item self-report inventory for use with children and adolescents from 7 to 18 years old. For each item, youth rate the frequency at which they experience a thought, feeling, or behavior related to anxiety from *never* to *always*. The BYI is used for screening, assessment, treatment planning, and measuring response to treatment. It takes approximately 5–10 minutes for a youth to complete. It can be purchased online at http://www.pearsonclinical.com/psychology/products/100000153/beck-youth-inventories-second-edition-byiii.html?Pid=015-8014-197#tab-pricing.

Screen for Childhood Anxiety-Related Disorders

Screen for Childhood Anxiety-Related Disorders (SCARED) was developed to screen children and adolescents aged 8 and older for anxiety disorders (Birmaher et al., 1999). It consists of 41 items that measure different types of anxiety based on the DSM, including general anxiety, separation anxiety, social phobia, school phobia, and physical symptoms of anxiety. The youth is asked to rate each item as 0 = *not true*, 1 = *somewhat or sometimes true*, or 2 = *very true or often true*. A caregiver report form is also available. The form takes approximately 5 minutes to complete. It can be downloaded free from http://www.wpic.pitt.edu/research under tools and assessments.

Case Studies

Here are some case studies of youth who experience some form of anxiety. In the next chapter, we will discuss evidence-based treatments and practices used to treat anxiety in children and adolescents. We will return to each of these youths to discuss the diagnoses, the different interventions they received, and the outcomes.

Andrea
Andrea was 7 when she was placed in foster care. She was removed from her mother because the mother's boyfriend was physically and sexually abusing her, and her mother was unable to protect her. Prior to the boyfriend moving into the home, Andrea was an average student. She was pleasant and got along well with her peers. One of her teachers made a report to Child Welfare Services because she noticed that Andrea had started coming to school with bruises on her body and had a significant change

in her schoolwork and behaviors. Andrea became irritable and angry with her peers, often without provocation. She stopped doing her homework, and in class she seemed to daydream rather than pay attention.

Andrea was placed in a home with three other foster children. She shared a room with another little girl. In the foster home, she continued to be irritable. She hardly interacted with the other children or her foster parents. She did not seem to have any interest in normal childhood activities. If someone walked up behind Andrea, she jumped. At night, she would wake up screaming as a result of having nightmares about her mother's boyfriend trying to find her and kill her.

Consider the following questions:

1. What symptoms was Andrea experiencing?
2. Based on the information provided, does she meet the criteria for an anxiety disorder? Explain. If she does which one?
3. Based on your current knowledge, what interventions would you suggest? Do you believe that she received the appropriate intervention or treatment?
4. Who should be included in Andrea's treatment planning and interventions?
5. What barriers might get in the way of effectively intervening with Andrea?
6. What suggestions, thoughts, or ideas do you have for the other members of Andrea's family?

Juan

Juan is a 14-year-old who was really late getting to school nearly every day of the week. Each morning before Juan left his house, he was compelled to count to 100 over and over for fear that something bad would happen to him if he did not. When Juan tried to ignore his thoughts and not count, he became more anxious and ended up having to count to 100 more times than usual. The same thing would happen if his mother tried to get him to leave the house on time to get to school. His mother did not know about his counting ritual. To her, it seemed that Juan was being resistant to going to school and not following her directions. She took Juan to the community mental health clinic for evaluation.

Try to answer the following questions:

1. What symptoms was Juan experiencing?
2. Based on the information provided, does he meet the criteria for an anxiety disorder? Explain. If he does, which one?
3. Based on your current knowledge, what interventions would you suggest?
4. Who should be included in Juan's treatment planning and interventions?
5. What barriers might get in the way of effectively intervening with Juan?
6. What suggestions, thoughts, or ideas do you have for the other members of Juan's family?

Andy

Andy is a 6-year-old. He is a very bright child. However, whenever he walked into a building, any building, he felt compelled to go into each restroom and touch the pipes under the sink. As can be imagined, this could take a considerable amount of time and was very embarrassing to his parents. It got to the point where they would not take him anywhere. He was either at school or at home. A doctor recommended putting Andy on medication to control his compulsions. Neither of his parents was comfortable with their son taking meds. They felt that it would be better to let him grow out of it.

When Andy went to school each day, he had to touch all the sink pipes before he went to his classroom. He was consistently late to class. His mother started driving him to school an hour early every day so he could complete his ritual before class started. It became a huge issue that Andy had to check the pipes in the girls' restroom and the teacher and staff restrooms, as well as the boys' restroom. At first, the school was very tolerant about Andy's need, but as he got older, the school did not feel that it was appropriate for him to go into the girls' and teachers' restrooms. They tried to stop Andy, which resulted in a huge anger outburst. His parents ended up removing him from school and home-schooling him. Andy became very isolated in his home.

Can you answer the following questions?

1. What symptoms was Andy experiencing?
2. Based on the information provided, does he meet the criteria for an anxiety disorder? Explain. If he does, which one?
3. Based on your current knowledge, what interventions would you suggest?
4. Who should be included in Andy's treatment planning and interventions?
5. What barriers might get in the way of effectively intervening with Andy?
6. What suggestions, thoughts, or ideas do you have for the other members of Andy's family?

Reggie

Reggie is a 15-year-old high school student. Reggie refused to attend any events such as dances or parties because he was afraid that he would do or say something embarrassing. When teachers asked him questions in front of the class, his face turned red. He would not answer the teacher's question for fear of not giving the correct answer or saying something stupid. Reggie even missed school on days when he was supposed to do a presentation in front of the class and instead accepted an F for the assignment. He felt that he was not as smart as the other students.

Consider the following questions.

1. What symptoms was Reggie experiencing?
2. Based on the information provided, does he meet the criteria for an anxiety disorder? Explain. If he does, which one?
3. Based on your current knowledge, what interventions would you suggest?
4. Who should be included in Reggie's treatment planning and interventions?
5. What barriers might get in the way of effectively intervening with Reggie?
6. What suggestions, thoughts, or ideas do you have for the other members of Reggie's family?

References

American Psychiatric Association. (2013). *Diagnostic and statistical manual of mental disorders* (5th ed.). Washington, DC: Author.

Beck, J. S., Beck, A. T., & Jolly, J. B. (2005). *Beck Youth Inventorie InventoriesSecond Edition for Children and Adolescents manual.* San Antonio, TX: PsychCorp.

Birmaher, B., Brent, D. A., Chiappetta, L., Bridge, J., Monga, S., & Baugher, M. (1999). Psychometric properties of the Screen for Child Anxiety Related Emotional Disorders (SCARED): A replication study. *Journal of the American Academy of Child and Adolescent Psychiatry, 38,* 1230–1236.

Blackford, J. U., & Pine, D. S. (2012). Neural substrates of childhood anxiety disorders: A review of neuroimaging findings. *Child and Adolescent Psychiatry Clinics of North America, 21*(3), 501–525.

Davis, M. (1992). The role of the amygdala in fear and anxiety. *Annual Review of Neuroscience, 15,* 353–375.

Hettema, J. M., Neale, M. C., & Kendler, K. S. (2001). A review and meta-analysis of the genetic epidemiology of anxiety disorders. *American Journal of Psychiatry, 158,* 1568–1578.

Hettema, J. M., Prescott, C. A., Myers, J. M., Neale, M. C., & Kendler, K. S. (2005). The structure of genetic and environmental risk factors for anxiety disorders in men and women. *Archives of General Psychiatry, 62,* 182–189.

Kaabi, B., Gelernter, J., Woods, S. W., Goddard, A., Page, G. P., & Elston, R. C. (2006). Genome scan for loci predisposing to anxiety disorders using a novel multivariate approach: Strong evidence for a chromosome 4 risk locus. *American Journal of Human Genetics, 78,* 543–553.

Kandel, E. R., Schwartz, J. H., & Jessell, T. M. (2000). *Principles of neural science* (4th ed.). New York: McGraw-Hill.

Kessler, R. C., Petukhova, M., Sampson, N. A., Zaslavsky, A. M., & Wittchen, H. U. (2012). Twelve-month and lifetime prevalence and lifetime morbid risk of anxiety and mood disorders in the United States. *International Journal of Methods in Psychiatric Research, 21*(3), 169–184.

Maron, E., Hettema, J. M., & Shlik, J. (2010). Advances in molecular genetics of panic disorder. *Molecular Psychiatry, 15,* 681–701.

Martin, E. I., Ressler, K. J., Binder, E., & Nemeroff, C. B. (2009). The neurobiology of anxiety disorders: Brain imaging, genetics, and psychoneuroendocrinology. *Psychiatric Clinics of North America, 32*(3), 549–575.

Merikangas, K. R., He, J. P., Burstein, M., Swanson, S. A., Avenevoli, S., Cui, C. B., . . . Swendse, J. (2010). Lifetime prevalence of mental disorders in US adolescents: Results from the National Comorbidity Survey Replication—Adolescent Supplement (NCS-A). *Journal of the American Academy of Child and Adolescent Psychiatry, 49*(10), 980–989.

National Institute of Mental Health (NIMH). (n.d.). Anxiety disorders. Retrieved from https://www.nimh.nih.gov/health/topics/anxiety-disorders/index.shtmlpart_145335

Perry, B. D. (1994). Neurobiological sequelae of childhood trauma: Post-traumatic stress disorders in children. In M. Murburg (Ed.), *Catecholamine function in posttraumatic stress disorder: Emerging concepts* (pp. 253–276). Washington, DC: American Psychiatric Press-.

Perry, B. D. (2006). Applying principles of neurodevelopment of clinical work with maltreated and traumatized children: The neurosequential model of therapeutics. In N. B. Webb (Ed.), *Working with traumatized youth in child welfare* (pp. 27–52). New York: Guilford Press.

Solomon, E. P., & Heide, K. M. (2005). The biology of trauma: Implications for treatment. *Journal of Interpersonal Violence, 20,* 51–60.

Spence, S. H., Barrett, P. M., & Turner, C. M. (2003). Psychometric properties of the Spence Children's Anxiety Scale with young adolescents. *Journal of Anxiety Disorders, 17,* 605–625.

Teicher, M. H., Anderson, S. L., Polcari, A., Anderson, C. M., Navalta, C. P., & Kim, D. M. (2003). The neurobiological consequences of early stress and childhood maltreatment. *Neuroscience and Biobehavioral Reviews, 27,* 33–44.

Terr, L. C. (1991). Childhood traumas: An outline and overview. *American Journal of Psychiatry, 148,* 10–20.

Van der Kolk, B. A. (1987). The separation cry and the trauma response: Developmental issues in the psychobiology of attachment and separation. In B. A. Van der Kolk (Ed.), *Psychological trauma* (pp. 31–62). Washington, DC: American Psychiatric Press.

Wehry, A. M., Katja Beesdo-Baum, K., Meghann, M., Hennelly, M. M., Connolly, S. D., & Strawn, J. R. (2015). Assessment and treatment of anxiety disorders in children and adolescents. *Current Psychiatry Reports, 17*(7), 591.

8

Treatment of Anxiety Disorders

The treatment of anxiety disorders is very similar to the treatment of depression. As with depression, anxiety is treated with psychotropic medications, various psychotherapies, or a combination of both. Research suggests that combing medication with a behavioral therapy to treat youth with severe anxiety disorders greatly improves the outcome and should be the standard of care (Taylor et al., 2018). Evidence-based interventions and practices for treating the different types of anxiety utilize cognitive-behavioral therapy (CBT) techniques such as teaching youth how negative thinking affects levels of anxiety, how to identify the physical aspects of anxiety, and how to change thoughts or use relaxation techniques to reduce anxiety. Unless children or adolescents are a danger to themselves or others or are significantly unable to function, psychotherapy is often the preferred first line of treatment. If after a few weeks psychotherapy is ineffective, medication is added to the treatment regimen.

Medication Treatment

Medications used to treat anxiety disorder include antianxiety medications and antidepressants. The most frequently prescribed antidepressants used in the treatment of anxiety are in the selective serotonin reuptake inhibitor (SSRI) class. These include fluoxetine (Prozac), sertraline (Zoloft), escitalopram (Lexapro), fluvoxamine (Luvox), paroxetine (Paxil), and citalopram (Celexa) (see Chapter 6 for a full discussion of antidepressants). Both Zoloft and Paxil are approved by the US Food and Drug Administration (FDA) for treating generalized anxiety disorder (GAD), panic disorder, obsessive-compulsive disorder, and social phobia. Venlafaxine (Effexor XR) and duloxetine (Cymbalta), both serotonin norepinephrine reuptake inhibitors (SNRI), have been found effective in treating anxiety disorders. Antidepressants used to treat anxiety in youth come with the same black-box warnings (the most serious

Understanding the Mental Health Problems of Children and Adolescents. Kirstin Painter and Maria Scannapieco,
Oxford University Press (2021). © Oxford University Press. DOI: 10.1093/oso/9780190927844.003.0008

medication warnings given by the FDA) as they do for treating depression due to the possibility that they may cause suicidal thoughts. Therefore, it is important to closely monitor any young person taking an antidepressant. Four to six weeks should be allowed to experience the full effect of the medications.

Another class of medications used to treat anxiety is the benzodiazepines (see Table 8.1). This class of drugs affects the central nervous system by enhancing the response of receptors in the brain to a neurotransmitter called *gamma-aminobutyric acid* (GABA), thereby negatively charging the neuron and making it resistant to excitation. Benzodiazepines are rarely used in treating anxiety disorders in youth because they have the potential for dependence. However, they are occasionally used to treat extreme levels of anxiety on a very short-term basis.

Some of the most commonly prescribed benzodiazepines are clonazapam (Klonopin), used mostly for treating social phobia and GAD; lorazepam (Ativan), used mostly for panic disorder; and alprazolam (Xanax), which is used for both panic disorder and GAD. A benefit of using benzodiazepines on a short-term basis is their relatively few side effects. The main side effects experienced by children and adolescents are drowsiness, sedation, and decreased mental acuity.

Table 8.1 Benzodiazepines for treating anxiety

Brand name	Generic name
Ativan	Lorazepam
Dalmane	Flurazepam
Klonopin	Clonazepam
Halcion	Triazolam
Librium	Chlordiazepoxide
Restoril	Temazepam
Serax	Oxazepam
Tranxene	Clorazepate
Valium	Diazepam
Xanax	Alprazolam

Psychotherapies and Anxiety

There are several manualized and nonmanualized evidence-based practices and interventions for anxiety. Most of the interventions are based on a combination of cognitive-behavioral, trauma, and social learning theories. Many of the interventions focus treatment on both the youth and the caregiver(s). Empirically supported practices focus on helping the youth identify negative thinking that leads to anxiety and on learning new skills to manage it. For caregivers, many of the interventions focus on education about anxiety and the role that problematic parenting styles can play in the youth's anxiety level. The goal is for caregivers to learn more effective ways of parenting. Some examples of existing evidence-based treatments are discussed in the following subsections.

Coping Cat

There are several manualized interventions based on cognitive-behavioral theory. Coping Cat is one example of a manualized cognitive-behavioral intervention for children aged 8–17 (Kendall, Choudhury, Hudson, & Webb, 2002; Kendall & Hedtke, 2006a, 2006b). The intervention consists of 16 sessions. These sessions focus on teaching youth about anxiety, helping them identify stress-inducing situations, and helping them develop coping skills. Coping Cat uses techniques common to CBT such as role-playing, relaxation training, self-reinforcement techniques, and practicing skills in real-life situations to help the youth develop the skills necessary for managing anxiety.

Once youth are able to identify the physical reactions related to the onset of anxiety, they can learn ways to manage the anxiety before it reaches a serious point. Youth are also taught to identify thinking errors (faulty beliefs) that lead to anxious feelings in order to change negative cognitions to more positive ones. The last eight sessions focus on practicing the new skills, first in imaginary stress-inducing situations, and then working up to practicing the skills in real-life stress-inducing situations as appropriate. This method is a form of an effective stress management technique called *systematic desensitization*.

Trauma-Focused Cognitive-Behavioral Therapy

Trauma-focused CBT (TF-CBT) is an evidence-based intervention appropriate for treating children and adolescents who have experienced abuse, neglect, or other traumatic experiences or have witnessed a traumatic event. Many adults believe that children are resilient and able to forget traumatic events. Rather than understanding the negative consequences of trauma, they have expectations of the child and how the child should behave. Research has found that young children are negatively affected by traumatic events and need a way to derive meaning from them. TF-CBT has been found effective in treating posttraumatic stress disorder. It is based on learning, behavioral, and cognitive theories. Using techniques of CBT and family therapies, treatment focuses on both the youth and a nonoffending caregiver, with emphasis on improving attachment and communication between them. Like CBT, TF-CBT is time-limited, lasting 12–18 sessions.

The key components of TF-CBT have been summarized by the mnemonic PRACTICE (Substance Abuse and Mental Health Services Administration, 2014).

- *Psychoeducation and parenting skills.* This component of treatment focuses on educating caregivers about the effects of abuse and trauma on children because caregivers who do not have this understanding often set unrealistic expectations for how their child should feel and behave. Research has found that problematic parenting styles contribute to a youth's anxiety. Caregivers who are overly protective often set limits on their children that are excessively restrictive and do not allow the children to experience developmentally appropriate situations in which to experience new situations and develop coping skills. Caregivers who have difficulty coping with their own anxiety model ineffective ways of coping for their children. Caregivers are taught more effective parenting skills, effective communication skills, and how to respond empathetically to their child's feelings.
- *Relaxation techniques.* Relaxation techniques are one of the most effective ways to manage stress and anxiety. Young people, especially younger children, feel a sense of accomplishment and empowerment through learning and using these techniques. Using a relaxation technique called

progressive muscle relaxation, youth learn to isolate their focus onto different parts of the body, to tense the muscles in that area, and then release all the tension. This continues until the entire body feels relaxed. *Focused breathing* is a relaxation technique that helps a youth take long, deep breaths and increasingly relax the body with each exhale. *Visual imagery* is another effective relaxation technique in which youth close their eyes and focus on being in a safe, comfortable environment such as lying in a meadow with the sun beaming down or floating on a magic carpet.

- Affective expression and regulation. The therapist works with both the child and caregiver to manage emotional reactions to places or situations that are reminders of the abuse. Rather than reacting in a destructive manner, they learn to identify and express their emotions verbally and to self-soothe.

- Cognitive coping and processing are taught to the youth and caregiver so that they connect their thoughts with their feelings and behaviors. The therapist helps them identify faulty beliefs (thinking errors) that result in unconstructive behaviors and methods of coping. They learn to reframe thinking errors with positive thoughts that will then lead to more positive behaving and coping.

- Trauma narrative and processing. Developing a trauma narrative is a key component in helping youth cope with their trauma. The therapeutic environment provides a safe place for children to process their experiences and make sense of the traumatic event(s). They can confront upsetting thoughts and feelings resulting from the event. When developing a trauma narrative, a therapist guides the caregiver and child through a series of questions to help them recreate the traumatic event(s) in some way. Young children often recreate the traumatic event through play or artwork.

- In vivo exposure, also known as systematic desensitization (discussed previously), is another key component of TF-CBT. After the youth learns coping and relaxation techniques, the therapist begins exposing him or her to places or situations that are reminders of the trauma, such as the room where the trauma took place. The therapist first helps the youth visualize the stress-inducing place or situation while helping him or her to practice the new coping and relaxation techniques. Once the youth is able to manage emotional reactions while visualizing the place or situation, the therapist gradually brings him or her closer and closer until he or she is able to manage emotional reactions when fully exposed to the stress-inducing place or situation.

- Conjoint parent/child sessions and Enhancing personal safety and future growth. During conjoint sessions, youths are able to share their trauma narratives with the caregiver. These joint sessions provide opportunities to normalize the anxiety experienced by the child. The caregiver learns the skills needed to provide positive affect and to encourage the child. The family learns skills to improve communication with each other. The final key component of TF-CBT is education and training to maintain the safety of the youth. Nonoffending caregivers are taught the skills needed to help their children develop the sense of safety that is important for overcoming anxiety. They learn to identify and avoid situations that could put their children in danger of abuse. Youth are taught skills that empower them to look after their personal safety as well.

Child–Parent Psychotherapy

Child–parent psychotherapy (CPP) is an empirically supported intervention aimed at treating very young children, from birth through age 6, who have experienced at least one traumatic event resulting in emotional, behavioral, and/or attachment problems (National Child Traumatic Stress Network, 2007). The overarching goal of CPP is to strengthen the attachment between child and caregiver(s) and return the child to a normal developmental path. This intervention has been evaluated and found effective across racially and ethnically diverse populations.

CPP is not a manualized intervention. Therefore, it can be more difficult to learn than some of the other empirically supported interventions. Clinicians providing CPP are usually master's-level social workers or psychologists with specialized training in mental health issues. To provide CPP, a clinician must receive face-to-face training and become certified as a CPP provider. For the certified CPP clinician, ongoing phone consultation and occasional booster sessions help increase fidelity to the model and provide support and guidance for dealing with difficult situations.

CPP is a didactic intervention based on attachment theory, and it also draws from psychodynamic, trauma, social learning, and cognitive-behavioral theories. Treatment includes key components of TF-CBT. During sessions, caregivers learn about the effects of trauma on behavior and functioning and how to respond empathetically and give their child positive affect. For example, a session might consist of a child playing while the therapist/counselor teaches the caregiver to pay attention to the child's play and respond in empathetic, supportive ways. When the child is very young, such as an infant, treatment focuses on providing the caregiver with the skills needed to provide a safe and loving environment. If caregivers have their own unresolved trauma issues, they are addressed in separate sessions.

Computerized Therapies

Two computerized CBT therapies for treating children experiencing anxiety (BRAVE for Children-Online and Camp-Cope-a-Lot: The Coping Cat) were developed and evaluated for their effectiveness in alleviating the symptoms of anxiety (March, Spence, & Donovan, 2009; Khanna & Kendall, 2010; respectively). Three computerized CBT therapies for treating adolescents experiencing anxiety (BRAVE for Teenagers-Online; Cool Teens; and Think, Feel, Do Feel) have also been developed and evaluated (Spence et al., 2011; Stallard et al., 2011; Wuthrich et al., 2012). All five programs show promise in alleviating or reducing symptoms of depression in children or adolescents.

Both BRAVE for Children-Online (March et al., 2009) and Camp-Cope-a-Lot (Khanna & Kendall, 2010) involve having the child complete sessions on a computer. BRAVE stands for Body signs, Relaxation, Active helpful thoughts, Victory over your fears, and Enjoy and reward yourself. The program consists of 10 very interactive sessions that use games, quizzes, puzzles, and animation examples aimed at teaching the child the needed skills to overcome fearful or worrying situations. Each session takes approximately an hour to complete. Children can complete the program in their own home and at their own pace. BRAVE was developed based on CBT techniques (e.g., learning to identify anxiety and stress, develop relaxation and problem-solving skills, and reframe negative thinking to more useful thinking). It includes two refresher sessions taken at 1 month and 3 months after completing BRAVE. There is a four-session program for parents of younger children experiencing anxiety. The child can have a personal BRAVE trainer throughout the program if needed. Brave can be purchased at http://www.brave-online.com/about-brave-online-program/.

Camp Cope-a-Lot Online is a 12-module computerized program that also uses CBT techniques. It is based on the Coping Cat program described earlier. The child completes the first six sessions independently, and the last six sessions are completed with a coach who is either a therapist or caregiver. The Camp Cope-a-Lot program is also very interactive, allowing the child to experience many different adventures all aimed at learning skills needed to overcome fearful or worrying situations. Camp Cope-a-Lot can be purchased at http://www.copingcatparents.com/Camp_Cope_A_Lot.

All of the computerized programs developed for adolescents follow similar techniques as those designed for children. Each program's content and activities were developed to be age-appropriate for teenagers. Cool Teens is an 8- to 12-week program that helps adolescents aged 11–17 develop coping skills to manage their anxiety. It contains eight multimedia modules that focus on CBT techniques. It was designed to target generalized anxiety disorder, social anxiety disorder, and other anxiety disorders. Cool Teens can be computer-based, self-guided, or clinician-assisted. BRAVE for Adolescents-Online is nearly identical to the BRAVE program developed for children. It was also developed based on CBT techniques (e.g., learning to identify anxiety and stress, develop relaxation and problem-solving skills, and reframe negative thinking to more useful thinking) and includes two refresher sessions taken at 1 month and 3 months after treatment.

Think, Feel, and Do (TFD) follows a three-pronged approach to CBT. It consists of six sessions on a CD-ROM and is based on the CBT workbook *Think Good—Feel Good* (Stallard et al., 2011). Each of the six sessions take approximately 30–45 minutes to complete. A facilitator, needing only minimal expertise in CBT, facilitates the program by discussing and elaborating on the program's content. The facilitator is present through the completion of each module to provide support and clarify anything that the youth does not understand. TFD uses multimedia with sounds, photos, cartoons, and music and, it is narrated to guide the teenager through the sessions.

Brave for Adolescents Online can be purchased at http://www.brave-online.com/about-brave-online-program/. Cool Teens can be purchased at https://www.c4tbh.org/program-review/cool-teens.

Case Studies

Andrea

Andrea is the 7-year-old who was placed in foster care because she had been physically and sexually abused by her mother's boyfriend, and her mother had been unable to protect her. Andrea was placed in a foster home where three other foster children lived. She isolated herself from the other children. She continued to isolate herself and did not participate in activities or develop any friendships in her new school. She continued to have nightmares and started wetting the bed. The foster family was at a loss about how to manage Andrea. They requested that she be removed from their home. Andrea was put into another foster home with foster parents who had been trained to manage children with emotional or behavioral problems. Child Protective Services paid for her to attend counseling with a therapist trained in TF-CBT. She was diagnosed with posttraumatic stress disorder.

The therapist asked to have Andrea's mother participate in the therapy sessions. Child Protective Services allowed the mother to participate, and the mother agreed. She wanted to have Andrea return home, and she had broken up with her boyfriend. Near the end of treatment, both the mother and Andrea had made great progress. The therapist advocated for Andrea to spend increasing increments of time at home to test how the two would do together. The therapist, case worker, mother, and Andrea met to develop a treatment plan that led to Andrea returning home to live. After Andrea spent 6 months at home, the Child Protective Services case was closed.

Juan

Juan is the 14-year-old who was really late getting to school nearly every day of the week. He could not leave his house until he had counted to 100 over and over for fear that something bad would happen to him if he did not. When Juan tried to ignore his thoughts and not count, he became more anxious and ended up having to count to 100 more times than usual. Juan's mother became frustrated with him and took him to the community mental health clinic for evaluation. Juan was evaluated by a psychiatrist who diagnosed him with obsessive-compulsive disorder and started him on a low dose of the medication venlafaxine (Effexor). Within 2 weeks, Juan's counting ritual had subsided considerably. Within 4 weeks, the ritual had ceased, and Juan began to function better in school.

Andy

Andy is the 6-year-old who felt compelled to go into each restroom in any building he entered and touch the pipes under the sink. His parents took him to a doctor who recommended medication. They refused to put him on medication. His compulsion resulted in problems in school that eventually led to his parent's home-schooling him and his becoming very isolated. Andy got to the point where he would not leave his house. If his parents tried to make him leave, he became very upset and screamed and yelled until they usually gave up and left him at home alone, even though he was so young. One evening when his parents were not home, Andy played with matches and set his bed on fire. The fire spread quickly. A neighbor saw smoke and called 911. When the firefighters arrived, they found Andy home alone and standing in the doorway crying. His room was completely burned, but he was not harmed. Child Protective Services was called.

Andy was allowed to stay with his parents as long as they agreed not to leave him alone and to participate in family therapy. His parents agreed. The therapist provided services in the family's home. They met with the therapist twice a week for an hour each time. The therapist diagnosed Andy with anxiety disorder not otherwise specified, meaning that he clearly had an anxiety disorder but did not meet the criteria for obsessive-compulsive disorder. The therapist provided Andy with CBT. Andy got to the point where he could leave the house. He learned to cope with and control the need to touch all the bathroom pipes in a building and was able to start leaving the house and going places with his family. He was discharged from therapy, and the Child Protective Services case was closed. It is not known if he ever returned to school or participated in age-appropriate activities with peers.

Reggie

Reggie is the 14-year-old who refused to attend any events such as dances or parties because he was afraid that he would do or say something embarrassing. He did not have any friends and began to exhibit symptoms of depression. He was diagnosed with social phobia and began CBT. He became less anxious but still had difficulty interacting with others and seemed depressed. After 5 weeks in counseling, his counselor referred him to a psychiatrist. The psychiatrist put him on the antidepressant paroxetine (Paxil). After a month on Paxil, Reggie was significantly less anxious and less depressed. The therapist continued to work with him and encouraged Andy to join the youth group at his church, which Andy did. He began to participate in church activities and developed some friendships. He began to feel more confident in school and stopped avoiding situations where he would be the center of attention, such as answering questions in class.

Study Questions

1. What do these real-life scenarios have in common?
2. What are the differences?
3. Now that you have learned what happened to each of the youths, do you have any different thoughts about how you would have handled the situation if you were the families' social worker?

References

Kendall, P. C., Choudhury, M., Hudson, J., & Webb, A. (2002). *The CAT project manual for the cognitive-behavioral treatment of anxious adolescents.* Ardmore, PA: Workbook Publishing.

Kendall, P. C., & Hedtke, K. (2006a). *Cognitive-behavioral therapy for anxious children: Therapist manual* (3rd ed.). Ardmore, PA: Workbook Publishing.

Kendall, P. C., & Hedtke, K. (2006b). *The Coping CAT workbook* (2nd ed.). Ardmore, PA: Workbook Publishing.

Khanna, M. & Kendall, P. (2010). Computer-assisted cognitive behavioral therapy for child anxiety: Results of a randomized clinical trial. *Journal of Consulting and Clinical Psychology, 78,* 737–745.

March, S., Spence, S. H., & Donovan, C. L. (2009). The efficacy of an internet-based cognitive-behavioral therapy intervention for child anxiety disorders. *Journal of Pediatric Psychology, 34,* 474–487.

National Child Traumatic Stress Network. (2007). Child parent psychotherapy fact sheet. Retrieved from http://www.nctsn.org/nctsn_assets/ pdfs/promising_practices /Child_Parent_Psychotherapy_CPP_fact_sheet_3-20-07.pdf

Spence, S. H., Donovan, C. L., March, S., Gamble, A., Anderson, R. E., Prosser, S., Kenardy, J. (2011). A randomized controlled trial of online versus clinic-based CBT for adolescent anxiety. *Journal of Consulting and Clinical Psychology, 79,* 629.

Stallard, P., Richardson, T., Velleman, S., Atwood, M. (2011). Computerized CBT (Think, Feel, Do) for depression and anxiety in children and adolescents: Outcomes and feedback from a pilot randomized controlled trial. *Behavioral Cognitive Psychotherapy*, *39*, 273–284.

Substance Abuse and Mental Health Services Administration. (2014). National registry of evidence-based programs and practices: Trauma-focused cognitive-behavioral therapy (TF-CBT). Retrieved from http://www.nrepp.samhsa.gov/viewintervention. aspx?id=135.

Taylor, J. H., Lebowitz, E. R., Jakubovski, E., Coughlin, C. G., Silverman, W. K., & Bloch, M. H. (2018) Monotherapy insufficient in severe anxiety? Predictors and moderators in the child/adolescent anxiety multimodal study. *Journal of Clinical Child & Adolescent Psychology*, *47*(2), 266–281.

Wuthrich, V. M., Rapee, R. M., Cunningham, M. J., Lyneham, H. J., Hudson, J. L., Schniering, C. A. (2012). A randomized controlled trial of the cool teens CD-ROM computerized program for adolescent anxiety. *Journal of the American Academy of Child and Adolescent Psychiatry*, *51*, 261–270.

9

Attention Deficit Hyperactivity Disorder

Attention deficit hyperactivity disorder (ADHD) is a neurodevelopmental disorder marked by problems with functioning or development characterized by inattention, hyperactivity, and impulsivity (American Psychiatric Association [APA], 2013); see Boxes 9.1, 9.2 and 9.3). Like anxiety disorders, ADHD is one of the most common mental health problems in youth. ADHD affects as many as 1 in 20 children (National Institute of Mental Health, 2012). The diagnosis of ADHD has increased at a rate of approximately 5 percent each year (APA, 2013). From 2003 through 2011, diagnosed ADHD increased 42 percent (Visser et al., 2014). The estimates for prevalence of ADHD by age are 2.7 percent for children aged 4 and 5, 9.5 percent for those aged 6–11, 11.8 percent for children aged 12–17, and 4 percent for 18-year-olds (Pastor, 2015). It affects both males and females, but it is more predominant in males (estimated at 12.9 percent of males compared to 4.3 percent of females) (Merikangas et al., 2010). The behaviors experienced are more severe and occur more frequently than would be expected for the developmental level of the child. Compared to youth without ADHD, children with ADHD tend to be significantly more restless, impatient, and active. The impulsive and hyperactive behaviors and inattentiveness impede a youth's success in school, relationships with peers, and family relationships.

Some children experience inattentiveness, some experience hyperactive or impulsive behaviors, and others experience a combination of both hyperactive/impulsive behavior and inattentiveness. Inattentiveness can interfere with a youth's ability to complete tasks such as homework or activities that require focus for some period of time. Children who experience problems with impulsiveness often get in trouble for doing things spontaneously. They may experience multiple trips to an emergency room for accidents related to inattentiveness or risky behavior associated with their impulsiveness.

Symptoms of ADHD usually appear between the ages of 3 and 6 (Kieling et al., 2010) but often go undiagnosed until children first begin school, which

Understanding the Mental Health Problems of Children and Adolescents. Kirstin Painter and Maria Scannapieco,
Oxford University Press (2021). © Oxford University Press. DOI: 10.1093/oso/9780190927844.003.0009

Box 9.1 Symptoms of inattention

Often does not give close attention to details or makes careless mistakes
in schoolwork, work, or other activities
Often has trouble keeping attention on tasks or play activities
Often does not seem to listen when spoken to directly
Often does not follow instructions and fails to finish schoolwork, chores,
or duties in the workplace (not due to oppositional behavior or failure
to understand instructions)
Often has trouble organizing activities
Often avoids, dislikes, or doesn't want to do things that take a lot of mental
effort for a long period of time (such as schoolwork or homework)
Often loses things needed for tasks and activities (e.g., toys, school
assignments, pencils, books, or tools)
Is often easily distracted
Is often forgetful in daily activities

Box 9.2 Symptoms of hyperactivity-impulsivity

Often fidgets with hands or feet or squirms in seat
Often gets up from seat when remaining in seat is expected
Often runs about or climbs when and where it is not appropriate
(adolescents or adults may feel very restless)
Often has trouble playing or enjoying leisure activities quietly
Often on the go or often acts as if driven by a motor
Often talks excessively

Box 9.3 Symptoms of impulsivity

Often blurts out answers before questions have been finished
Often has trouble waiting for a turn
Often interrupts or intrudes on others (e.g., butts into conversations or
games)

is the first time they are expected to remain in their seat, focus on tasks, and
follow rules throughout the day. Teachers are often the first to notice the
symptoms because the child has trouble following rules, has difficulty with
completing tasks, or seems to space out. ADHD is the most common reason
for children, particularly boys, to be referred to a mental health professional.

Referral is due to the disruption that can go along with the impulsive behavior and the short attention span associated with the disorder.

Youth with inattentive symptoms are easily distracted. A noise in another room or in the school hall can easily distract their attention from tasks.
Classrooms with lots of decorations can be very distracting. These youth have
difficulty maintaining focus on people talking to them. They may appear to
be daydreaming. Rapid processing of information and following directions
are very challenging. Faced with a request involving compound instructions,
a 12-year-old child experiencing ADHD may have difficulty processing the
information and following through with the task. For instance, 12-year-old
children without ADHD who were told to pick up their toys, take them to
their room, and put them where they belong would be able to process the information and follow through with the request. A child with ADHD might
not be able to process the information and therefore might not complete all
of the tasks. Adults may incorrectly associate their behavior with oppositional defiant disorder.

Youth with ADHD who predominantly experience symptoms of inattention may go undiagnosed. They are not disruptive in class and can get along
with other children. Teachers and parents may feel that they lack initiative to
do well in school or that they are lazy. The ADHD is overlooked because we
typically picture a hyperactive child when we think of ADHD. Inattention
can fly under the radar.

Youth experiencing hyperactive symptoms have difficulty sitting still and
appear to be in constant motion. They tend to squirm in their seats or have
to continually stand up. They talk nonstop and seem to get into everything
around them. They have trouble waiting to take their turn in games, waiting
in line for a drink at a water fountain, or waiting to get their lunch. They become bored easily and jump from one activity to another, unable to focus
for more than a few minutes on any task that is not enjoyable, thus making
it very difficult for them to complete tasks. They have difficulty focusing on
details and turn in sloppy or incomplete work. Without structure and help,
they forget things such as completing their homework or taking it back to
school. Children experiencing hyperactivity and impulsiveness can also be
overlooked as they may be thought to have a behavioral problem and just
lack discipline.

Dealing with a child who has ADHD can be very challenging and requires
a significant amount of patience. It can be frustrating to have a child or student who exhibits challenging behaviors without considering consequences

or shows emotions without restraint. It can be very difficult for the youth with ADHD as well. Because of their impulsive behaviors, other kids may not want to play with them, leaving them to become isolated and left out of pro-social activities. Getting in trouble constantly for not sitting still, blurting out answers, or exhibiting other problem behaviors during school can result in constant trips to the principal. The problem is not that they do not want to follow rules; following rules is often beyond their control.

Being unsuccessful in school and unable to make good grades can be an-other source of frustration for children with ADHD. Approximately 40–60 percent of youth with ADHD have co-occurring learning disabilities. Others have normal or above normal IQs, but still struggle in school due to their symptoms. Both have the potential of failing classes or entire grades. Self-esteem can be significantly damaged. Youth end up being disciplined for making bad grades and told that they are just not trying hard enough. All of these negatives in their lives can result in depression, drug or alcohol abuse, or developing relationships with oppositional-defiant or antisocial peer groups.

Causes

The exact causes of ADHD are not yet known. Prior to technologies such as magnetic resonance imaging (MRI), ADHD was thought to be caused by en-vironmental factors, with inconsistent parenting being commonly blamed. Current research is focused on possible linkages between ADHD and bio-logical, genetic, environmental, and nutritional causes (National Institute of Mental Health, 2012). In the area of nutrition, the general public has com-monly believed that giving children too much sugar makes them hyperactive and causes ADHD. Researchers have conducted extensive research on the correlation between sugar and ADHD. To date, there has been no evidence that links sugar to ADHD. Giving a child too much sugar does not cause ADHD (Millichap & Yee, 2012). Most recently, research has emerged identi-fying food additives as a cause or contributor in the development of ADHD. As with sugar, there is no empirical evidence to support food additives as a cause or contributor to ADHD (Nigg, Lewis, Edinger, & Falk, 2012). Research on possible connections between nutrition and ADHD continues to be a focus.

Environmental factors being studied as possible causes or contributors to the development of ADHD include exposure to high levels of lead and in utero exposure to cigarette smoke and alcohol. There is some evidence suggesting that children exposed to high levels of lead, found in the paint of old buildings, experience higher risks of developing ADHD than other children (Millichap, 2008). There is also empirical evidence suggesting that children born to mothers who drank alcohol or smoked cigarettes while pregnant experience a higher prevalence of ADHD (Froehlich et al., 2009; Nomura, Marks, & Halperin, 2010).

Genetics research has found a familial link to ADHD (Faraone & Mick, 2010; Gizer, Ficks, & Waldman, 2009). Twin studies have found that ADHD tends to run in families. Children with a parent, uncle, or grandparent with ADHD are more likely to develop ADHD than is a child with no familial history. Researchers are currently studying several genes that have been identified as possible contributors to ADHD. Researchers hope that identifying genes that cause ADHD will allow treatments to be targeted specifically to those genes prior to the onset of ADHD, thus preventing its onset.

Attention Deficit Hyperactivity Disorder and the Brain

Researchers are actively studying delays and abnormalities in brain development of youth with ADHD (see, e.g., Gilliam et al., 2011; Shaw et al., 2012). Research on the brain has found that children diagnosed with ADHD experience normal brain development, but the development in the frontal cortex is delayed on average by 3 years (Shaw, Eckstrand, et al., 2007). This area of the brain plays a part in cognitive functioning related to the ability to control impulsive behavior, focus attention, make sound judgments, solve problems, and exhibit socially appropriate behaviors.

Another part of the brain, the motor cortex, has been found to mature faster than normal in children with ADHD. The motor cortex is involved in the planning, control, and execution of actions and behavior. There is some belief that differences in the development of the frontal and motor cortexes play a role in the restlessness and fidgetiness that accompanies ADHD.

Other studies on the brain have found that children with ADHD who carry a particular version of a gene that is responsible for brain development have thinner brain tissue in areas of the brain responsible for controlling attention. As they move into puberty, the brain tissue becomes normal and the symptoms of ADHD improve (Shaw, Gornick, et al., 2007). Youth with this particular version of the gene have been found to have higher IQ and better clinical outcomes than youth with other versions of the same gene.

Diagnosing Attention Deficit Hyperactivity Disorder

As with all other mental health disorders, ADHD is diagnosed following a thorough psychosocial evaluation and after ruling out other plausible causes for the presentation of symptoms. A person is first diagnosed with ADHD and then a specifier (i.e., predominantly inattentive, hyperactive, impulsive, or a combination of all three) is added to further define the symptoms. To be diagnosed with ADHD, youth aged 16 and younger must experience at least six symptoms in one of the specifiers; five symptoms are required for diagnosing adolescents 17 and older. Onset of symptoms must be by age 12. The child or adolescent must experience significant functional impairment for at least 6 months across two or more settings (i.e., home, school, and work).

Parents are not good informants of their child's behavior while in school; therefore, the *Diagnostic and Statistical Manual of Mental Disorders* (DSM-5) suggests that clinicians obtain information from more than one adult source (Castellanos, 2011). To determine if a person fully meets all the criteria, assessment includes investigation across life domains and seeks to determine if the home, school, work, or other environment is unusually stressful; how the person functions across settings; the duration, frequency, and context of symptoms; and the appropriateness of behaviors for the developmental age of the person.

A thorough medical history, family history, and physical examination are important to rule out physical, developmental, and mental health disorders or conditions that have symptoms that either mimic ADHD symptoms or are comorbid with ADHD. If other disorders or conditions are not properly ruled out, another serious problem may be missed or misdiagnosed as ADHD. In addition, if comorbid conditions are not identified and go untreated, ADHD symptoms may be exacerbated. Disorders found to commonly co-occur with ADHD are autism spectrum disorder, sleep disorders, oppositional defiant disorder, learning disorders, and anxiety disorders (Barkley, 2006; Reale et al., 2017). Children and adolescents with combined symptoms of ADHD and severe impairment are more likely to have a comorbid psychiatric diagnosis. Oppositional defiant disorder is comorbid in about half of children and adolescents with combined presentation and a quarter of those with predominantly inattentive presentation (APA, 2013). Common disorders and conditions with symptoms that mimic ADHD are listed in Table 9.1.

Prior to DSM-5, a person with an intellectual or developmental disability was exempt from being diagnosed with ADHD. In reviewing the literature, the workgroup concluded that there is clear evidence that ADHD and autism spectrum disorders are commonly comorbid with one another (Castellanos, 2011).

Assessment Tools

Child Behavior Checklist

The Child Behavior Checklist (CBCL) is a measurement tool with good psychometric properties that assesses for child and adolescent behavioral and emotional problems. There are several versions of the CBCL that are designed to help a clinician to get a full picture from multiple informants of the types of symptoms experienced and the intensity, duration, and situations in which the problems are experienced (Achenbach, 1991; Achenbach & Ruffle, 2000). The CBCL for ages 1½–5 (CBCL 1½–5) includes the Parent Report Form and a Caregiver-Teacher Report Form. The CBCL 6–18 includes the Parent Report Form, Teacher Report form, and a Youth Self-Report Form for youth ages 11 through 18. The forms are completed based on a youth's behaviors using the response options of "0" (*not true*), "1" (*somewhat or sometimes true*), or "2" (*very true or often true*) to statements such as "too fearful or anxious," "gets teased a lot," and "feels worthless or inferior." The CBCL consists of the Internalizing Problems Scale (i.e., Anxious/Depressed, Withdrawn/Depressed, and Somatic Complaints) and the Externalizing Problems Scale (i.e., Rule-Breaking Behavior and Aggressive Behavior). A total composite problem score is given which also includes Social Problems, Thought Problems, and Attention Problems for a total of eight subscales. The CBCL can be hand- or computer-scored. It can be purchased at https://aseba.org/.

Table 9.1 Common disorders and conditions with symptoms that mimic attention deficit hyperactivity disorder (ADHD)

Disorder	Shared symptoms	Symptoms to differentiate from ADHD
Bipolar disorder	Decreased concentration Inattention Hyperactivity	ADHD—may have mood lability, but it is distinct from a manic episode Bipolar D/O—symptoms are episodic and must last at least 4 days and are accompanied by elevated mood, grandiosity, and other symptoms of bipolar
Depressive disorders	Decreased concentration Inattention	DO—Poor concentration is only prominent during depressive episode
Autism spectrum disorder (ASD)	Impaired social skills Distraction Inattention Difficult to manage behaviors	ADHD—Impairment due to inability to manage major transitions due to impulsivity or poor self-control ASD—Social disengagement, isolation, indifference to facial and tonal communication
Conduct disorder (CD)/ Oppositional defiant disorder (ODD)	Poor educational Attainment	Difficulty sustaining attention, impulsivity, and forgetting instructions ODD/CD—Resist tasks due to not conforming to others demands
Intermittent explosive disorder (IED)	High levels of impulsive behavior	Serious aggression in IED, and lack of attention problems
Anxiety disorders	Poor concentration	ADHD—Inattention due to attraction to external stimuli, new activities, or preoccupation; restlessness is not due to worry and rumination Anxiety—Inattention is due to worry and rumination
Sleep disorders	Inattentiveness Forgetfulness Disorganization Behavior problems	Full sleep assessment for comorbidity or differential diagnosis
Learning disorders (LD)	Inattentiveness	LD—Inattention; does not have impairment outside of academic work. It is a result of frustration, limited ability, or lack of interest
Phenylketonuria (PKU)	Hyperactivity Delayed development Behavioral, emotional and social problems	PKU—tend to have lower IQ, symptoms fully present by age 2, smaller head size, genetic differences ADHD—Visual-spatial deficits

(Continued)

Table 9.1 *Continued*

Disorder	Shared symptoms	Symptoms to differentiate from ADHD

Posttraumatic stress disorder (PTSD)	Hypervigilance
	Inattention
	Detachment
	Irritability
	Anger outbursts
	Distraction
	Restlessness
	Impatience
	Impulsiveness
	Difficulty concentrating
	  Limited future
	  orientation
		Thorough assessment should include a detailed history of trauma, family history, and child's development, behavior, and attachment in order to assess for differential or comorbid diagnosis.

From Scannapieco & Painter (2018).

ADHD Rating Scale–5 for Children and Adolescents

The ADHD Rating Scale–5 is another psychometrically sound assessment tool that determines the frequency and severity of ADHD symptoms and level of impairment in youth aged 5–17. The tool includes a home, parent-report version, and a teacher-report school version. It is available in English and Spanish and is available in a child version (5–10) and an adolescent version (11–17). The manual, *ADHD Rating Scale–5 for Children and Adolescents: Checklists, Norms, and Clinical Interpretation* (DuPaul, Power, & Anastopoulos, 2016), can be purchased for around $150. Anyone who purchases the manual has permission to reproduce the forms and score sheets for repeated use. The versions, developed based on the DSM diagnostic criteria for ADHD, include two symptom subscales (Inattention [9 items] and Hyperactivity–Impulsivity [9 items]) and a Total Scale (18 items). The ADHD Rating Scale–5 assesses six domains of impairment (relationships with significant others, peer relationships, academic functioning, behavioral functioning, homework performance, and self-esteem). Each scale takes approximately 5 minutes to complete. https://www.guilford.com/books/ADHD-Rating-Scale-5-for-Children-and-Adolescents/DuPaul-Power-Anastopoulos-Reid/9781462524877

Case Studies

Following are some case studies for youth experiencing disorders similar to those discussed in this chapter. Following each case study is a list of questions for review. In the next chapter, we will explore evidence-based treatments and practices for ADHD. We will return to the case studies presented in this chapter to learn about the actual types of interventions provided to these youths.

Eric

Eric is a 10-year-old boy living with his grandmother. Before he came to live with her at age 7, his grandmother reported that he was removed from his mother's care by Child Protective Services as a result of physical abuse. Eric had no contact with his father or his father's family. Child Protective Services allowed his mother to visit as long as his grandmother was present.

Eric had significant difficulty in school. He was antsy and could not remain seated. He refused to do his schoolwork, and he did not get along with the other children. He did not have any friends and did not participate in any activities with other kids. By the age of 10, he had been kicked out of two elementary schools, the last one for stabbing another student with a pencil.

Eric's grandmother took him to a community mental health center when he moved in with her. She reported that he had tried to hang himself twice, had killed a puppy, and was all over the place. Eric received medication for ADHD and depression and attended counseling once a week. His grandmother met with the therapist at the end of every appointment to give an update on his week. Each week for nearly 3 years, Eric's grandmother reported that he continued to be out of control and to experience episodes. When his counselor tried to talk with Eric about his mother and his suicide attempts, all he would say was that he did not remember. When asked about why he continued to have episodes at home, he would say something negative about himself.

Consider the following questions:

1. What symptoms was Eric experiencing?
2. Does he meet the criteria for a diagnosis of any of the types of ADHD? Explain. If he does, which type?

3. Based on your current knowledge, what interventions would you suggest? Do you believe that the appropriate intervention or treatment was provided?
4. Who should be included in the treatment planning and interventions?
5. What barriers might get in the way of effectively intervening?
6. What suggestions, thoughts, or ideas do you have for the other members of his family?

Peter

When Peter was 12 years old and in the seventh grade, he had difficulty focusing in class. He was failing all of his classes and tested below his grade level on standardized tests. In class, Peter was the class clown. He constantly made jokes and did things to make classmates laugh. He would not remain seated. When teachers tried to redirect him, he became oppositional. He was sent to the office for his behaviors and for disturbing class on a regular basis.

Peter also had problems with his behavior at home. He lived with his mother, who gave birth to him when she was 16. He never met his father. Peter's mother could not manage his oppositional behaviors as Peter grew older. Peter stayed out past curfew and roamed the streets. He refused to help his mother around the house. She had trouble getting him up to go to school. Every morning there was a fight to get him out of bed. Peter often arrived at school late or was absent altogether. The truant officer for the school ticketed Peter's mother for not getting him to school each day and for not getting him there on time. Both Peter's teachers and his mother were frustrated.

The school strongly suggested that Peter's mother take him to a doctor to get him started on Ritalin so that he would not be suspended for the remainder of the school year. She did not want him to take Ritalin because she had heard bad things about it. She heard that it would stunt his growth for life and that it would lead to his abusing drugs and alcohol. She took him to see a counselor who met with both of them once a week. The counselor worked with Peter's mother to develop a behavioral system whereby Peter would earn privileges for good behavior and consequences for bad behavior. Peter's behaviors did not improve. If his mother grounded him, he walked out of the house and stayed out. His mother did not know what to do and asked the counselor for help. The counselor said that his mother needed to stick to the behavioral system, not give in to Peter's behavior, and that Peter would eventually improve. This did not happen.

Following are some questions for review:

1. What symptoms was Peter experiencing?
2. Does he meet the criteria for a diagnosis of any of the types of ADHD? Explain. If he does, which type?
3. Based on your current knowledge, what interventions would you suggest? Do you believe the appropriate intervention or treatment was provided?
4. Who should be included in the treatment planning and interventions?
5. What barriers might get in the way of effectively intervening?
6. What suggestions, thoughts, or ideas do you have for the other members of his family?

References

Achenbach, T. M. (1991). *Manual for the Child Behavior Checklist/4–18 and 1991 Profile*. Burlington, VT: University of Vermont, Department of Psychiatry.

Achenbach, T. M., & Ruffle, T. M. (2000). Behavioral/emotional problems and competencies: The Child Behavior Checklist and related forms for assessing. *Pediatrics in Review, 21*, 265 doi:10.1542/pir.21-8-265

American Psychiatric Association. (2013). *Diagnostic and statistical manual of mental disorders* (5th ed.). Washington, DC: Author.

Barkley, R. A. (2006). *Attention–deficit hyperactivity disorder: A handbook for diagnosis and treatment* (3rd ed.). New York: Guilford.

Castellanos, F. X. (2011). ADHD in 2011: Update on research, medication treatment, and diagnostic controversies. Retrieved from http://www.thebalancedmind. org/adhd-in-2011-update-on-research-medication-treatment-and-diagnostic-controversies?

DuPaul, G. J., Power, T. J., & Anastopoulos, A. D. (2016). *ADHD Rating Scale-5 for children and adolescents: Checklists, norms, and clinical interpretation*. New York: Guilford.

Faraone, S. V., & Mick, E. (2010). Molecular genetics of attention deficit hyperactivity disorder. *Psychiatric Clinics of North America, 33*, 159–180.

Froehlich, T. E., Lanphear, B. P., Auinger, P., Hornung, R., Epstein, J. N., Braun, J., & Kahn, R. S. (2009). Association of tobacco and lead exposures with attention-deficit/hyperactivity disorder. *Pediatrics, 124*, 1054–1063.

Gilliam, M., Stockman, M., Malek, M., Sharp, W., Greenstein, D., Lalonde, F., . . . Shaw, P. (2011). Developmental trajectories of the corpus callosum in attention-deficit/ hyperactivity disorder. *Biological Psychiatry, 69*, 839–846.

Gizer, I. R., Ficks, C., & Waldman, I. D. (2009). Candidate gene studies of ADHD: A meta-analytic review. *Human Genetics, 126*, 51–90.

Kieling, C., Kieling, R. R., Rohde, L. A., Frick, P. J., Moffitt, T., Nigg, J. T., . . . Castellanos, F. X. (2010). The age at onset of attention deficit hyperactivity disorder. *American Journal of Psychiatry, 167*, 14–16.

Merikangas, K. R., He, J. P., Burstein, M., Swanson, S. A., Avenevoli, S., Benjet, C., Georgiades, K., Swendsen, J. (2010). Lifetime prevalence of mental disorders in US adolescents: Results from the National Comorbidity Study-Adolescent Supplement (NCS-A). *Journal of the American Academy of Child and Adolescent Psychiatry, 49*(10), 980–989.

Millichap, J. G. (2008). Etiologic classification of attention-deficit/hyperactivity disorder. *Pediatrics, 121*, 358–365.

Millichap, J. G., & Yee, M. M. (2012). The diet factor in attention-deficit/hyperactivity disorder. *Pediatrics, 129*, 330–337.

National Institute of Mental Health. (2012). Attention deficit hyperactivity disorder (NIH Publication No. 12-3572). Retrieved from http://www.nimh.nih.gov/health/ publications/attention-deficit-hyperactivity-disorder/index.shtml

Nigg, J. T., Lewis, K., Edinger, T., & Falk, M. (2012). Meta-analysis of attention-deficit/ hyperactivity disorder or attention-deficit/hyperactivity disorder symptoms, restriction diet, and synthetic food color additives. *Journal of American Academy of Child and Adolescent Psychiatry, 51*, 86–97.

Nomura, Y., Marks, D. J., & Halperin, J. M. (2010). Prenatal exposure to maternal and paternal smoking on attention deficit hyperactivity disorders symptoms and diagnosis in offspring. *Journal of Nervous and Mental Disease, 198*, 672–678.

Pastor, P. N., Duran, C., & Reuben, C. (2015). QuickStats: Percentage of children and adolescents aged 5–17 years with diagnosed Attention-Deficit/Hyperactivity Disorder (ADHD), by race and Hispanic ethnicity: National Health Interview Survey, United States, 1997–2014. *Morbidity and Mortality Weekly Report (MMWR), 64*(33), 925. doi:10.15585/mmwr.mm6433a11

Reale, L., Bartoli, B., Cartabia, M., Zanetti, M., Costantino, M. A., Canevini, M. P., Termine, C., & Bonati, M.(2017). Comorbidity prevalence and treatment outcome in children and adolescents with ADHD. *European Child & Adolescent Psychiatry, 26*(12), 1443–1457.

Scannapieco, M. A., & Painter, K. (2018). Attention deficit hyperactivity disorder. In J. C. Raines (Ed.), *Evidence-Based Practice in School Mental Health: Addressing DSM-5 Disorders in Schools* (pp. 61–90). New York: Oxford University Press.

Shaw, P., Eckstrand, K., Sharp, W., Blumenthal, J., Lerch, J. P., Greenstein, D., . . . Rapoport, J. L. (2007). Attention-deficit/hyperactivity disorder is characterized by a delay in cortical maturation. *Proceedings of the National Academy of Sciences of the United States of America, 104*(49), 19649–19654.

Shaw, P., Gornick, M., Lerch, J., Addington, A., Seal, J. Greenstein, D., et al. (2007). Polymorphisms of the dopamine D4 receptor, clinical outcome, and cortical structure in attention-deficit/hyperactivity disorder. *Archives of General Psychiatry, 64*, 921–931.

Shaw, P., Malek, M., Watson, B., Sharp, W., Evans, A., & Greenstein, D. (2012). Development of cortical surface area and gyrification in attention-deficit/hyperactivity disorder. *Biological Psychiatry, 72*, 191–197.

Visser, S., Danielson, M. L., Bitsko, R. B., Holbrook, J. R., Kogan, M. D., Ghandour, R. M., Perou, R., & Blumberg, S. J. (2014). Trends in the Parent-report of Health Care Provider Diagnosed and Medicated ADHD: United States, 2003–2011. *Journal of American Academy of Child and Adolescent Psychiatry, 53*(1), 34–46.

10

Treatment of Attention Deficit Hyperactivity Disorder

There are many treatments for attention deficit hyperactivity disorder (ADHD). Each person with ADHD has different needs, so no one treatment fits all. Treatment for ADHD can take the form of behavior therapy, family therapy, social skills training, parent skills training, psychotherapy, and medication. Education and supportive therapies are helpful for a family dealing with a child with ADHD. These treatments can help a child or adolescent experience significant improvement in symptoms and daily functioning and help caregivers understand and cope with the illness. A combination of medication and other therapies can be the most effective means of improving symptoms of ADHD and level of functioning. Even with treatment, symptoms may take time to improve. Some youth experience a decrease of symptoms with or without treatment when they enter adolescence. Others carry the symptoms into adulthood. It is also important to recognize that the side effects of untreated ADHD, such as a youth's feelings of failure, low self-esteem, depression, and social isolation, may cause more problems than the disorder itself. It is always important to promote a youth's strengths and instill a sense of competence.

Psychotropic Medications

Although controversial, psychotropic medication is most often the first line of treatment. The most commonly prescribed medications for treating ADHD are stimulants. Several stimulant medications have been approved by the US Food and Drug Administration (FDA) for children and adolescents and have been found to be effective in managing attentive and impulsive symptoms in up to 80 percent of youth (National Institute of Mental Health, 2012). Imaging studies of the brain have found that neurotransmitters in the brains of persons with ADHD are reabsorbed prematurely into the neuron,

Understanding the Mental Health Problems of Children and Adolescents. Kirstin Painter and Maria Scannapieco,
Oxford University Press (2021). © Oxford University Press. DOI: 10.1093/oso/9780190927844.003.0010

keeping messages from being delivered to receptors. Stimulant medications act in the central nervous system, increasing neurotransmitters such as dopamine or norepinephrine in the brain and slowing their reabsorption so that messages can transmit effectively. This provides a calming effect and helps reduce impulsive behavior and improve attention span.

Although stimulant medications have been found to be highly effective in treating the symptoms of ADHD, there has been and continues to be significant controversy about their use in children and adolescents. Stimulant medications are classified as schedule II drugs under the Controlled Substances Act (CSA; PL 91–513, 1970), which was enacted into law by Congress as Title II of the Comprehensive Drug Abuse Prevention and Control Act of 1970. As specified under the CSA, schedule II substances are those that meet the following criteria (CSA Schedules, 2014):

- The drug or other substance has a high potential for abuse
- The drug or other substance has currently accepted medical use in treatment in the United States or currently accepted medical use with severe restrictions
- Abuse of the drug or other substance may lead to severe psychological or physical dependence

Schedule II drugs are highly monitored by the US Drug Enforcement Administration (DEA), the governmental entity with authorization to provide oversight for controlled substances. The CSA requires anyone who handles controlled substances to be registered and authorized by the DEA to ensure secure storage and maintain inventories and records of any transaction that involves controlled substances.

Only persons authorized through the DEA can prescribe stimulant medications. Due to the addictive nature of these medications, there is concern about the potential for later substance abuse. Research has not found a link to future substance abuse for children treated for ADHD with stimulants. However, stimulant medications are commonly sold on the street and abused for nonmedical reasons. A study conducted in 2011 and funded through the National Institute of Drug Abuse (NIDA) found that methylphenidate (Ritalin) was used for nonmedical reasons by 1.3 percent of eighth graders, 2.6 percent of tenth graders, and 2.6 percent of twelfth graders in the study. Amphetamine combination (Adderall) was abused by 1.7 percent of eighth graders, 4.6 percent of tenth graders, and 6.5 percent of twelfth graders in the study. It is also not uncommon for caregivers with addictions to take their children to the doctor to get prescriptions for these controlled substances so that they can take the medication themselves.

The long-term effects of stimulant medications are not known. There is evidence that youth experience stunted growth (in both height and weight) while taking stimulants (American Academy of Pediatrics, 2001). Some research suggests that the stunted growth resolves once the medication has been stopped, but this issue continues to be studied. Other long-term consequences of taking these medications are not yet known.

All medications have potential minor and serious side effects. Most people experience no side effects or very minimal side effects from medications, including stimulants. When side effects are experienced, they usually dissipate after a few days or weeks. Only a very small percentage of people experience serious side effects from a medication. Most often, serious side effects result from a combination of the medication and another physical or mental health problem. All medications should be taken as prescribed under the supervision of a medical health professional. If any side effects are experienced, the treating physician should be notified immediately.

Serious side effects from stimulant medications, including increased blood pressure and heart rate and even sudden death, have been found in children with heart problems. Stimulants also have the potential to worsen or result in new psychiatric problems. In some persons they have been reported to cause new or worsened aggressive behavior, hostility, psychotic symptoms, and thought problems. It is always important for a treating physician to be aware of this history. Youth with a history or family history of suicide, bipolar disorder, or depression should be evaluated and monitored closely. Each medication also has the potential to result in other side effects. Common FDA-approved stimulant medications and side effects are listed in Table 10.1.

There are three FDA-approved, nonstimulant, nonaddictive medications for treating ADHD, and these provide an alternative treatment for ADHD. The first nonstimulant medication approved was atomoxetine (Strattera). It has been found to cause serious side effects in a small population of those studied in clinical trials (i.e., stunted growth, suicidal thoughts and actions, heart-related problems, and serious liver damage) in addition to the more common side effects of decreased appetite, nausea or vomiting, dizziness, mood swings, and drowsiness. The two newer nonstimulant medications approved for treating ADHD are clonidine (Catapres) and guanfacine

Table 10.1 Medications for attention deficit hyperactivity disorder (ADHD)

Trade name	Generic name	Dosage form	FDA-approved age	Common side effects
Adderall	Amphetamine	Tablet	3 years and older	Seizures Blurred vision
Adderall XR	Amphetamine (extended release)	Extended release	6 years and older	Headache Stomach ache Trouble sleeping Decreased appetite Nervousness Dizziness
Dexedrine	Dextroamphetamine	Capsule (extended release)	3 years and older	Fast heartbeat Decreased appetite Tremors Headache Trouble sleeping Dizziness Stomach upset Weight loss Dry mouth
Dextrostat	Dextroamphetamine	Tablets	3 years and older	Fast heartbeat Tremors Trouble sleeping Stomach upset Dry mouth Decreased appetite Headache Dizziness Weight loss
Concerta	Methylphenidate (long acting)	Tablet (extended release)	6 years and older	Stomach upset Dry mouth Decreased appetite Headache Dizziness Weight loss Nervousness Trouble sleeping Anxiety

(Continued)

Table 10.1 *Continued*

Trade name	Generic name	Dosage form	FDA-approved age	Common side effects
				Irritability
				Increased sweating
Ritalin	Methylphenidate	Tablet	6 years and older	Loss of appetite
				Abdominal pain
Ritalin SR	Methylphenidate (extended release)	Tablet (extended release)		Weight loss
				Insomnia
				Tachycardia
Ritalin LA	Methylphenidate (long acting)	Long acting		
Daytrana	Methylphenidate	Patch	6 years and older	Redness, small bumps, or itching where applied
				Poor appetite
				Nausea
				Vomiting
				Stomach pain
				Weight loss
				Tics
				Trouble sleeping
				Mood swings
				Dizziness
Metadate ER	Methylphenidate	Tablet (extended release)	6 years and older	Loss of appetite
				Abdominal pain
Metadate CD	Methylphenidate	Capsule (extended release)		Weight loss
				Insomnia
				Tachycardia
				Headache
				Nervousness
				Trouble sleeping
				Dizziness
Strattera	Atomoxetine	Capsule	6 years and older	Nausea
				Vomiting
				Fatigue
				Decreased appetite
				Abdominal pain
				Drowsiness

Table 10.1 *Continued*

Trade name	Generic name	Dosage form	FDA-approved age	Common side effects
Vyvanse	Lisdexamfetamine dimesylate	Capsule	6 years and older	Anxiety
				Decreased appetite
				Nausea
				Diarrhea
				Dizziness
				Dry mouth
				Trouble sleeping
				Upper stomach pain
				Vomiting
				Irritability
Focalin	Dexmethylphenidate	Capsule	6 years and older	Abdominal pain
				Fever
Focalin XR	Dexmethylphenidate	Extended release		Allergic reactions
				Nausea
				Decreased appetite
				Seizures

(Tenex). Both of these medications are commonly used to treat high blood pressure. Extended-release forms of the medications are thought to improve ADHD by affecting the part of the brain that controls attention and impulsivity.

It is important to watch for serious side effects and changes in behaviors when taking any medication. When a medication does not seem to be reducing the symptoms of ADHD, it is important to advocate for an alternative treatment. However, it is also necessary to allow medications enough time to affect symptoms. Some medications act faster than others. As always, it is important to work closely with a treating physician to determine the best treatment for a child or adolescent. Psychotropic medications have not been found to normalize behavior in youth with ADHD. Even with medication, youth continue to experience poor academic achievement and problems functioning.

Psychotherapy

Psychotherapy can be effective in helping manage the behavioral symptoms that are experienced with ADHD. "Psychotherapy" is often used as a generic term referring to mental health treatment in the form of talking to a mental health provider. There are other terms commonly used to mean the same thing, such as "counseling," "talk therapy," or "therapy." There are many approaches to psychotherapy. These approaches differ based on the individual, the individual's family, and the problem being treated. Milder symptoms of ADHD may be responsive to psychotherapy without the use of medications. Psychotherapy may also be indicated when medications are not effective.

Psychotherapeutic interventions for treating ADHD commonly use techniques such as teaching caregivers parenting skills to manage problem behaviors, teaching youth social skills to manage impulsive or aggressive behaviors and to interact in more socially appropriate ways, or using family therapies aimed at addressing issues across the family system that contribute to problem behavior. Many of the evidence-based practices and treatments incorporate one or all of these types of interventions.

Defiant Teen and Defiant Children

Defiant Teen and Defiant Children, developed by Russell A. Barkley (2006), are examples of two skills training curricula that integrate evidence-based practices for managing youth with ADHD. Barkley developed the curricula based on research that supports each procedure utilized throughout the manual. The program provides a structured methodology for training parents to manage problem behavior in children and adolescents. The skills are meant to be taught sequentially because each new skill is built on previous skills. These skills training curricula provide the family training in parental management skills, help in understanding the underlying correlates of social learning of childhood defiant behavior, and aid in the use of positive attention as a means to improve parental management skills and competence in dealing with behavior problems, particularly noncompliant or defiant behavior. Guidelines for therapists in conducting each step of the program, assessment materials, and handouts are included.

The child curriculum consists of 10 self-contained training units and the adolescent version contains 18 units. The units can be incorporated into family therapy or parent counseling and can be offered individually or in a group format. Each session follows a standardized pattern. The overarching goal of the curricula is to improve family harmony by meeting the following objectives:

- Increase parental knowledge of the causes of childhood defiant behavior
- Improve caregiver use of positive attention
- Teach caregivers to provide clear guidance, rules, and instruction to their children
- Teach caregivers to provide swift, fair, and just discipline for inappropriate behavior

The first half of both curricula consists of teaching caregivers a series of behavior management tactics to employ with their child. The curricula follow the same core components for managing challenging youth behavior (see Box 10.1). Both curricula include the Skills Development and Enhancement Model, which focuses on teaching parents about causes of problem behaviors and developing specific parenting skills. The adolescent version includes Graduated Problem-Solving and Communication Training, which teaches parents and adolescents methods of proper problem-solving and communication skills for negotiating through conflict.

Defiant Teen and Defiant Children are examples of curricula based on evidence-based practices, but they are not considered evidence-based treatments. Providers are not required to participate in any training by the developer. The following subsections will provide a few examples of evidence-based treatments for ADHD.

Challenging Horizons Program

The Challenging Horizons Program (CHP) is an empirically supported, school-based treatment program developed for students aged 6–17 who are experiencing ADHD (Evans, Langberg, Raggi, Allen, & Buvinger, 2005; Langberg et al., 2006). This program combines behavioral and cognitive interventions with supportive counseling. It targets social impairment, family conflict, and academic problems. The goals of CHP are to improve academic achievement, confidence, motivation, attendance, and behaviors. Providers of CHP must participate in 15 hours of off-site training and

---

Box 10.1 Core components of Defiant Child and Defiant Teen curricula

---

Skills Development and Enhancement Model

Impose immediate positive or negative consequences in response to the child's behavior

Impose consequences that are specific to the behavior being addressed

Make all consequences predictable, contingent, and discriminate

Establish incentive programs for rewarding the appropriate alternative behavior before punishing negative behaviors

Make consequences consistent across settings, over time, and between caregivers

Anticipate problematic behaviors and develop methods that will reduce the probability of those problems developing

Recognize and modify unreasonable beliefs, thoughts, and expectations that caregivers have about their child

Recognize that family interactions are reciprocal and change the parent's unilateral view that either they caused the problem or the problem is the teen's fault.

Graduated Problem-Solving and Communication Training

Gradually allow the youth increased developmentally appropriate independence

Distinguish behaviors and consequences that are negotiable from those that are nonnegotiable

Involve adolescents in problem solving for negotiable issues

Maintain good communication between caregivers and youth

Develop realistic expectations of family hierarchy.

---

ongoing supervision; schools providing CHP must be accredited annually. Accredited sites are required to adhere to a set of core components:

- Low student-to-staff ratio
- An environment that is safe and engaging and provides social reinforcement, tangible rewards, and clear and consistently enforced rules
- Training in enabling skills, such as organization
- Training in specific educational skills, such as math and reading
- Emphasis on improving social skills
- Emphasis on goal-setting and improving self-regulation of behavior
- Parental involvement through group parent training and weekly reports

- Participation in continuous quality improvement assisted by manuals, preservice training, on-site supervision and feedback using fidelity forms, and empirical evaluation of CHP activities

Two versions of CHP have been developed, evaluated, and found to be effective for managing symptoms and behaviors associated with ADHD. In the after-school model, counselors and trained providers meet with groups of 5–20 students with ADHD two to three times a week. A ratio of one staff person for every two to three group members is required to ensure that students receive individual help and attention. During the group sessions, students receive training in organizational skills, problem-solving skills, study skills, assignment tracking, note taking, pro-social skills, and self-monitoring of behaviors. Counselors maintain regular contact with teachers and caregivers to monitor progress. The second version of CHP, the consulting model, is provided by school staff such as teachers or counselors trained in CHP. Individual sessions are conducted with students during the school day and focus on the same goals as the after-school version.

Parenting with Love and Limits

Parenting with Love and Limits (PLL; Sells, 1998) is a widely used evidence-based practice that combines group and family therapies. It was developed for treating youth aged 10–18 with severe emotional and behavioral problems, including ADHD. Families participate in six 1- to 2-hour didactic group sessions with as many as six other families. Sessions are led by two trained therapists. Each session focuses on a specific topic aimed at teaching caregivers new information and skills designed to reestablish their parental authority through consistent limits and a loving relationship. During the first hour, parents and youth meet together. They split into separate groups during the second hour. Table 10.2 shows the topics and goals of each session.

Families also participate in individual family therapy sessions. The number of family therapy sessions in which a family participates depends on the level of family problems. It can range from three sessions for families whose children have moderate behavioral problems to as many as 20 sessions for families whose child exhibits more severe behavioral problems. During and between therapy sessions, parents and youth practice skills to enhance what they have learned.

Agencies/programs that provide PLL must be licensed annually. The cost for annual licensing is approximately $1,500 per family served plus travel expenses. Providers receive a 5-day training session, regular telephone consultation, annual on-site consultation, and videotaped therapist supervision.

Table 10.2 Session agenda for Parenting with Love and Limits

Weekly topic	Goals of session
Week 1: Understanding why your teen misbehaves	To teach caregivers the reasons why teens act out and to prevent teens from regaining control.
Week 2: Button pushing	To teach youth and caregivers how and why button pushing creates family conflict and how to identify buttons that escalate fights.
Week 3: Why traditional behavioral contracts fail and the art of negotiation	To teach families how to negotiate and design their own rewards.
Week 4: Writing new contracts and the use of emotional warm-ups	To teach parents how to develop behavioral contracts and how to present the contracts to their children. To teach youth how to reduce conflict and enhance relationships.
Week 5: Pulling it all together	To teach parents how to use creative consequences to stop problem behaviors and how to create a Positive Teen Report Certificate and use it to catch children acting positively.
Week 6: Restoring lost nurturance and tenderness (if needed)	To educate families on reactive attachment and to teach them how the fine line between love and dislike works and why there is a current lack of nurturance.
Week 7 and beyond: Ongoing coaching (if needed)	To reduce problems at home and school and with the law.

Case Studies

Eric

Eric is the 10-year-old who was removed from his mother's care by Child Protective Services for physical abuse and placed with his grandmother. Eric had no contact with his father or his father's family. He was allowed to see his mother as long as his grandmother was present.

In school, Eric was antsy and could not remain seated. He refused to do his schoolwork and did not get along with the other children. He did not have any friends and did not participate in any activities with other kids. By the age of 10 he had been kicked out of two elementary schools, the last one for stabbing another student with a pencil.

When Eric moved in with his grandmother, she took him to a community mental health center. She reported that he had tried to hang himself twice and was all over the place. Eric received medication for ADHD and depression and attended counseling once a week. His grandmother met with the therapist at the end of every appointment to give an update on his week. Each week for nearly 3 years, Eric's grandmother reported that he continued to be out of control and to experience episodes. When his counselor tried to talk with Eric about his mother and his suicide attempts, all he would say was that he did not remember. When asked why he continued to have episodes at home, he would say something negative about himself.

Eric's counselor moved out of the area, and Eric met with a new counselor. After looking through his records, the new counselor decided that she needed more information from other sources. She met with Eric's teachers and principal. He had been transferred to this school after being expelled from another school. His teachers reported that Eric's behavior had improved considerably; they felt that the improvement was due to the expectation that he could behave appropriately. They chose not to listen to the problems he had experienced at past schools. They all felt that he was very bright and reported that he was doing very well academically, going from failing to making the honor roll.

After meeting with Eric's teachers and principal, Eric's counselor scheduled a meeting at his grandmother's house and requested that his mother attend. The counselor noticed that Eric's behavior with his grandmother was very erratic and that his grandmother seemed to say things that set him off. He acted lovingly and appropriately with his mother. The counselor felt that it would be important for the family to have in-home services and to include his mother in the treatment as well.

The family was referred into wraparound and in-home skills training services. The wraparound team consisted of Eric, his grandmother, his mother, his English teacher, and his Child Protective Services case worker. In wraparound meetings, Eric's mother reported that she wanted Eric to eventually move back with her. The grandmother became very angry at this idea and refused to attend any more wraparound meetings or skills training sessions. The rest of the team continued to meet and devised a wraparound plan that included increasing contact between Eric and his mother and monitoring how things went. When he was with his mother, Eric behaved very well. The skills trainer noted that Eric's mother was working very hard and incorporating skills that she had learned in sessions. Eric ended up returning to live with his mother. He was taken off all medications and continued to do well in school, make friends, and participate in pro-social activities. After a year, Child Protective Services closed his case.

Peter

Peter is the 12-year-old seventh grader who was failing all of his classes and tested below his grade level on standardized tests. He was the class clown who made jokes and did things to make classmates laugh. He teachers were unable to redirect him, and he became oppositional. He was sent to the office for his behaviors and for disturbing class regularly.

Peter also had problems with his behavior at home. He lived with his mother, who gave birth to him when she was 16. Peter's mother could not control his behaviors. He broke curfew regularly and roamed the streets. He refused to help his mother around the house. She had trouble getting him up to go to school. His mother was ticketed for not getting him to school each day and for not getting him there on time.

The school strongly suggested that Peter's mother take him to a doctor to get him started on Ritalin so that he would not be suspended for the remainder of the school year. His mother did not want him to take Ritalin because she had heard bad things about it. Instead, she took him to see a counselor who met with both of them once a week. The counselor worked with his mother to develop a behavioral system whereby Peter would earn privileges for good behavior and consequences for bad behavior. The behavioral plan was ineffective in managing Peter's behaviors. Finally, his mother decided to take him to see a psychiatrist, who prescribed Adderall. The Adderall helped Peter focus at school and stop squirming around. He continued to get in trouble at home and school.

Study Questions

1. What do these real-life scenarios have in common?
2. What are the differences?
3. After learning what happened to each of the youths, do you have any different thoughts on how you would have handled the situation if you were the families' social worker?

References

American Academy of Pediatrics. (2001). Clinical practice guideline: Treatment of the school-aged child with attention deficit/hyperactivity disorder. *Pediatrics, 108,* 1033–1044.

Barkley, R. A. (2006). *Attention-deficit/hyperactivity disorder: A handbook for diagnosis and treatment* (3rd ed.). New York: Guilford.

Controlled Substances Act of 1970, Pub. L. No. 91–513 § 84 Stat. *1242* (1970).

CSA Schedules. (2014). Retrieved from http://www.drugs.com/csa-schedule.html

Evans, S. W., Langberg, J., Raggi, V., Allen, J., & Buvinger, E. (2005). Development of a school-based treatment program for middle school youth with ADHD. *Journal of Attention Disorders, 9,* 343–353.

Langberg, J., Smith, B. H., Bogle, K. E., Schmidt, J. D., Cole, W. R., & Pender, C. A. (2006). A pilot evaluation of small group Challenging Horizons Program (CHP): A randomized trial. *Journal of Applied School Psychology, 23,* 31–58.

National Institute of Mental Health. (2012). Attention deficit hyperactivity disorder (NIH Publication No. 12–3572). Retrieved from http://www.nimh.nih.gov/health/publications/attention-deficit-hyperactivity-disorder/index.shtml

Sells, S. P. (1998). *Treating the tough adolescent: A step-by-step, family-based guide.* New York: Guilford.

11

Oppositional Defiant Disorder and Conduct Disorder

Oppositional defiant disorder (ODD) and conduct disorder (CD) are disruptive behavioral disorders. Because of their prevalence and the disruption that they cause, not only to children's lives, but also to the lives of those around them, they are also two of the most problematic mental health disorders of childhood and adolescence. They are more prevalent in males than they are in females at a ratio estimated at anywhere from 3:1 to 9:1 (Loeber, Burke, Lahey, Winters, & Zera, 2000). Both disorders are referred to as *externalizing disorders* in that their symptoms are characterized by acting-out behaviors and defiance of authority. Youth who develop CD or ODD often have experienced physical abuse, sexual abuse, neglect, poverty, and/or family dysfunction; therefore, youth in the juvenile justice and child welfare systems are highly susceptible to developing one of these disorders (Farmer, Compton, Burns, & Robertson, 2002).Youth with these disorders are often those who are moved from foster home to foster home, who end up in residential treatment, or who come in contact with the juvenile justice system due to the difficulties and challenges that their behaviors pose. Left untreated, these externalizing disorders can develop into chronic delinquency that will disrupt positive development and can follow the youth into adulthood (Farmer et al., 2002; Hill, Coie, Lochman, & Greenberg, 2004). The result could be criminal activity, unemployment, substance abuse, ineffective parenting, and relationship problems. The children of these youth are then at risk of becoming the next generation in the juvenile justice, mental health, and child welfare systems. If we identify and treat these problems early, we are not only improving the lives of these youth, but we are helping to stop a generational cycle of abuse and neglect, criminal activity, or other problems. The first step in this process is identifying and understanding the problem.

Understanding the Mental Health Problems of Children and Adolescents. Kirstin Painter and Maria Scannapieco,
Oxford University Press (2021). © Oxford University Press. DOI: 10.1093/oso/9780190927844.003.0011

Oppositional Defiant Disorder

ODD is a less severe behavioral disorder than CD; however, it is still disruptive to a youth's functioning and development and very challenging to those around him or her. Youth with ODD are characterized by inflexibility, negative mood, and hostility (American Psychiatric Association [APA], 2013). Their overall view of life tends to be negative. They focus on the negative aspects of themselves, others, and situations rather finding the positive aspects. These youth often have poor problem-solving and coping skills and thus respond to the environment and others in negative ways. Youth experiencing symptoms of ODD can be highly irritable and respond to even small problems or things that bother them with intense anger. Their intense anger and hostile response are often used to control others. One consequence of this way of responding is poor relationships with peers, teachers, and family.

Signs of ODD are usually evident before the age of 8 (APA, 2013). A child with ODD is one who *consistently* refuses to comply with requests from authority figures or does not comply within a reasonable amount of time or to the degree expected. For example, when a caregiver requests the child to do something, such as clean his or her bedroom, the child generally refuses to comply and responds by screaming and yelling things such as "This is unfair, I hate you!" The child may finally go to his or her room, but rather than cleaning it as expected, he or she will push all the dirty clothes under the bed instead of putting them in the dirty clothes hamper. This is the child who is prone to throwing temper tantrums or even possibly making physical threats in order to get his or her way. This is not the child who occasionally does not want to clean his or her room. This is the child whose response to requests is extreme for the situation. When confronted with a task with which he or she is struggling or that he or she perceives as too difficult, the child tends to give up and move on to another activity. If someone pushes him or her to complete the task—for example, to finish homework—he or she will respond by screaming and yelling, hitting objects, or engaging in other extreme behavioral responses rather than working through the problem.

These behaviors may sound like normal youth behavior. However, for a diagnosis of ODD, the behaviors must be occurring at a level that is more intense or frequent than would be expected for a youth at the same developmental stage (APA, 2013). To those around the youth, everything seems to be spiraling out of control. The problems rise to a level that is seriously affecting the youth's functioning, relationships, or success in school and causing sig-nificant stress for caregivers.

Diagnosing Oppositional Defiant Disorder

The *Diagnostic and Statistical Manual of Mental Disorders* (DSM) spells out the criteria for a diagnosis. As specified in the DSM, to be diagnosed with ODD, a youth must be younger than 18 and exhibit four or more of the fol-lowing behaviors for at least 6 months:

- Often loses temper
- Often argues with adults
- Often actively defies or refuses to comply with adults' requests or rules
- Often deliberately annoys people
- Often blames others for his or her mistakes or misbehavior
- Is often touchy or easily annoyed by others
- Is often angry and resentful
- Is often spiteful or vindictive

The DSM emphasizes that a youth must have a persistent pattern of angry and irritable mood along with vindictive behavior. The behaviors identi-fied in the DSM as characteristic of ODD are divided into three symptom clusters: angry/irritable, touchy/easily annoyed by others, and angry/re-sentful. The intensity is specified based on age, with the requirement that those younger than 5 experience symptoms almost every day and those who are 5 or older experience symptoms at least once a week.

There are no blood tests, brain scans, or other biological tests that can be conducted to diagnose ODD. To make the diagnosis, a mental health pro-fessional must interview a youth face to face and obtain reliable information from others, such as a caregiver, teacher, or other person involved with the youth. The evaluation should explore the youth's development, the family history of mental health and substance abuse problems, and the youth's func-tioning at school and home and in the community. The mental health pro-fessional should explore whether the youth may have another problem that is the true explanation for the behavior. It is not uncommon for depressed youth, particularly males, to express their depression in a way that looks like ODD. It is also likely that there is a coexisting issue, such as attention deficit hyperactivity disorder (ADHD) or a learning disability, that confounds the problem. It is essential for a correct diagnosis or diagnoses to be made. This is not possible without an in-depth evaluation. Effective treatment is impossible without targeting the correct problem or coexisting conditions.

It is important not to blame the youth or the caregiver if progress in treatment is not being made because the treatment may not have been directed at the right problem.

Conduct Disorder

ODD is often seen as a precursor to CD and/or substance abuse. Approximately a third of youth with ODD go on to develop CD (Dickstein, 2010). The good news is that approximately two-thirds of youth do not develop CD and may simply grow out of the problem behaviors. Children and teens with CD are thought of by the general public as juvenile delinquents rather than as youth with a mental illness. As previously stated, CD is a more serious and disruptive behavioral disorder than ODD. Youth with CD exhibit patterns of violating the rights of others and/or violating social rules (APA, 2013). Often a lack of empathy or remorse accompanies these behaviors. If asked why they do certain things, youth with CD will often respond that they were bored. They lack the ability to read social cues. For instance, a happenstance eye glance in their direction may be misinterpreted as confrontational and trigger a strong reaction, such as threatening behavior. Youth with CD are more likely to abuse illegal substances and engage in risk-taking behavior. These youth typically have significant juvenile justice involvement. Violations of rules and of other people, lack of empathy or remorse, and inability to read social cues result in significant levels of impairment in daily functioning, particularly in relationships.

Diagnosing Conduct Disorder

As with ODD, CD is diagnosed through a face-to-face diagnostic interview with a mental health professional and not with a blood test or brain scan. To receive a diagnosis of CD, a person must be younger than 18 and have exhibited three or more behaviors in the past 12 months (at least one in the past 6 months) that involved aggression against people or animals, serious violation of rules, destruction of property, and/or deceitfulness or theft. The DSM (APA, 2013) identifies behaviors under each of these four categories:

1. Aggression against people and animals
   a. Often bullies, threatens, or intimidates others;
   b. Often initiates physical fights;
   c. Has used a weapon that can cause serious physical harm to others;
   d. Has been physically cruel to people;
   e. Has been physically cruel to animals;
   f. Has stolen while confronting a victim (e.g., mugging, purse snatching, extortion, or armed robbery);
   g. Has forced someone into sexual activity.
2. Destruction of property
   a. Has deliberately engaged in fire-setting with the intention of causing serious damage;
   b. Has deliberately destroyed others' property (other than by fire setting).
3. Deceitfulness or theft
   a. Has broken into someone else's house, building, or car;
   b. Often lies to obtain goods or favors or to avoid obligations (i.e., cons others);
   c. Has stolen items of nontrivial value without confronting a victim (e.g., shoplifting, but without breaking and entering or forgery).
4. Serious violations of rules
   a. Often stays out at night despite parental prohibitions, beginning before age 13;
   b. Has run away from home overnight at least twice while living in parental or parental surrogate home (or once without returning for a lengthy period);
   c. Is often truant from school, beginning before age 13.

The DSM includes the specifiers "*with*" or "*without callous and unemotional traits.*" For the specifier "with callous and unemotional traits," two or more of the following characteristics should be persistently evident for at least 12 months and in more than one setting or relationship (APA, 2013):

- *Lack of remorse or guilt*: Does not feel bad or guilty when he or she does something wrong (except if expressing remorse when caught and/or facing punishment).
- *Callousness and lack of empathy*: Disregards and is unconcerned about the feelings of others.
- *Lack of concern about performance*: Does not show concern about poor/problematic performance at school or work or in other important activities.
- *Shallow or deficient affect*: Does not express feelings or show emotions to others except in ways that seem shallow or superficial (e.g., emotions are not consistent with actions; can turn emotions on or off quickly) or when they are used for gain (e.g., to manipulate or intimidate others).

Although people may continue to carry a diagnosis of CD past the age of 18 even if they do not fully meet the criteria, most often the diagnosis will change to antisocial personality disorder (APD). CD and APD share many similarities (APA, 2013). APD is a chronic disorder. Someone with the disorder perceives situations and relates to others in an abnormal, destructive manner. These are the adults who have been sent to prison for committing severe acts of violence and who lack remorse for their actions. All youth with CD do not go on to have antisocial disorder as adults; however, evidence suggests that they are at a high risk because personality disorders are thought to have roots in childhood delinquency (Farmer et al., 2002; Hill et al., 2004). Children whose behaviors early on involve violence and aggression against others are at the highest risk for APD. As children age, their behaviors may become more aggressive and violent and occur more frequently. The differences between those who do and those who do not go on to exhibit criminal activity as adults are the level and type of intervention they receive as youth and the age at which they receive it.

Causes and Correlates of Oppositional Defiant Disorder and Conduct Disorder

Many risk factors contribute to the development of ODD or CD. Youth who have experienced child abuse or neglect or who have caregivers with similar oppositional or criminal traits and characteristics have a higher risk of developing one of these disorders. No single factor results in the disorders;

rather it is the culmination of risk factors that come together (Henggeler, Schoenwald, Rowland, & Cunningham, 2002). These factors include caregiver, youth, community, and peer group characteristics.

Caregiver Characteristics

Studies of both ODD and CD have reported that the heritability rate of both disorders ranges anywhere from 61 to 74 percent (Herdon & Iacono, 2005; Hicks, Krueger, Iacono, McGue, & Patrick, 2004; Lahey & Waldmand, 2012). Many caregiver characteristics place youth at risk of developing ODD or CD (Dickstein, 2010; Fergusson, Lynskey, & Horwood, 1993; Frick et al., 1992). Caregivers experiencing high levels of stress with low educational levels, lack of social support, and inability to cope with or manage the stress often respond by lashing out at others around them or retreating from others. Studies have found a strong correlation between youth problem behaviors and maternal depression, stress, or marital discord (Christensen, Phillips, Glasgow, & Johnson, 1983; Dumas, Gibson, & Albin, 1989; Fergusson et al., 1993; Nigg & Hinshaw, 1998). When a mother is experiencing depression, she is more likely to be neglectful of her children due to a lack of interest or ability to parent. Children from neglectful households are characterized by poorer adjustment than those from other types of households. They are more likely to use drugs and alcohol and participate in delinquent behavior.

Research has also found a strong association between parental and child externalizing disorders, suggesting a familial transmission. Specifically, caregivers who lack concern for societal rules and lack empathy have a high probability of having children who develop similar temperamental characteristics. It is not unknown for parents to take a child with negative acting-out behavior to see a mental health professional and to report difficulty in understanding where their children's behavior comes from right after yelling at the check-in staff about what they perceived as a long wait to see the counselor.

Caregivers (usually paternal) with antisocial disorder are more likely to have children who develop ODD or CD than are other caregivers. APD is similar to CD in that people with the disorder violate societal rules and the rights of others. They perceive situations abnormally and thus behave in an abnormal manner, such as with violence. Adults with APD likely had CD as youth.

Another of the major causes of noncompliance, defiance, and social aggression is poor, ineffective, inconsistent, and indiscriminant child or teen management by parents, often combined with unusually harsh or extreme disciplinary methods and poor monitoring of teen activities (Henggeler, Schoenwald, Borduin, Rowland, & Cunningham, 1998; Henggeler et al., 2002). Parents with an authoritarian parenting style are directive and controlling and exhibit low levels of comfort and warmth to their children. Their punishment style tends to be severe and often physically abusive. This style of parenting has been linked to aggression, poor self-confidence, internalized distress, and social withdrawal in children. Children living in authoritarian households are not allowed to experience the natural consequences of their behaviors.

On the other extreme is the permissive style of parenting. Permissive parents can be very loving; some want to be their child's friend rather than parent. However, they do not provide or possibly cannot provide structure or discipline and thus they allow their children to exhibit impulsive or other behaviors without any consequence. Children living in households with a permissive form of parenting may exhibit impulsive, aggressive behavior and a lack of social responsibility.

Youth Characteristics

Children are all born with unique temperaments that affect how they interact and respond to the world. *Temperament* differs from *personality* in that temperament is a core characteristic. It is consistent across time. Personality is a combination of life experiences and core characteristics. The temperament of youth who develop ODD or CD tends to be negative and inflexible. This temperament results in their experiencing problems in adapting to different situations. They exhibit poor social skills and/or problem-solving skills. They often have difficulty managing their own behavior, resulting in heightened reactions that are more extreme than would be expected for the situation. These characteristics can exacerbate problems in relationships between the child and caregivers, peers, and teachers. People often find themselves frustrated with the child's behavior and react to it in ways that are not consistent with their normal behavior. Children or teens having certain temperaments and cognitive characteristics are more prone to exhibit coercive-aggressive behavior and noncompliance than are other teens or children.

Peer and Community Characteristics

The larger contextual events surrounding a family, both internal and external, create or contribute to increased risk of a youth developing ODD or CD. A vast amount of research exists on the influence of peer groups on youth behavior (Henggeler et al., 1998, 2002). A child or teen who hangs out with friends who abuse substances and participate in criminal and delinquent behavior is more likely to interact with these same behaviors than a youth who has friends who participate in pro-social activities. Understandably, caregivers of youth who participate in pro-social activities will not want their children to be involved with youth known to be delinquent for fear that they will negatively influence their child. This makes it more difficult for youth with a history of delinquency to change to a peer group that would be a positive influence.

The community surrounding a youth also has a great influence on the development of problem behaviors. Communities that lack opportunities for youth to participate in pro-social activities such as organized sports or the Boy or Girl Scouts have also been linked to youth problem behavior due to boredom. Youth who live in communities with high levels of crime and violence are at an increased risk of becoming involved in criminal and violent activity.

Youth spend much of their time in a school setting. School settings can have a significant influence on youth behavior. Schools with rigid rules and negative teacher–student interactions can have a negative effect on youth behavior. Many youth with a behavior disorder also have a learning disability. Placement in an appropriate educational setting with teachers who are knowledgeable and skilled, not only in dealing with the learning disability, but also in managing behavioral problems in the classroom, is imperative. It can take a certain temperament to work with youths with CD.

The Brain, Oppositional Defiant Disorder, and Conduct Disorder

CD and ODD are both associated with neurocognitive impairments (i.e., lower IQ, deficit in executive functioning) related to abnormalities in underlying brain mechanisms (Noordermeer, Luman, & Oosterlaan, 2016). Findings of research on abnormalities in the brains of youth with CD could change the way we think about its development. The emerging evidence suggests that antisocial and aggressive behavior is attributable to these abnormalities rather than to peer pressure (Passamonti et al., 2010; Sterzer, Stadler, Poustka, & Kleinschmidt, 2007). Evidence suggests that youth with CD have abnormalities in brain structures and functioning that contribute to its onset and associated behaviors (Fairchild et al., 2011; Passamonti et al., 2010; van Goozen & Fairchild, 2006; van Goozen, Fairchild, Snoek, & Harold, 2007). More recent studies are finding that adolescents with CD experience abnormal neural activity when processing the facial expressions of others (Fairchild, van Goozen, Calder, Stollery, & Goodyer, 2009). Impairment to the frontal lobe results in poor impulse control, difficulty learning from past experiences, and difficulty planning for the future (Fairchild, van Goozen, Stollery, et al., 2009). Decreased serotonin and cortisol levels and decreased gray matter in the amygdala have also been found in youth with CD. These differences may explain their lack of fear, decreased ability to control aggressive and impulsive behaviors, and inability to recognize emotional reactions of others. When youth are unable to understand others' reactions, particularly distress, they are unable to exhibit empathy. Studies have found that youth who have callous and unemotional traits have less activity in their amygdala than other youth with CD and are those exhibiting lack of empathy for others (Marsh et al., 2008).

Noordermeer et al. (2016) conducted a systematic review and meta-analysis of research that used structural and functional magnetic resonance imaging (MRI) to study the brain of youth with ODD and CD. They reported that there is strong evidence of specific abnormalities in the amygdala of youth with ODD and CD. Their study supported the growing research that brain abnormalities in youth with ODD and CD are associated with problem-solving, self-control emotion processing, and error monitoring.

Comorbidity with Other Disorders

The most common disorder found to be comorbid (or commonly occurring together) with both ODD and CD is ADHD (APA, 2013; National Institute of Mental Health, 2012). It is believed that nearly 50 percent of youth with ODD also have ADHD, and as many as 30 percent of boys and 55 percent of girls with CD also experience ADHD (National Institute of Mental Health, 2012). Depression has also been found to be linked to both ODD and CD.

Some youth experiencing depression may exhibit symptoms of ODD or CD and have the problem with depression undiagnosed. Youth with a dual diagnosis of CD and ADHD have been found to be more aggressive than youth with CD alone. Conduct disorder is often found to be comorbid with several other mental health, substance use/abuse, and learning disorders (National Institute of Mental Health, 2012). Youth with CD have been found to begin use/abuse of alcohol and drugs at an earlier age than other youth and are more likely to use more types of substances. The most common learning disability found to be comorbid with CD is language impairments, affecting as many as 25 percent of youth with CD.

Implications for Foster Youth

As we know, youth in the child welfare system are at a higher risk than other children of having or developing CD or ODD due to the high correlation of these disorders with physical abuse, neglect, poverty, and family dysfunction. Think about the characteristics of caregivers who come in contact with the child welfare system. Many possess characteristics correlated with a child or teen developing ODD or CD. Caregivers coming in contact with the child welfare system are most likely the ones experiencing high levels of stress and having poor coping skills and/or a mental health problem, such as major depression or bipolar disorder.

Although youth in the foster care system do possess many of the risk factors associated with ODD and CD, it is for this very reason that we must be careful in assessing these disorders. We should not jump to the conclusion that a youth who is acting out has one of these disorders and ignore other plausible causes of this behavior. There are many reasons for acting-out behavior. The youth may be responding to the stress of being removed from home, siblings, school, and friends and placed in an unfamiliar setting with strangers. It is understandable that a child or teenager, even one who normally can cope with stress, would act out in response to such an extreme change in his or her life. It is important to remember that different youth will respond in different ways based on their own characteristics, such as temperament, stress management skills, and coping skills. Given time and positive support, these acting-out behaviors may cease. At the same time, if the youth is not provided support and time to deal with what is happening to him or her, the behaviors may persist even to the point of developing into one of these externalizing disorders.

Sometimes youth experiencing other mental health disorders may exhibit acting-out behaviors that are masking the true mental health problem. This can be particularly true for males with depression. Females tend to exhibit the symptoms we picture when thinking about depression. Males, on the other hand, sometimes exhibit anger and acting-out behavior in response to depression. It is also important to understand that ODD and CD are often comorbid with other mental health problems. Common mental health problems that can coexist with ODD or CD are depression, anxiety, ADHD, learning disabilities, or one or more other problems.

It is important for social workers to ensure that all children or teenagers entering child welfare receive a trauma-informed, comprehensive, psychosocial, emotional, behavioral, educational, and biological assessment in order to provide them with the best care possible. Acting-out behaviors attract attention because of the irritation they cause case workers, service providers, and foster parents. If our response to the youth's behavior is to keep moving him or her from foster home to foster home or into residential placement, the youth has been set up for failure. If we do not identify the correct problem(s), chances are that any interventions provided will not be successful. A child presenting with ODD symptoms should have a comprehensive evaluation. It is important to look for other disorders that may be present, such as ADHD, learning disabilities, mood disorders (depression, or bipolar disorder), and anxiety disorders. It may be difficult to improve the symptoms of ODD without treating the coexisting disorder.

Case Studies

The following are some case studies of youth experiencing behavioral problems. To protect their privacy, we will not use their real names. As you read each story, think about the symptoms being exhibited and which disorder you believe the youth is experiencing. All of these youths were diagnosed with either ODD or CD. They each received a different form of intervention, and their lives took completely different paths. Their case studies will be continued in Chapter 12.

Tim

Tim is a 13-year-old boy. He lives with his mother and 11-year-old sister in a public housing apartment complex. His father died when he was 7. Tim's mother, Jean, has an intellectual disability with an IQ under 90. He and his sister both have normal IQs. The family survives on Jean's Social Security check and the Social Security checks that Tim and his sister receive due to the death of their father.

Jean did well with raising her children when they were young. She ensured that they had clean clothes, ample food, and safe housing and that they went to school every day. She belonged to a church that provided her with support. As Tim grew older, he stopped listening to his mother. He told her that she was stupid and that he did not have to do what she said. He tormented his sister both verbally and physically. He stayed out past his curfew and hung out with friends. His first run-in with the juvenile justice system came when he and his friends were caught breaking into the school and destroying property. His mother did not know what to do to control his behavior. His second encounter with the juvenile justice system occurred when a young girl in the neighborhood reported that he had been sexually abusing her. Tim was adjudicated and mandated to attend outpatient sex offender treatment. While he was completing his treatment, it was reported that he was abusing a neighborhood boy. The judge ordered him into an inpatient sex offender treatment program. He received intensive individual and group therapy for the year he remained in the program. He was then discharged to return home.

Consider the following questions:

1. What symptoms was Tim experiencing?
2. Based on the information provided, does he meet the criteria for a diagnosis of either CD or ODD? Explain. If he does, which one?
3. Based on your current knowledge, what interventions would you suggest? Do you believe that he received the appropriate intervention or treatment?
4. Who should be included in Tim's treatment planning and interventions?
5. What barriers might get in the way of effectively intervening with Tim?
6. What suggestions, thoughts, or ideas do you have for the other members of Tim's family?

Tracy

Tracy is an 8-year-old girl. She had always exhibited difficult behavior, such as throwing a tantrum when she did not get her way, but her negative and acting-out behaviors became increasingly unbearable. She was getting in trouble at school more frequently. She talked back to her teachers and sometimes refused to do her work. Many of the children in her classroom did not like her because she made fun of them or tried to get them in trouble by telling the teacher that they had started a fight with her. When a teacher confronted her about lying, Tracy started yelling and said that she did not lie. She walked out of her classroom and down the hall. The teacher caught up with her, and they walked together to the principal's office. She received a 3-day in-school suspension. At home she was mean to her little brother. Often, when her mother asked her to put her school books and toys in her room or to do some other chore, Tracy would reply, "I will do it when my favorite show is over." If her mother pressed her, she would sometimes comply; however, more often, she would scream and yell and run to her room and slam the door. Tracy's mother was at her wits' end and took her to see a counselor.

Write your answers to the following questions:

1. What symptoms was Tracy experiencing?
2. Does she meet the criteria for either CD or ODD? Explain. If she does, which one?
3. Based on your current knowledge, what interventions would you suggest? Do you believe that she received the appropriate intervention or treatment?
4. Who should be included in Tracy's treatment planning and interventions?
5. What barriers might get in the way of effectively intervening with Tracy?
6. What suggestions, thoughts, or ideas do you have for the other members of her family?

James

James is a 17-year-old living with both his parents in a middle-class neighborhood. When his father was not home, James talked back and cursed at his mother, refused to follow her rules, and threatened to hurt her. His father had more control over James's behavior. He was a large man with an explosive anger that at times became physical. James was afraid of his father. James's father worked a night shift and was not home much when James was home. James walked out of the house at any time of the night he chose and hung out with friends. They drank alcohol, smoked marijuana, and huffed glue. At school he was a bully. He was suspended and placed in an alternative school for beating up other students, skipping school, and defying his teachers. One evening, his mother tried to stop him from leaving the house. James beat her severely. Her face was bloody and so swollen that it was unrecognizable. When her husband returned home from work, he found her on the kitchen floor and called 911. James was not at home. His mother was taken to the hospital with broken ribs and bruises that covered her body. The police located James and took him to the juvenile detention center. When questioned about the incident, he at first lied and said that he did not beat up his mother. When he finally admitted to it, he said that it was his mother's fault for never shutting up.

James spent 3 months in juvenile detention. He was discharged to return home with an ankle monitor and strict instructions from the judge that he would be sent to a more restrictive lockup facility until he turned 21 if he did not comply with his probation or had any more incidences of trouble.

Think about the following questions:

1. What symptoms was James experiencing?
2. Does he meet the criteria for CD or ODD? Explain. If he does, which one?
3. Based on your current knowledge, what interventions would you suggest? Do you believe that the appropriate intervention or treatment was provided?
4. Who should be included in the treatment planning and interventions?
5. What barriers might get in the way of effectively intervening?
6. What suggestions, thoughts, or ideas do you have for the other members of James's family?

Dale

Dale is a 16-year-old who has been in and out of the juvenile justice system since the age of 13 for causing bodily harm to others, theft, and use of illegal drugs. He is failing in school. He spent several months in alternative school. He was placed in residential care for a year. As is common, the residential care center was located hundreds of miles from his home and his mother. While he was in care, his mother had little participation in treatment other than a monthly meeting with the social worker to discuss his progress. His mother was a single parent. Dale did not know his father.

While in the residential treatment center, Dale received intensive treatment that included daily group therapy and weekly individual counseling. He was taught stress management, anger management, and problem-solving and decision-making skills. He also attended a 12-step group on the center's campus. Dale was put into a behavioral system whereby he could earn increased privileges and freedoms on the residential treatment center campus. He went to school on campus with teachers trained to understand mental health problems. Because the classes were smaller than those found in the typical classroom, he received more individual attention. He was also diagnosed with a reading disorder for which he received help. Dale's problem behaviors improved significantly after 6 months in the center. Within 9 months, he had moved to the least restrictive unit on the campus, allowing him more freedom. For the next 3 months, he maintained good behavior and utilized the new skills he had learned. After a year in treatment, he was discharged to return home and went back to his old school.

Write your answers to the following questions:

1. What symptoms was Dale experiencing?
2. Does he meet the criteria for either CD or ODD? Explain. If he does, which one?
3. Based on your current knowledge, what interventions would you suggest? Do you believe that the appropriate intervention or treatment was provided?
4. Who should be included in the treatment planning and interventions?
5. What barriers might get in the way of effectively intervening?
6. What suggestions, thoughts, or ideas do you have for the other members of Dale's family?

References

American Psychiatric Association. (2013). *Diagnostic and statistical manual of mental disorders* (5th ed.). Washington, DC, Author.

Christensen, A., Phillips, S., Glasgow, R. E., & Johnson, S. M. (1983). Parental characteristics and interactional dysfunction in families with child behavior problems: A preliminary investigation. *Journal of Abnormal Child Psychology, 11*, 153–166.

Dickstein, D. P. (2010). Oppositional defiant disorder. *Journal of the American Academy of Child and Adolescent Psychiatry, 49*, 435–436.

Dumas, J. E., Gibson, J. A., & Albin, J. B. (1989). Behavioral correlates of maternal depressive symptomology in conduct-disordered children. *Journal of Consulting and Clinical Psychology, 57*, 516–521.

Fairchild, G., Passamonti, L., Hurford, G., Hagan, C. C., von dem Hagen, E. A., van Goozen, S. H., . . . Calder, A. J. (2011). Brain structure abnormalities in early-onset and adolescent-onset conduct disorder. *American Journal of Psychiatry, 168*, 624–633.

Fairchild, G., van Goozen, S. H., Calder, A. J., Stollery, S. J., & Goodyer, I. M. (2009). Deficits in facial expression recognition in male adolescents with early-onset or adolescence-onset conduct disorder. *Journal of Child Psychology and Psychiatry, 50*, 627–636.

Fairchild, G., van Goozen, S. H., Stollery, S. J., Aitken, M. R., Savage, J., Moore, S. C., & Goodyer, I. M. (2009). Decision making and executive function in male adolescents with early-onset or adolescence-onset conduct disorder and control subjects. *Biological Psychiatry, 66*, 162–168.

Farmer, E. M. Z., Compton, S. N., Burns, B. J., & Robertson, E. (2002). Review of the evidence base for treatment of childhood psychopathology: Externalizing disorders. *Journal of Consulting and Clinical Psychology, 70*, 1267–1302.

Fergusson, D. M., Lynskey, M. T., & Horwood, L. J. (1993). The effect of maternal depression on maternal ratings of child behavior. *Journal of Abnormal Child Psychology, 21*, 245–269.

Frick, P. J., Lahey, B. B., Loeber, R., Stouthamer-Loeber, M., Christ, M. A. G., & Hanson, K. (1992). Familial risk factors to oppositional defiant disorder and conduct disorder: Parental psychopathological and maternal parenting. *Journal of Consulting and Clinical Psychology, 60*, 49–55.

Henggeler, S. W., Schoenwald, S. K., Borduin, C. M., Rowland, M. D., & Cunningham, P. B. (1998). *Multisystemic treatment of antisocial behavior in children and adolescents.* New York: Guilford Press.

Henggeler, S. W., Schoenwald, S. K., Rowland, M. D., & Cunningham, P. B. (2002). *Serious emotional disturbance in children and adolescents: Multisystemic therapy.* New York: Guilford Press.

Herndon, R. W., & Iacono, W. G. (2005). The familial transmission of antisocial behavior from parent to child. *Psychological Medicine, 35*, 1815–1824.

Hicks, B. M., Krueger, R. F., Iacono, W. G., McGue, M., & Patrick C. J. (2004). Family transmission and heritability of externalizing disorders: a twin family study. *Archives of General Psychiatry, 61*, 922–928.

Hill, L. G., Coie, J. D., Lochman, J. E., & Greenberg, M. T. (2004). Effectiveness of early screening for externalizing problems: Issues of screening accuracy and utility. *Journal of Consulting and Clinical Psychology, 72*, 809–820.

Lahey, B. B., & Waldman, I. D. (2012). Annual research review: phenotypic and causal structure of conduct disorder in the broader context of prevalent forms of psychopathology. *Journal of Child Psychology and Psychiatry, 53(5)*, 536–557.

Loeber, R., Burke, J. D., Lahey, B. B., Winters, A., & Zera, M. (2000). Oppositional defiant and conduct disorder: A review of the past 10 years, part I. *Journal of the American Academy of Child and Adolescent Psychiatry, 39*(12), 1468–1484.

Marsh, A. A., Finger, E. C., Mitchell, D. G. V., Reid, M. E., Sims, C., Kosson, D. S., . . . Blair, R. J. R. (2008). Reduced amygdala response to fearful expressions in children and adolescents with callous-unemotional traits and disruptive behavior disorders. *American Journal of Psychiatry, 165*, 712–720.

National Institute of Mental Health. (2012). Attention deficit hyperactivity disorder (NIH Publication No. 12–3572). Retrieved from http://www.nimh.nih.gov/health/publications/attention-deficit-hyperactivity-disorder/index.shtml

Nigg, J. T., & Hinshaw, S. P. (1998). Parent personality traits and psychopathology associated with antisocial behaviors in childhood attention-deficit hyperactivity disorder. *Journal of Child Psychology and Psychiatry, 39*, 145–159.

Noordermeer, S. D, Luman, M., & Oosterlaan, J. (2016). A systematic review and meta-analysis of neuroimaging in oppositional defiant disorder (ODD) and conduct disorder (CD) taking attention-deficit hyperactivity disorder (ADHD) into account. *Neuropsychology Review, 26*(1), 44–72.

Passamonti, L., Fairchild, G., Goodyer, I. M., Hurford, G., Hagan, C. C., Rowe, J. B., & Calder, A. J. (2010). Neural abnormalities in early-onset and adolescence-onset conduct disorder. *Archives of General Psychiatry, 67*, 729–738.

Sterzer, P., Stadler, C., Poustka, F., & Kleinschmidt, A. (2007). A structural neural deficit in adolescents with conduct disorder and its association with lack of empathy. *Neuroimage, 37*, 335–342.

van Goozen, S. H., & Fairchild, G. (2006). Neuroendocrine and neurotransmitter correlates in children with antisocial behavior. *Hormones and Behavior, 50*, 647–654.

van Goozen, S. H., Fairchild, G., Snoek, H., & Harold, G. (2007). The evidence for a neurobiological model of childhood antisocial behavior. *Psychological Bulletin, 133*, 149–182.

12

Treatment for Conduct Disorder and Oppositional Defiant Disorder

The good news is that there are effective interventions in existence for oppositional defiant disorder (ODD) and conduct disorder (CD). However, interventions found to be effective are not effective for everyone. A percentage of the population will not be responsive to these treatments. The earlier the mental health problem is treated, the better the likelihood that the treatment will be successful. That does not mean that intervention with older teenagers who may have been exhibiting the signs and symptoms of one of these disorders for several years will not be effective. Treatment may be more challenging with an older youth, but success is still possible.

Many evidence-based interventions have been highly researched and recognized as evidence-based treatments (EBTs) for both of these externalizing disorders (Burns, Hoagwood, & Mrazek, 1999; Child and Adolescent Mental Health Division, 2004; Farmer, Compton, Burns, & Robertson, 2002). These EBTs share many of the same components. Many of them use combinations of one or more heavily researched practices found to be effective. These practices may be focused on working individually with caregivers, working with the youth, working with caregivers and youth together, or working with the peer group or community.

Evidence-Based Practices with Youth

Practices found to be effective in improving the functioning of youth experiencing CD or ODD are geared toward those youth characteristics often associated with these disorders (Burns et al., 1999; Child and Adolescent Mental Health Division, 2004; Farmer et al., 2002; Waldron & Turner, 2008). Skills training aimed at helping youth identify their normal ways of reacting and learning more effective ways of solving problems or coping with frustrations and the ups and downs of life can help them better

Understanding the Mental Health Problems of Children and Adolescents. Kirstin Painter and Maria Scannapieco, Oxford University Press (2021). © Oxford University Press. DOI: 10.1093/oso/9780190927844.003.0012

maneuver through problems and better adapt to different situations. Because many youth have difficulty with relationships, communication skills and social skills training have been found to be effective in helping them interact more appropriately and positively with peers and authority figures. Self-regulation is another skill that youth can learn to manage their behavior and reduce extreme reactions to minor situations.

Although medication is not a first-line treatment for ODD and CD, it is sometimes prescribed to control some of the more distressing symptoms. Some mental health professionals consider this a form of "chemical restraint," meaning that the medication is used to slow the youth down so that he or she cannot get into as much trouble. Others would consider medication appropriate to treat problems such as aggressive behavior. Either way, medication alone will not be effective in treating ODD or CD. Medication can be effective in treating symptoms related to coexisting conditions such as attention deficit hyperactivity disorder, anxiety, and mood disorders.

Evidence-Based Practices with Caregiver(s)

Improving parental management skills in dealing with noncompliant or defiant behavior is a practice that is used across all EBTs for externalizing disorders (Burns et al., 1999; Child and Adolescent Mental Health Division, 2004; Farmer et al., 2002). Well-meaning social workers sometimes tell parents to set boundaries and give consequences for problem behavior. These are things that parents can and should do, but if they are not done correctly or in conjunction with other interventions, the youth's behavior and family functioning can and most likely will get worse. Before a parent disciplines a child, the parent and child must first have positive interactions. Sometimes the first step to changing a youth's problem behavior is to teach a parent to praise and use positive reinforcement for good behavior and to spend time doing something fun with the child. Many people may see this as counterintuitive; however, children are more likely to respond to discipline from someone with whom they have a positive relationship and someone who gives them positive reinforcement for good behaviors.

Providing support for caregivers raising a child with either ODD or CD has been found to be helpful. It can be very difficult for parents/caregivers to deal with extreme problem behaviors. They will need support and understanding. They will also need to learn to take time for themselves doing enjoyable activities and building their own stress-relieving skills. Involving other adults such as a coach can be helpful.

Evidence-Based Practices with Youth and Caregivers Together

The most effective interventions found for ODD and CD involve a systemic approach. That is, the intervention should not treat only the child or youth; instead, interventions should be focused on all the risk factors discussed in the previous chapter: individual youth characteristics, environmental characteristics, peer group characteristics, and caregiver characteristics (Burns & Hoagwood, 2002; Child and Adolescent Mental Health Division, 2004). If treatment is focused only on the youth and not on other aspects of the youth's life, the intervention will be neither effective nor sustaining.

Evidence-Based Treatments

There are many existing EBTs geared at externalizing mental health problems. The following are a few of the most heavily researched and disseminated.

Parent–Child Interaction Therapy

Parent–child interaction therapy (PCIT) is a highly researched, evidence-based family intervention for young children aged 2–7 with behavior disorders. It was developed by Sheila Eyberg based on the idea that optimal parenting and interactions between a caregiver and a child are correlated with better child outcomes (Eyberg, Boggs, & Algina, 1995; Funderburk & Eyberg, 2011). PCIT uses concepts from play therapy, attachment theory, and social learning theory aimed at teaching caregivers to parent using positive nurturing and appropriate limit setting (authoritative parenting style).

PCIT consists of two phases. During both phases, the caregiver plays with the child for approximately an hour while the therapist observes the interactions, usually from behind a two-way mirror, and coaches the caregiver, usually through an earpiece. This allows the therapist to witness the

caregiver's interactions with the child first-hand and to provide immediate feedback and instruction on better ways to respond. During phase 1
of PCIT (child-directed interaction), the therapist focuses on instructing
the caregiver how to interact with and respond to the child, with the child
as the center of attention. The second phase (parent-directed interaction)
focuses on teaching the caregiver effective discipline skills. Through this
coaching, caregivers learn strategies for reinforcing their child's positive
behaviors and for setting limits without being harsh or negative.

Functional Family Therapy

Functional family therapy (FFT) was developed in 1972 as a strengths-
based, family-focused intervention aimed at at-risk youth aged 10–18 who
are experiencing acting-out behaviors and substance abuse problems, including those diagnosed with ODD or CD (Alexander, Barrett Waldron,
Robbins, & Neeb, 2013; Gordon, Graves, & Arbuthnot, 1995). Evaluation
of FFT has found it to be highly effective in reducing youth problem
behaviors and family conflict, improving family communication, and
improving parenting skills. FFT has been successfully implemented in
child welfare, juvenile justice, and mental health service systems. Facilities
wanting to be FFT providers must participate in extensive training.
Implementation of FFT is highly monitored.

FFT consists of five major pretreatment and intervention components
aimed at reducing risk factors and building protective factors: engagement
in change, motivation to change, relational/interpersonal assessment
and planning for behavior change, behavior change, and generalization.
Therapists work with families for an average of 12 sessions over a 3- to
4-month period. During the behavior change phase, therapists work with
youth and their families on improving communication skills, improving
coping, modeling and prompting positive behavior, caregiver parenting
skills, and any other area identified as a need.

Multisystemic Therapy

Multisystemic therapy (MST) is an evidence-based intervention that
was developed for the treatment of juvenile offenders (Henggeler, 1999,

2003; Henggeler, Melton, Smith, Schoenwald, & Hanley, 1993; Henggeler, Schoenwald, Borduin, Rowland, & Cunningham, 1998; Henggeler, Schoenwald, Rowland, & Cunningham, 2002). It is a community-based treatment that has achieved favorable long-term outcomes including reduced out-of-home placement and increased school attendance for children and adolescents presenting with serious clinical problems and their families. It takes a social ecological approach to assessment and treatment and utilizes empirically supported goal-oriented treatments, such as cognitive-behavioral therapy, family therapies, or parent training. Assessment focuses on identifying all of the risk factors contributing to a youth's emotional and behavioral problems, and interventions are aimed at all identified sources. Interventions may focus on the youth, caregivers, school environment, peer group, or many other possible influences on the youth's problems.

MST interventions occur in the youth's natural environment, such as in the home or community, and require active efforts from the caregivers to reach treatment goals. It is the responsibility of the therapist and provider agency to ensure that treatment goals are being met and that families are actively engaged in the treatment process. If goals are not being met, the therapist must reassess the situation, change the treatment strategy, or seek new ways to engage the family.

To become an MST provider, an agency must become licensed and agree to adhere to the fidelity of MST. Each MST clinician maintains a caseload of four to six families, allowing time to continuously assess outcomes and provide an intensive level of treatment to the family in its home and community. Services are problem-focused and time-limited, lasting from 4 to 6 months. The MST therapist or a member of the therapist's team is available 24 hours a day, 7 days a week to help the family work through any crisis that may arise. An on-site supervisor provides regularly scheduled weekly clinical supervision to the MST team and monitors the therapist's adherence to MST fidelity. In addition to on-site supervision, each MST team and supervisor works closely with an assigned consultant from MST Services who monitors MST fidelity and helps the team overcome treatment barriers and develop treatment strategies. More information on MST or how to become a certified provider can be found at http://mstservices. com.

Multidimensional Treatment Foster Care

Multidimensional treatment foster care (MTFC) is an evidence-based treatment that was developed as a cost-effective alternative to regular foster care placements, residential treatment, or incarceration of youth who have severe behavior problems (Leve, Fisher, & Chamberlain, 2009; Westermark, Hansson, & Olsson, 2011). Early evidence suggests that it is effective in reducing substance abuse among teenagers as well (Smith, Chamberlain, & Eddy, 2010). Youth are placed in foster homes with highly trained and well-supported foster parents for approximately 6–9 months. While youth are in the placement, they receive skills training, supportive therapy, school-based behavioral interventions, and supportive mentoring. The foster parents implement a structured plan that has been designed by a program supervisor with input from a treatment team consisting of a family therapist, an individual therapist, and a child skills trainer.

The biological family (or other caregiver) receives supportive family therapy to prepare for the youth's return to the home and parenting skills training to learn to provide close supervision, set fair and consistent limits, and provide consistent consequences for problem behaviors. The caregiver and youth have sessions and home visits together to allow the caregiver time to practice skills and receive feedback before the youth returns home permanently. MTFC can only be provided by programs that are certified or are receiving clinical supervision from TFC Consultants, Inc.

Case Studies

Let's return to the case studies of the youth from Chapter 11. You will see the diagnosis and any additional interventions that they received. Finally, you will see the outcome for each youth.

Tim
Tim is the 13-year-old boy living with his mother and 11-year-old sister in a public housing apartment complex. His father is deceased and his mother has an intellectual disability with an IQ under 90. Tim and his sister both have normal IQs.

Tim refused to listen to his mother and tormented his sister. He had several encounters with the juvenile justice system. He was adjudicated as a sex offender and started counseling. He reoffended and was ordered into an inpatient sex offender treatment program where he received intensive individual and group therapy. Tim was diagnosed with CD. When he was released from the sex offender treatment program, he returned home with his mother and sister. He remained on probation under a specialized probation unit. He is now 15 years old and his sister is 13.

When Tim first returned home, there was a honeymoon period. He followed his mother's rules and left his sister alone. As time passed, Tim began to pick up the delinquent behavior he exhibited prior to his adjudication. He ignored his mother's requests. His probation officer met with him weekly. If Tim missed the curfew set by the judge or skipped school, his probation officer sent him to juvenile detention. Tim reoffended by sexually abusing a 7-year-old neighbor. He was sentenced by a judge to remain in a state juvenile facility until he turned 18.

Tracy

Tracy is the 8-year-old girl who was exhibiting negative and acting-out behaviors. She got in trouble at school, talking back to her teachers and sometimes refusing to do her work. The other children in her classes did not like her because she was a bully. She did not always follow the rules at home. Tracy often screamed and yelled, ran to her room, and slammed the door. Tracy's parents were at their wits' end. Her mother took her to see a counselor. The counselor diagnosed Tracy with ODD. Tracy attended therapy for an hour each week, working with her therapist on anger management, coping, and problem-solving and social skills. After a few months, there were no noticeable changes in Tracy's behaviors at school or home. The therapist discharged Tracy from treatment.

Over the next 2 years, Tracy continued to exhibit behavioral problems. Once again at her wits' end, Tracy's mother sought help. The family was referred to receive wraparound treatment. Tracy and her parents, with guidance from the facilitator, helped to decide who they wanted to include on their family team. Team members initially included Tracy, her parents, a younger sister, a schoolteacher, and her mother's best friend, whom Tracy really liked. The wraparound facilitator guided the team through a process of identifying the family's strengths and needs and developing a wraparound (service) plan. The team identified formal and informal community services and supports to address the needs of the child and family. Tracy's parents received help with their parenting skills twice a week in their own home from a trained therapist. Her mother started attending a support group with other parents of children experiencing problems similar to Tracy's.

Tracy's teacher helped implement a behavior plan at school whereby Tracy could earn time to play video games or do other things she enjoyed. A daily report was e-mailed to Tracy's parents. If she had a good report, she was allowed to stay up and watch television for an extra 30 minutes. If she had a bad day, she was not allowed to watch her favorite shows that night.

Tracy started equestrian therapy in which she was assigned a horse to groom, feed, and ride a couple of times a week. As part of the therapy, she learned how to take responsibility for her actions and problem-solving and coping skills. Tracy loved riding and taking care of the horse. Her self-esteem improved. She also attended a weekly skills training group with other children. Tracy's behaviors changed considerably. She made a friend at school with whom she ate lunch and had sleepovers.

James

James is the 17-year-old who lived with his parents in a middle-class neighborhood. He was afraid of his father's explosive anger, but intimidated his mother when his father was at work. James hung out with a group of peers who abused drugs and alcohol. He was a bully to others. James was placed in detention for 3 months after he severely beat his mother, landing her in the hospital. He was diagnosed with CD while in detention. He was discharged to return home with strict orders from the judge that he would be sent to a more restrictive lockup facility until he turned 21 if he did not comply with his probation or had any more incidents of trouble. His family was offered MST; the parents agreed, but James was not so agreeable.

The MST therapist worked mostly with James's parents, helping them to manage James's behaviors. James refused to speak with the therapist. The therapist worked with his parents on being partners in dealing with James's behaviors and worked with his father on managing his own explosive temper. The family learned how to spend positive time together, and they incorporated a family dinner night on Sunday evenings.

James was very negative and continued to be defiant for the first 2 months of MST. As part of his probation, he was ordered not to hang out with his old friends, to attend school regularly, and not to use drugs or alcohol. His probation officer worked with the MST therapist and his parents to enforce the rules. He tested James for drug use on an intermittent basis. He put James on an ankle monitor for breaking curfew and hanging out with his old friends.

The MST therapist worked with James and his parents to develop a behavior plan. James loved listening to hard rock and had always wanted to play guitar. A behavioral plan was set up whereby James could earn a new electric guitar and lessons that would be purchased through flexible funds offered as a component of MST. James was able to earn the guitar and lessons. Through the music studio where he took lessons, he met some other guys and they started a band. James's behavior at home and school completely changed. The MST therapist stopped working with the family after 5 months. The next summer, James's mother sent a thank you letter to the MST therapist. James graduated from high school. His behaviors had changed, and he was enrolled in a technical school.

Dale

Dale is the 16-year-old who was placed in residential care for a year. He was diagnosed with CD. While he was in care, his parents had limited participation in treatment other than a monthly meeting with the social worker to discuss his progress. Dale received intensive treatment and skills training. Dale was put on a behavioral system whereby he could earn increased privileges and freedoms on the residential treatment center campus. He went to school on campus with teachers trained to understand mental health problems. Within 9 months, Dale's behaviors improved to the point where he was moved to the least restrictive unit on the campus, allowing him more freedom. After a year in treatment, he was discharged to return home and went back to his old school.

When Dale returned home, he utilized his new skills and did his best to follow rules and do well in school. His mother was very harsh and her reactions were unpredictable. Dale felt that, no matter what he did, his mother would yell or hit him. In the larger classroom setting, he began to struggle to keep up with others. Within 6 months, he was back to getting in trouble, using drugs, and hanging out with his old friends. He stole a car and ended up back in the detention center. As an alternative to sending him back to the residential treatment center or keeping him locked up in the detention center, he and his mother were referred to a MTFC pilot being implemented using grant funding. He was placed in a foster home with trained foster parents, in his community. This time, both he and his mother received help together and individually. An advocate helped get him into the correct educational setting. His mother was referred to a psychiatrist who diagnosed her with bipolar disorder and prescribed a mood stabilizer. She received skills training to help her better cope with stress and anxiety. After 3 months, Dale began having home visits. After 6 months, he returned home to live with his mother and was reportedly doing well.

Study Questions

1. What do these real life scenarios have in common?
2. What are the differences?
3. Now that you have learned what happened to each of the youths, do you have any different thoughts on how you would have handled the situation if you were the families' social worker?

References

Alexander, J. F., Barrett Waldron, H., Robbins, M. S., & Neeb, A. A. (2013). *Functional family therapy for adolescent behavior problems.* Washington, DC: American Psychological Association.

Burns, B. J., & Hoagwood, K. (Eds.). (2002). *Community treatment for youth: Evidence-based interventions for severe emotional and behavioral disorders.* New York: Oxford University Press.

Burns, B. J., Hoagwood, K., & Mrazek, P. J. (1999). Effective treatment for mental disorders in children and adolescents. *Clinical Child and Family Psychology Review, 2,* 199–254.

Child and Adolescent Mental Health Division. (2004). *Evidence-based Service Committee: Biennial report: Summary of effective interventions for youth with behavioral and emotional needs.* Honolulu: Hawaii Department of Health.

Eyberg, S., Boggs, S., & Algina, J. (1995). Parent-child interaction therapy: A psychosocial model for the treatment of young children with conduct problem behavior and their families. *Psychopharmacology Bulletin, 3,* 83–91.

Farmer, E. M. Z., Compton, S. N., Burns, B. J., & Robertson, E. (2002). Review of the evidence base for treatment of childhood psychopathology: Externalizing disorders. *Journal of Consulting and Clinical Psychology, 70,* 1267–1302.

Funderburk, B. W., & Eyberg, S. (2011). Parent–child interaction therapy. In J. C. Norcross, G. R. VandenBos, & D. K. Freedheim (Eds.), *History of psychotherapy: Continuity and change* (2nd ed., pp. 415–420). Washington, DC: American Psychological Association.

Gordon, D., Graves, K., & Arbuthnot, J. (1995). The effect of functional family therapy for delinquents on adult criminal behavior. *Criminal Justice and Behavior, 22,* 60–73. doi:10.1177/0093854895022001005

Henggeler, S. W. (1999). Multisystemic therapy: An overview of clinical procedures, outcomes, and policy implications. *Child Psychology and Psychiatry Review, 4,* 4–9.

Henggeler, S. W. (2003). Multisystemic therapy: An evidence-based practice for serious clinical problems in adolescents. *NAMI Beginnings, 3*(Fall), 8–10.

Henggeler, S. W., Melton, G. B., Smith, L. A., Schoenwald, S. K., & Hanley, J. H. (1993). Family preservation using multisystemic treatment: Long-term follow-up to a clinical trial with serious juvenile offenders. *Journal of Child and Family Studies, 2,* 283–293.

Henggeler, S. W., Schoenwald, S. K., Borduin, C. M., Rowland, M. D., & Cunningham, P. B. (1998). *Multisystemic treatment of antisocial behavior in children and adolescents.* New York: Guilford.

Henggeler, S. W., Schoenwald, S. K., Rowland, M. D., & Cunningham, P. B. (2002). *Serious emotional disturbance in children and adolescents: Multisystemic therapy.* New York: Guilford.

Leve, L., Fisher, P., & Chamberlain, P. (2009). Multidimensional treatment foster care as a preventive intervention to promote resiliency among youth in the child welfare system. *Journal of Personality, 77,* 6.

Smith, D., Chamberlain, P., & Eddy, M. (2010). Preliminary support for multidimensional treatment foster care in reducing substance use in delinquent boys. *Journal of Child & Adolescent Substance Abuse, 19,* 343–358.

Waldron, H. B., & Turner, C. W. (2008). Evidence-based psychosocial treatments for adolescent substance abuser. *Journal of Clinical Child and Adolescent Psychology, 37,* 238–261.

Westermark, P. K., Hansson, K., & Olsson, M. (2011). Multidimensional treatment foster care (MTFC): Results from an independent replication. *Journal of Family Therapy, 33,* 20–41. doi:10.1111/j.1467–6427.2010.00515.x

13

Bipolar Disorder

Bipolar disorder (BD), also known as *manic depression*, is a category of mood disorders. In the fifth edition of the *Diagnostic and Statistical Manual of Mental Disorders* (DSM-5) BD appears in the section titled "Bipolar and Related Disorders" (American Psychiatric Association [APA], 2013). BD is a brain disorder that results in severe changes in a person's mood and energy level. It affects an estimated 1–3 percent of youth (Birmaher, 2013). As its name implies, it is characterized by extreme highs (mania) and/or extreme lows (major depression, as discussed in Chapter 5). Between episodes, some people experience lingering symptoms, whereas others may be symptom free (Goodwin & Jamison, 2007). Medication(s) control the symptoms of BD; however, there is currently no cure. We hope that ongoing research will someday result in a cure, but, for now, it is a lifelong, chronic illness.

Researchers estimate that people experience the symptoms of BD for a median of 6 years before receiving treatment (Drancourt et al., 2012). When BD goes untreated in children and adolescents, they can experience social, emotional, and academic impairments. However, with treatment people can recover and live happy, healthy, productive lives (Kessler et al., 2005; National Depressive and Manic-Depressive Association, 2001). In this chapter we will discuss bipolar I disorder, bipolar II disorder, and cyclothymia (APA, 2013).

Signs and Symptoms

Mania and Hypomania

Mania is an abnormally heightened state of energy and mood. It is far more extreme than the emotion that a person would normally expect to experience when happy or excited. Mania causes serious problems, to the point that it interferes with a person's ability to function in daily life. According to the DSM, symptoms of mania include

Understanding the Mental Health Problems of Children and Adolescents. Kirstin Painter and Maria Scannapieco,
Oxford University Press (2021). © Oxford University Press. DOI: 10.1093/oso/9780190927844.003.0013

- Excessive energy, restlessness, racing thoughts, and rapid talking
- Denial that anything is wrong
- Extremely happy feelings
- Being easily irritated
- Little need for sleep
- Unrealistic belief in one's ability
- Poor judgment
- Sustained, unusual behavior
- Increased sex drive
- Substance abuse
- Aggressive behavior
- Paranoia

During a manic episode, someone may go days without needing any sleep or may be overly restless. The person may experience excessive energy and do things such as clean the entire house from top to bottom for hours on end. During a manic episode, a person may experience a combination of symptoms. She may be more talkative than usual, have pressured speech, and have racing thoughts or flight of ideas, where she moves from topic to topic and the topics do not connect together. Poor judgment, increased sex drive, and extreme risk-taking behaviors have also been found to accompany mania. Any of these issues alone can be a serious problem. Someone in a manic episode may be overly sexually promiscuous, putting him or her at high risk of contracting a sexually transmitted disease or experiencing an unwanted pregnancy. It is common for someone experiencing mania to go on wild spending sprees and max out their own credit cards or credit cards stolen from others, purchasing things they do not need or that seem irrational. They often leave themselves or someone else in significant debt. As an example, one young adult stole her parent's credit cards and car. She went on a spending spree purchasing several high-end designer purses, pairs of shoes, and expensive jewelry. By the time her parents realized what happened and contacted the credit card companies, their daughter had purchased thousands of dollars in merchandise. The family ended up filing charges on their daughter with the hopes that she could get treatment rather than going to jail. Their daughter ended up with a felony on her record and jail time until the family finally convinced the court to transfer her to a psychiatric hospital on an involuntary commitment.

Delusional thinking and inflated self-esteem are often symptoms of mania. Some people experiencing a manic episode truly believe that they are famous movie stars, members of royalty, religious figures, a famous singer, the best baseball player in the world, or any number of other beliefs. At times, a person experiencing mania may be extremely irritable for no reason or show unusual behavior for an extended period. Aggressive behavior, substance abuse, and extreme feelings of paranoia are other common symptoms. When I was a social worker in a psychiatric hospital, a 16-year-old male patient was admitted to the hospital on many occasions involuntarily due to experiencing a manic episode during which he became highly agitated and put himself in dangerous situations. He did things such as jump off the roof of his parents' house into the pool. Fortunately, he did not miss. He was pulled over by police on several occasions during a manic episode because he was driving wildly at extremely fast speeds. He became very argumentative with his family. He threw furniture and punched holes in the wall. When admitted to the hospital, he would scream and curse at staff and other patients. Once stabilized on medication, his personality was completely different. He was friendly, funny, and kind.

Another patient was admitted to the hospital during a period of mania. When she was brought in by police, she was wearing a full-length fur coat in the middle of summer that she had just purchased, had a feather boa around her neck, and was carrying an urn. She believed she was a member of royalty and expected others to treat her as royalty. She would wander around the hospital unit talking to everyone she could, addressing them as her subjects. When asked about the urn, she said it was for her husband who was not deceased; it was for when he died. These are just some examples of real-life people and the ways in which their mania manifested.

At the end of a manic episode, a person experiences a crash. Some people describe their crash as the end of good times. During a manic episode, many people report feeling on top of the world, as if they can do anything; this is followed by crashing, during which they sleep long hours and wake up unable to function. They have expended all their energy. Mania can feel exhilarating and exciting; going into the crash can feel as if one has fallen into a black hole of sadness and despair that will never end. It is common for people to abuse substances to try to find their "high" again or to stop taking their medication when stabilized because they feel "down" when really they are at a level of functioning that is normal for people without BD.

Hypomania is similar to mania, but the symptoms are not as intense and disruptive to daily life. With hypomania, there a clear change from a person's normal mood that persists most of the day, every day for at least 4 consecutive days. According to the DSM, hypomania is a distinct period of "abnormally and persistently elevated, expansive, or irritable mood and abnormally and persistently increased activity or energy." In addition, there must be three or more (four if the mood is only irritable) of the following symptoms that are not due to substance abuse:

- Inflated self-esteem or grandiosity
- Decreased need for sleep (e.g., feels rested after only 3 hours of sleep)
- More talkative than usual or pressure to keep talking
- Flight of ideas or subjective experience that thoughts are racing
- Distractibility
- Increase in goal-directed activity (at work, at school, or sexually) or psychomotor agitation
- Excessive involvement in activities that have a high potential for painful consequences (e.g., engaging in unrestrained buying sprees, sexual indiscretions)
- The episode is associated with an unequivocal change in functioning that is uncharacteristic of the person when not symptomatic
- The disturbance in mood and the change in functioning are observable by others
- The episode is not severe enough to cause marked impairment in social or occupational functioning or to necessitate hospitalization.

Psychotic symptoms do not occur with hypomania. When experiencing an exhilarated mood, a person can feel quite good and not perceive the hypomania as a problem. Others might find it fun to be around a person who is having a hypomanic episode. People often describe the feeling as being high but in control. They experience excessive energy. Ideas come faster. They may feel more creative, more confident, less shy, and/or more productive. If not treated, a hypomanic episode may transform into a severe manic or depressive episode (Goodwin & Jamison, 2007). Both manic and depressive symptoms can interfere with school performance. For youth experiencing mania, the risk-taking, impulsiveness, and erratic behaviors can become disciplinary problems. Racing thoughts and inability to concentrate interfere with the ability to focus on work. Relationships with peers are very likely to become problematic. The inability to comprehend others' facial expressions can lead to misunderstanding of social cues and can be a recipe for getting into arguments and fights.

Causes

The etiology of BD is not completely known; however, there does seem to be evidence that the cause includes a combined genetic, environmental, and biochemical relationship. BD has been found to run in families (Lin et al., 2006). Children who have a parent or other close relative with BD are more likely to develop it than are children with no family history of the disorder (Nurnberger & Foroud, 2000). Some estimates report that as many as 4–24 percent of persons who have a first-degree biological relative with bipolar I, 1–5 percent of persons with a first-degree relative with bipolar II, and 4–24 percent of persons with a first-degree relative with major depression also have BD. When one parent has BD, it is estimated that the risk to the child is anywhere from 15 to 30 percent. This risk increases from 50 to 75 percent when both parents have BD. Studies of twins and adoptions provide strong evidence of a genetic connection to BD, but they also suggest that environment plays a role. With fraternal twins, if one twin has BD, the risk that the other child will also develop it ranges from 15 to 25 percent. With identical twins, the risk is estimated to be 40 to 70 percent (Craddock & Jones, 1999).

Approximately 60 percent of adult patients with BD experienced mood symptoms before the age of 20, with 10 to 20 percent of those experiencing the symptoms before the age of 10 (Egeland, Hostetter, Pauls, & Sussex, 2000; Lish, Dime-Meenan, Whybrow, Price, & Hirschfeld, 1994; Loranger & Levine, 1978).

Research has found that bipolar I and bipolar II are equally likely to occur among different races, ethnicities, and genders (Gonzalez et al., 2007; Manchia et al., 2008; Tsuchiya, Byrne, & Mortensen, 2003). In bipolar I, males are more likely to experience mania as a first symptom. Females are more likely to experience major depression as a first symptom. Research suggests that bipolar I is more common in men and bipolar II is more common in women (Merikangas et al., 2011). In general, women experience more major depressive symptoms than do men throughout the course of the disease. Women are at risk of developing symptoms following childbirth, particularly psychotic symptoms. Sometimes women will experience their first episode of mania or major depression postpartum. This episode often includes psychosis. When a woman is premenstrual, she can experience a worsening of manic or depressive symptoms. Men are more prone to hypomania than depression and experience as many or more hypomanic episodes as major depressive episodes.

Drug and alcohol abuse occur in more than half of people diagnosed with BD (Bizzarri et al., 2007; Strakowski et al., 1998). If a person is predisposed to BD, abusing drugs or alcohol can increase the likelihood of developing it. Sometimes youth self-medicate with alcohol or drugs in order to feel normal.

Bipolar Disorder and the Brain

Bipolar spectrum disorders are considered brain disorders. Scientists have been studying the brain in an effort to find the biological correlates to BD. As discussed previously, norepinephrine, serotonin, and dopamine are the neurotransmitters involved in the functioning of the brain and body. Research suggests that abnormalities in serotonin and dopamine are contributors to BD (Soares & Mann, 1997a, 1997b). Ongoing studies have found that the brain of a child with BD does not perform in the same ways as it does in a healthy child (Gogtay et al., 2007; Soares & Mann, 1997a, 1997b). Through a noninvasive technique that allows scientists to measure brain functioning (magnetoencephalography), differences between children with BD and other children have been found in the areas of the brain that direct attention to identifying environmental signals and organize behavior. Imaging studies have helped identify different brain activity patterns and connections associated with the symptoms of BD. For instance, children with BD have been found to have difficulty in identifying facial expressions in others. It is believed by the scientific community that this may be an inherited trait that affects children with BD and other children who have a first-degree relative with the disorder. Findings of genomic studies suggest that multiple genes on a chromosome are associated with BD (Group PGCBDW, 2011), and there is some evidence that BD, schizophrenia, and autism share genetic risk (Lichtenstein et al., 2009; Sullivan et al., 2012). This shared genetic risk is discussed in Chapter 15.

A link between BD and altered genes has also been found through research. The altered gene that seems to have the most correlation with BD is located in the axons in a region of the brain responsible for controlling the firing of neurons. As science continues to advance our knowledge of BD, it will allow for preventative interventions, improved treatments, and, hopefully, a cure.

Diagnosing Bipolar Disorder

The diagnosis of BD is based on patient self-reports and reports from family members or other persons who have witnessed abnormal behavior. In addition to the psychiatric evaluation, a physical exam, including a complete laboratory panel, should be conducted to rule out a general medical condition or substance abuse as the underlying cause of symptoms.

As stated earlier in this chapter, BD is really a category of mood disorders rather than one singular disorder. The commonality across these categories is the presence of one or more incidents of an abnormally elevated energy level, called mania or hypomania. Depending on the type of BD a person develops, he or she may experience depressive episodes as well. Both manic and depressive episodes are often separated by periods of normal mood that can last weeks, months, or even years in some persons. For some persons, depression and mania may rapidly alternate, a condition known as *rapid cycling*. In addition to the types and intensities of symptoms experienced, a key factor in meeting the criteria for BD is that the symptoms cause significant distress or impairment across daily functioning.

Bipolar I

To meet the criteria for bipolar I, a person must have experienced one or more manic episodes. With bipolar I, experiencing a depressive episode is not required for the diagnosis; however, depressive episodes frequently occur.

Bipolar II

Bipolar II disorder is characterized by a history or occurrence of a hypomanic episode and at least one episode meeting the criteria for major depression. Hypomania is characterized by the same symptoms as mania, such as increased energy, but in less extreme forms. Because of this, bipolar II is more difficult to diagnose than bipolar I. Hypomania can appear similar to a period of successful, high productivity; thus, it is less likely to be reported than depressive episodes.

Cyclothymia

Cyclothymia is characterized by a presence or history of hypomanic episodes with periods of depression that do not meet criteria for major depressive episodes. A diagnosis of cyclothymia requires the presence of numerous hypomanic episodes intermingled with depressive episodes. A person with cyclothymia experiences more moderate cycling of moods. These mood changes interfere with a person's functioning, but they appear to the observer to be a personality trait.

The DSM-5 includes specifiers that further describe the symptoms, identify the correct treatments, and provide information about the course and prognosis of the disorder (APA, 2013). Here is a list of the specifiers along with a brief description of each:

- With anxious distress: Describes if the person experiences feeling keyed up/tense, is unusually restless, or has a feeling or fear that something awful may happen or they may lose control
- With mixed features: Describes if the person experiences a hypomanic or manic episode along with features of symptoms typically found in a depressive episode or if the person experiences a depressive episode along with symptoms that include features of hypomania or mania
- With rapid cycling: Describes if there have been at least four mood episodes (mania, hypomania, major depressive) in the previous 12 months that met the full criteria
- With melancholic features: Describes when a person is in a such a low state of a depressive episode that he or she cannot react with any feelings of pleasure
- With atypical features: Describes when the symptoms occur with mood reactivity. For example, the person's mood may brighten when good things happen, they may gain weight or have an increase in appetite, they may sleep more than usual, or they may have a heavy, almost paralyzing feeling in their arms and legs (cannot occur with catatonia)

- With mood-congruent psychotic feature: Describes when a person has delusions or hallucinations that reflect the person's mood
- With mood-incongruent psychotic features: Describes when a person has delusions or hallucinations that do not reflect the person's mood
- With catatonia: Describes when the person experiences catatonic symptoms (i.e., rigidity or stupor), erratic and extreme movements, repetition or echoing of words
- With peripartum onset: Describes when the onset of any of the symptoms occur during the 4 weeks following childbirth
- With seasonal pattern: Describes when periods of depression tend to occur and remit during certain times of the year
- Specify: Remission status if all criteria are not currently met for a manic, hypomanic, or major depressive episode.

Bipolar Disorder in Children and Adolescents

Diagnosing BD in children and adolescents is more difficult than diagnosing it in adults. Children and adolescents can experience the same symptoms as adults; however, they often experience symptoms that present differently. The developmental stage of the youth has to be taken into account when making a diagnosis. Early signs of BD in youth can include somatic complaints, exaggerated mood swings, dramatic changes in feelings and opinions, and emotional lability wherein the youth exhibits intense emotional overreaction to a situation such as temper tantrums, shouting, breaking things, and crying (Egeland et al., 2000; Geller et al., 2002). Not that long ago, BD was believed to emerge in late adolescence or adulthood. Although symptoms of BD more often emerge after childhood, it is now recognized that they can begin in early childhood. Children as young as 6 years can be diagnosed with BD. Prevalence estimates of childhood-onset BD range from less than 1 percent to 2.5 percent (Merikangas et al., 2011; Stringaris, Santosh, Leibenluft, & Goodman, 2010). Prevalence rates of bipolar in adolescents are close to those found in adults, which are estimated at 4.4 percent in the United States (Merikangas et al., 2011).

There is debate among healthcare providers and others as to whether the increased prevalence of BD in children and young teens is accurate or whether it is being wrongly or overly diagnosed. On one side of the argument, it is believed that children are finally being accurately diagnosed because mental health professionals are more knowledgeable of the disorder in children. Those making this argument assert that earlier identification and earlier access to appropriate treatment can result in a better trajectory of the disorder. The other side of the argument is that BD is overdiagnosed in children and teenagers. People in this camp believe it to be the latest fad in psychiatry rather than accurate early diagnosis. Some in this camp believe that we, as a society, are using BD as a crutch or a label to explain away inappropriate behaviors that would have been dealt with through discipline in the past. The answer to this debate probably lies somewhere in the middle. What is known is that children can develop BD, and, if it is identified and treated early, they can experience better outcomes and functioning.

When youth experiences mania, their behaviors may seem erratic and oppositional. Youth often take risks without thinking because their thoughts move rapidly, not allowing them time to consider the consequences. They may also feel indestructible and supreme. Common risk-taking behavior includes drug and alcohol use, dangerous stunts, and illegal behavior. An increased sex drive or obsession with sex can be a symptom of mania. Coupling that with risk-taking behavior can result in the youth having unprotected sex.

Both manic and depressive symptoms can interfere with school performance. For youth experiencing mania, the risk-taking, impulsiveness, and erratic behaviors can become disciplinary problems. Racing thoughts and inability to concentrate interfere with the ability to focus on work. Relationships with peers are very likely to become problematic. The inability to comprehend others' facial expressions can lead to misunderstanding of social cues and can be a recipe for getting into arguments and fights.

Research suggests that people who begin experiencing symptoms of BD during early childhood have more severe symptoms and a poorer trajectory of the disorder than those who begin experiencing symptoms in early adulthood (Bellivier, Golmard, Henry, Leboyer, & Schurhoff, 2001; Carter, Mundo, Parikh, & Kennedy, 2003; Hamshere et al., 2009; Kessler et al., 2005; Perlis et al., 2004). The onset of BD before the age of 13 is associated with increased lifetime repeated episodes of both depressive and manic symptoms and suicide attempts (Perlis et al., 2004). Hamshere and colleagues (2009) reported that in early childhood children are more likely to experience manic symptoms and rapid mood cycling. These cycles are seen as unpredictable, alternating between behavior that is aggressive and behavior that is silly. A child may appear to have an extremely short temper at times or experience unusually irritable moods resulting in explosive temper tantrums or rages that may last several hours. These is not the normal silliness or irritability that a child would ordinarily exhibit. Younger children who develop BD often experience audio and visual hallucinations.

Several studies show that youth with anxiety or major depressive disorders are more likely to develop BD than youth who never experience these disorders (Krishnan, 2005; Mueser et al., 1998). Youth who experience multiple recurrences of major depression are 10 to 15 percent more likely to develop bipolar I disorder than are other youth (Bellivier et al., 2003; Bellivier, Golmard, Henry, Leboyer, & Schurhoff, 2001). Although those who experience an anxiety or depressive disorder are at higher risk of developing BD than persons in the general population, it must be noted that the majority of children and teens with anxiety disorders do not develop BD.

There is emerging scientific evidence to suggest an association between child maltreatment (physical, sexual, and emotional abuse and neglect) and increased risk of developing BD (Etain et al., 2010; Garno, Goldberg, Ramirez, & Ritzler, 2005; Palmeir-Claus et al., 2016; Watson et al., 2014). Research also suggests that people who experience child maltreatment have more severe symptoms of BD and poorer clinical outcomes than people who did not experience child maltreatment (Agnew-Blais, 2016). Not only is there evidence to suggest that they experience more severe symptoms, there is also evidence to suggest that they have more frequent mood swings

Common symptoms of early-onset BD in young children include

- Bed wetting (especially in boys)
- Night terrors
- Rapid or pressured speech
- Obsessional behavior
- Excessive daydreaming
- Compulsive behavior
- Motor and vocal tics
- Learning disabilities
- Poor short-term memory
- Lack of organization
- Fascination with gore or morbid topics
- Hypersexuality
- Manipulative behavior
- Bossiness

- Lying
- Suicidal thoughts
- Destruction of property
- Paranoia

Differential Diagnosis

Other psychiatric and substance use disorders have symptoms that overlap or appear similar to those of BD, as do some physical health conditions such as thyroid disease, thus complicating accurate diagnosis. For example, a caregiver takes his or her 13-year-old to a mental health clinic for assessment. The youth is easily irritated, aggressive, and denies having any problems. Are these symptoms related to major depression, oppositional defiant disorder (ODD), a substance abuse problem, typical teenage behavior, or something else? The symptoms could be related to any of these problems, and a comprehensive, thorough assessment is warranted to rule out other diagnoses.

How do you differentiate between someone experiencing depression who has BD versus someone who has major depressive disorder (MDD), given that the symptoms and presentation of the depression are the same for both disorders? One key thing to look for is periods of mania or hypomania and severe mood changes. If there is at least one episode with mania, it is easier to identify because mania causes marked impairment in daily functioning. Since hypomania is not as severe and does not cause marked impairment, it can be more difficult to identify. The developmental level of the youth can complicate identifying mania or hypomania, but particularly hypomania. However, with hypomania the behaviors exhibited still must go well beyond what one would normally expect given the developmental level of the youth.

Many of the symptoms of BD share commonalities with the symptoms of attention deficit hyperactivity disorder (ADHD) and/or ODD. Youth experiencing mania may become easily distracted, hyperactive, and/or impulsive, which can appear more like ADHD. Severe acting-out and aggressive behaviors can appear to be an oppositional disorder. Researchers have found that if irritability is related to mania, it will almost always manifest with elation, which is far beyond normal happiness (Merikangas et al., 2011).

If a child with BD is misdiagnosed as having ADHD or depression, depending on the symptoms, there can be dangerous consequences. Someone predisposed to BD who takes the stimulant Ritalin or an antidepressant such as Prozac or Zoloft can experience extreme manic and/or psychotic behaviors. Accurate diagnosis is imperative. It should also be noted that children may start out with symptoms of one type of BD and later switch to symptoms of another type of the disorder (Birmaher et al., 2006).

Substance use/abuse is both a risk factor for and often comorbid with BD, particularly bipolar I (e.g., Feingold et al., 2015; Gibbs et al., 2015; Hunt, Malhi, Cleary, Lai, & Sitharthan, 2016; Kenneson, Funderburk, & Maisto, 2013; Salloum & Brown, 2017; Schepis & Hakes, 2013). The effects of substance use/abuse can mimic, provoke, or worsen mood symptoms and complicate BD diagnosis due to the similarity of the presentation of each. Additionally, comorbidity with substance use/abuse disorders occurs in more than half of the people who have BD (Bizzarri et al., 2007; Hunt et al., 2016; Strakowski et al., 1998). It is common for youth who experience symptoms of BD to self-medicate with alcohol or drugs in order to feel "normal." Looking at symptoms over the course of the illness and at the person's family history can play a key role in determining an accurate diagnosis or co-occurrence of diagnoses. It is difficult to know which came first, the substance abuse or the onset of BD. To make an accurate diagnosis, it is important to monitor someone when the substance(s) are out of the person's system. One teenager went away to college for the first time. She began having symptoms of mania and psychosis. Her parents signed her into a psychiatric hospital. A drug screen found that she had marijuana and opioids in her system. She was diagnosed with a substance use disorder, but her psychiatrist wanted to rule out other possible problems and kept her in the hospital for observation. After the substances were out of her system, psychotic and manic symptoms did not dissipate. If her symptoms were solely related to the substance use, they would have cleared once they were no longer in her system. She was started on a mood stabilizer and an antipsychotic. Her symptoms improved after a few weeks. Unfortunately, after she was discharged, she discontinued her medication and went back to using marijuana and opioids, and her symptoms returned, requiring her to be hospitalized again.

Disruptive Mood Dysregulation Disorder

A new diagnostic category called *disruptive mood dysregulation disorder* (DMDD) has been added to the DSM-5 to capture those youth who experience significant difficulties, such as severe temper outbursts and extreme irritability, but do not have the classic symptoms of mania/hypomania or characteristics such as a family history of BD. The symptoms of both BD and ODD have many similarities with DMDD; however, there are distinct differences as well (APA, 2013), and it is these distinct differences between the disorders that prompted research resulting in the addition of the new diagnosis. Youth with ODD exhibit extreme defiant behavior directed toward persons in authority; however, the duration and intensity do not meet the same threshold as the symptoms associated with DMDD. DMDD differs from BD in that the symptoms are constant rather than episodic. The symptoms of DMDD occur at least two to three times a week and last for at least a year. Many youth who fit into this new diagnostic category are those who were historically being diagnosed with BD not otherwise specified (NOS) because they were experiencing extreme problems that did not meet the criteria for ODD or BD. The criteria listed in the DSM-5 (APA, 2013) for DMDD include the following:

1. Severe recurrent temper outbursts that are grossly out of proportion, in intensity or duration, to the situation.
   a. The temper outbursts are manifested verbally and/or behaviorally, such as in the form of verbal rages or physical aggression toward people or property.
   b. The temper outbursts are inconsistent with developmental level.
2. The temper outbursts occur, on average, three or more times per week.
3. An irritable or angry mood is exhibited between temper outbursts:
   a. Nearly every day, for most of the day, the mood between temper outbursts is persistently irritable or angry.
   b. The irritable or angry mood is observable by others (e.g., parents, teachers, and peers).
4. Criteria 1–3 have been present for 12 or more months without three or more consecutive months without the symptoms of criteria 1–3.
5. Criterion 1 or 3 is present in at least two settings (at home, at school, or with peers) and must be severe in at least one setting.
6. The diagnosis should not be made for the first time before age 6 or after age 18.
7. The onset of criteria 1 through 5 is before the age of 10.
8. There has never been a distinct period lasting more than 1 day during which an abnormally elevated or expansive mood was present most of

the day, and the abnormally elevated or expansive mood was accompanied by the onset, or worsening, of mania.

The behaviors do not occur exclusively during an episode of MDD and are not better accounted for by another mental disorder. The symptoms are not due to the effects of a drug or to a general medical or neurological condition.

Assessment Tools

Over the past several years, there has been an increased focus on evidence-based assessment (EBA) using a multitiered systems of support (MTSS) framework to diagnose BD (Pendergast, Youngstrom, Ruan-Iu, & Beysolow, 2018). The MTSS framework aids clinicians in systematically incorporating information from multiple informants and data sources. Incorporating multiple data sources improves the likelihood of accurately diagnosing BD. One EBA diagnostic protocol for assessing BD in youth is the Alexian Brothers diagnostic protocol (Youngstrom et al., 2005). This protocol includes five steps. The first step involves screening for the presence of mania using the parent version of the Child Mania Rating Scale (CMRS). The CMRS-P is a parent report measure designed and tested specifically to assess for the symptoms of mania in pediatric BD (Pavuluri, Henry, Devineni, Carbray, & Brimaher, 2006). The CMRS-P is structured based on the DSM diagnostic criteria for mania. There are two versions of the CMRS-P, a 21-item and a 10-item, both having good psychometric properties (Pavuluri et al., 2006). CMRS-P is quick and easy to administer. Not only is it sensitive to detecting symptoms of mania, it also differentiates between symptoms of ADHD and mania.

The next two steps involve establishing an estimate of the likelihood of the youth having BD and evaluating for symptoms specific to BD that do not overlap with the criteria of other diagnoses (i.e., decreased need for sleep, unstable self-esteem and grandiosity, hypersexuality, elated mood, pressured speech, racing thoughts, and goal-directed activity). In step two, the results from the CMRS-P, the base rate of pediatric BD, and family history of BD are combined to determine the likelihood that the youth has BD. An in-depth description for calculating step two is beyond the scope of this book. To learn more about this step in the CMRS-P, see Youngstrom and Duax (2005) and Washburn, West, and Heil (2011). Step four involves assessing for evidence of a history of episodes of the symptoms (retrospectively), and step five focuses on assessing for the mood episodes prospectively.

Washburn and Youngstrom recommend using an assessment tool such as the National Institute of Mental Health Life Chart Method (NIMH-LCM) to document lifetime mood episodes, both retrospectively (completed using monthly ratings) and prospectively (using daily methods) (Denicoff et al., 2000). There is both a clinician-completed and a self-rated version of the NIMH-LCM. NIMH-LCM includes a chart for both retrospective and prospective documenting of mood. Levels of severity of mood states are rated from −4 (severe and incapacitating depression) to −1 (slight or mild depression) and +1 (mild mania) to +4 (severe mania). A score of 0 indicates that the mood is balanced and there is no evidence of depression or mania.

We presented the Alexian Brothers diagnostic protocol due to the importance of using multiple data sources to obtain and accurate diagnosis. Specifically, screening for mania, conducting an assessment of the classic symptoms of BD, obtaining the family history, and conducting a thorough investigation of the youth's history of mood problems are all important when assessing for BD. A thorough, careful assessment can reduce the likelihood of making an incorrect diagnosis that could have serious negative consequences in treating the wrong problem.

Case Studies

The following are some case studies of youth with symptoms similar to those discussed in this chapter. Chapter 14 will explore evidence-based treatments and practices for BD. We will then return to the case studies presented in this chapter to learn of the actual interventions provided.

Tina

Tina is a 13-year-old who always made good grades, had lots of friends, and loved sports. Her behavior suddenly changed. She began having trouble sleeping, often pacing around the house throughout the night. She was unable to sleep more than 2 hours a night for several days, but she claimed she did not feel tired.

At times her mood was overly happy and the next minute it seemed angry and irritable. She would curse at others for no known reason. She started talking rapidly about a lot of different things, but mainly she boasted about how much smarter and more popular she was than everyone else. During school, her behaviors were very disruptive. She would talk over the teacher about things not related to the class.

Her parents became concerned that she was using drugs. They did not know how to handle the situation. The final straw for them was when she stole their car and went for a ride even though she was not old enough to drive. The police stopped her for speeding. When they learned that she was not old enough to drive, they took her to the juvenile detention center. Her parents were able to convince the judge to drop the charges and allow them to take her to a hospital for drug and alcohol treatment.

When Tina was taken in for treatment, the doctor ordered a toxicology screening to determine what drugs she had been taking. Tina denied using drugs or alcohol. Her toxicology report came back negative for drugs and alcohol. She was transferred to the psychiatric adolescent unit of the hospital and, with parental consent, was started on Depakote against her will. Her parents did not want her to take the medication, but they did not know what else to do. After spending 3 weeks in the hospital, Tina was discharged and returned home to her normal life and school. She was given a follow-up appointment with her psychiatrist.

Consider the following questions:

1. What symptoms was Tina experiencing?
2. Does she meet the criteria for a bipolar diagnosis? Explain. If she does, which one?
3. Based on your current knowledge, what interventions would you suggest? Do you believe that the appropriate intervention or treatment was provided?
4. Who should be included in the treatment planning and interventions?
5. What barriers might get in the way of effectively intervening?
6. What suggestions, thoughts, or ideas do you have for the other members of her family?

Jack

When Jack was 7 years old, his parents noticed changes in his mood and behaviors over the course of several months. One minute, he would act silly and say silly things. He would make weird faces, laugh hysterically out of the clear blue, and run around the house. The next minute he would begin crying and tell his parents that he hated himself because he was ugly and stupid. He would apologize over and over for things that he perceived he did wrong, but which were in reality of no consequence. He went through periods of not needing sleep and exhibiting an extreme level of energy. During these times, he would start an activity and then move on to another activity without finishing the first. At other times, he would isolate himself in his room and not show any interest in playing video games or playing with friends. He would hit his baby sister, punch a wall, or exhibit other unprovoked aggressive behaviors. He told his parents he did these things because the voices were telling him to do bad things.

Jack's parents became frustrated with Jack's behavior, believing he was doing these things to get attention. Punishment did not seem to change his behaviors. One day, he choked his baby sister, bruising her neck. His mother called the police. The police said that they could not do anything to help because Jack was only 7 years old; they told her to call social services because he was a danger to his sister. Social services helped the parents find a residential facility where Jack was admitted for long-term care.

Write your answers to the following questions:

1. What symptoms was Jack experiencing?
2. Does he meet the criteria for a bipolar diagnosis? Explain. If he does, which one?
3. Based on your current knowledge, what interventions would you suggest? Do you believe that the appropriate intervention or treatment (if any) was provided?
4. Who should be included in the treatment planning and interventions?
5. What barriers might get in the way of effectively intervening?
6. What suggestions, thoughts, or ideas do you have for members of his family?

References

Agnew-Blais, D. (2016). Childhood maltreatment and unfavourable clinical outcomes in bipolar disorder: A systematic review and meta-analysis. *Lancet Psychiatry, 3*, 342–349.

American Psychiatric Association (APA). (2013). *Diagnostic and statistical manual of mental disorders* (5th ed.). Washington, DC, Author.

Bellivier, F., Golmard, J. L., Henry, C., Leboyer, M., & Schurhoff, F. (2001). Admixture analysis of age at onset in bipolar I affective disorder. *Archives of General Psychiatry, 58,* 510–512.

Bellivier, F., Golmard, J. L., Rietschel, M., Schultze, T. G., Malafosse, A., Preisig, M., . . . Lebover, M. (2003). Age at onset in bipolar I affective disorder: Further evidence for three subgroups. *American Journal of Psychiatry, 160,* 999–1001.

Birmaher, B. (2013). Bipolar disorder in children and adolescents. *Child and Adolescent Mental Health, 18*(3). Retrieved June 28, 2018, from https://www.ncbi.nlm.nih.gov/pmc/articles/PMC3835470/

Birmaher, B., Axelson, D., Strober, M., Gill, M. K., Valeri, S., Chiappetta, L., . . . Keller, M. (2006). Clinical course of children and adolescents with bipolar spectrum disorders. *Archives of General Psychiatry, 63,* 175–183.

Bizzarri, J. V., Sbrana, A., Rucci, P., Ravani, L., Massei, G. J., Gonnelli, C., . . . Cassano, G. B. (2007). The spectrum of substance abuse in bipolar disorder: Reasons for use, sensation seeking and substance sensitivity. *Bipolar Disorder, 9,* 213–220.

Carter, T. D., Mundo, E., Parikh, S. V., & Kennedy, J. L. (2003). Early age at onset as a risk factor for poor outcome of bipolar disorder. *Journal of Psychiatric Residency, 37,* 297–303.

Craddock, N., & Jones, I. (1999). Genetics of bipolar disorder. *Journal of Medical Genetics, 36,* 585–594.

Denicoff, K. D., Leverich, G. S., Nolen, W. A., Rush, S. L., McElroy, P. E., Keck, T., . . . Post, R. M. (2000). Validation of the prospective NIMH-Life-Chart Method (NIMH-LCM-p) for longitudinal assessment of bipolar illness. *Psychological Medicine, 30*(6), 1391–1397.

Drancourt, N., Etain, B., Lajnef, M., Henry, C., Raust, A., Cochet. B., . . . Bellivier, F. (2012). Duration of untreated bipolar disorder: Missed opportunities on the long road to optimal treatment. *Acta Psychiatrica Scandinavica, 127*(2), 136–144.

Egeland, J.A., Hostetter, A.M., Pauls, D.L., & Sussex, J.N. (2000). Prodromal symptoms before onset of manic-depressive disorder suggested by first hospital admission histories. *Journal of the American Academy of Child and Adolescent Psychiatry, 39*(10), 1245–1252.

Etain B., Mathieu, F., Henry, C., Raust, A., Roy, I., Germain, A., Leboyer, M., & Bellivier, F. (2010). Preferential association between childhood emotional abuse and bipolar disorder. *Journal of Trauma and Stress, 23,* 376–383.

Feingold, D., Weiser, M., Rehm, J., & Lev-Ran, S. (2015). The association between cannabis use and mood disorders: A longitudinal study. *Journal of Affective Disorders, 172,* 211–218.

Garno, J. L., Goldberg, J. F., Ramirez, P. M., & Ritzler, B. A., (2005). Impact of childhood abuse on the clinical course of bipolar disorder. *British Journal of Psychiatry, 186,* 121–125.

Geller, B., Zimerman, B., Williams, M., Delbello, M. P., Frazier, J., & Beringer, L. (2002). Phenomenology of prepubertal and early adolescent bipolar disorder: Examples of elated mood, grandiose behaviors, decreased need for sleep, racing thoughts and hypersexuality. *Journal of Child and Adolescent Psychopharmacology, 12*(1), 3–9.

Gibbs, M., Winsper, C., Marwaha, S., Gilbert, E., Broome, M., & Singh, S. P. (2015). Cannabis use and mania symptoms: A systematic review and meta-analysis. *Journal of Affective Disorders, 171,* 39–47.

Gogtay, N., Ordonez, A., Herman, D. H., Hayashi, K. M., Greenstein, D., Vaituzis, C., . . . Rapoport, J. L. (2007). Dynamic mapping of cortical development before and after the onset of pediatric bipolar illness. *Journal of Child Psychology and Psychiatry, 48,* 852–862.

Gonzalez, J. M., Thompson, P., Escamilla, M., Araga, M., Singh, V., Farrelly, N., . . . Bowden, C. L. (2007). Treatment characteristics and illness burden among European Americans, African Americans, and Latinos in the first 2,000 patients of the systematic treatment enhancement program for bipolar disorder. *Psychopharmacological Bulletin, 40,* 31–46.

Goodwin, F. K., & Jamison, K. R. (2007). *Manic-depressive illness: Bipolar disorders and recurrent depression* (2nd ed.). New York: Oxford University Press.

Group PGCBDW. (2011). Large-scale genome-wide association analysis of bipolar disorder identifies a new susceptibility locus near ODZ4. *Nature Genetics, 43,* 977–983.

Hamshere, M. L., Gordon-Smith, K., Forty, L., Jones, L., Caesar, S., Fraser, C., . . . Smith, D. J. (2009). Age-at-onset in bipolar-I disorder: Mixture analysis of, 1369 cases identifies three distinct clinical sub-groups. *Journal of Affective Disorders, 116,* 23–29.

Hunt, G. E., Malhi, G. S., Cleary, M., Lai, H. M., & Sitharthan T. (2016). Prevalence of co-morbid bipolar and substance use disorders in clinical settings, 1990–2015: Systematic review and meta-analysis. *Journal of Affective Disorders, 206,* 331–349.

Kenneson, A., Funderburk, J. S., & Maisto, S. A. (2013). Substance use disorders increase the odds of subsequent mood disorders. *Drug and Alcohol Dependence, 133,* 338–343.

Kessler, R. C., Berglund, P., Demler, O., Jin, R., Merikangas, K. R., & Walters, E. E. (2005). Lifetime prevalence and age-of-onset distributions of DSM-IV disorders in the National Comorbidity Survey Replication. *Archives of General Psychiatry, 62,* 593–602.

Krishnan, K. R. (2005). Psychiatric and medical comorbidities of bipolar disorder. *Psychosomatic Medicine, 67*(1), 1–8.

Lichtenstein, P., Yip, B. H., Bjork, C., Pawitan, Y., Cannon, T. D., Sullivan, P. F., & Hultman, C. M. (2009). Common genetic determinants of schizophrenia and bipolar disorder in Swedish families: A population-based study. *Lancet, 373,* 234–239.

Lin, P. I., McInnis, M. G., Potash, J. B., Willour, V., MacKinnon, D. F., DePaulo, R., & Zandi, P. P. (2006). Clinical correlates and familial aggregation of age at onset in bipolar disorder. *American Journal of Psychiatry, 163,* 240–246.

Lish, J. D., Dime-Meenan, S., Whybrow, P. C., Price, R. A., & Hirschfeld, R. M. (1994). The national Depressive and Manic-depressive Association (DMDA) survey of bipolar members. *Journal of Affective Disorders. 31*(4), 281–294.

Loranger, A. W., & Levine, P. M. (1978). Age at onset of bipolar affective illness. *Archives of General Psychiatry, 35*(11), 1345–1348.

Manchia, M., Lampus, S., Chillotti, C., Sardu, C., Ardau, R., Severino, G., & Del Zompo, M. (2008). Age at onset in Sardinian bipolar I patients: Evidence for three subgroups. *Bipolar Disorders, 10,* 443–446.

Merikangas, K. R., Jin, R., He, J. P., Kessler, R. C., Lee, S., Sampson, N. A., . . . Zarkov, Z. (2011). Prevalence and correlates of bipolar spectrum disorder in the world mental health survey initiative. *Archives of General Psychiatry, 68,* 241–251.

Mueser, K. T., Goodman, L. B., Trumbetta, S. L., Rosenberg, S. D., Osher, C., Vidaver, F. C., . . . Foy, D. W. (1998). Trauma and posttraumatic stress disorder in severe mental illness. *Journal of Consulting and Clinical Psychology, 66,* 493–499.

National Depressive and Manic-Depressive Association. (2001). Living with bipolar disorder: How far have we really come? [Community survey]. Retrieved from http://www.dbsalliance.org/pdfs/bphowfar1.pdf

Nurnberger, J. I., Jr., & Foroud, T. (2000). Genetics of bipolar affective disorder. *Current Psychiatry Reports, 2*, 147–157.

Palmier-Claus, J. E., Berry, K., Bucci, S., Mansell, W., & Varese, F. (2016). Relationship between childhood adversity and bipolar affective disorder: Systematic review and meta-analysis. *British Journal of Psychiatry, 209*, 454–459.

Pavuluri, M. N., Henry, D. B., Devineni, B., Carbray, J. A., & Birmaher, B. (2006). Child mania rating scale: Development, reliability, and validity. *Journal of the American Academy of Child and Adolescent Psychiatry, 45*(5), 550–560.

Pendergast, L. L., Youngstrom, E. A., Ruan-Iu, L., & Beysolow, D. (2018). The nomogram: A decision-making tool for practitioners using multitiered systems of support. *School Psychology Review, 47*(4), 345–359.

Perlis, R. H., Miyahara, S., Marangell, L. B., Wisniewski, S. R., Ostacher, M., DelBello, M. P., . . . Nierenberg, A. A. (2004). Long-term implications of early onset in bipolar disorder: Data from the first 1000 participants in the systematic treatment enhancement program for bipolar disorder (STEP-BD). *Biological Psychiatry, 55*, 875–881.

Salloum, I. M., & Brown, E. S. (2017). Management of comorbid bipolar disorder and substance use disorders. *American Journal of Drug and Alcohol Abuse, 43*, 366–376.

Schepis, T. S., & Hakes, J. K. (2013). Dose-related effects for the precipitation of psychopathology by opioid or tranquilizer/sedative nonmedical prescription use: Results from the national epidemiologic survey on alcohol and related conditions. *Journal of Addiction Medicine, 7*, 39–44.

Soares, J. C., & Mann, J. J. (1997a). The anatomy of mood disorders: Review of structural neuroimaging studies. *Biological Psychiatry, 41*, 86–106.

Soares, J. C., & Mann, J. J. (1997b). The functional neuroanatomy of mood disorders. *Journal of Psychiatric Residency, 31*, 393–432.

Strakowski, S. M., Sax, K. W., McElroy, S. L., Keck, P. E., Jr., Hawkins, J. M., & West, S. A. (1998). Course of psychiatric and substance abuse syndromes co-occurring with bipolar disorder after a first psychiatric hospitalization. *Journal of Consulting and Clinical Psychology, 59*, 465–471.

Stringaris, A., Santosh, P., Leibenluft, E., & Goodman, R.(2010). Youth meeting symptom and impairment criteria for mania-like episodes lasting less than four days: An epidemiological enquiry. *Journal of Child Psychology and Psychiatry, 51*(1), 31–38.

Sullivan, P. F., Magnusson, C., Reichenberg, A., Boman, M., Dalman, C., Davidson, M., . . . Lichtenstein, P. (2012). Family history of schizophrenia and bipolar disorder as risk factors for autism. *Archives of General Psychiatry, 69*, 1099–1103.

Tsuchiya, K. J., Byrne, M., & Mortensen, P. B. (2003). Risk factors in relation to an emergence of bipolar disorder: A systematic review. *Bipolar Disorders, 5*, 231–242.

Washburn, J. J., West, A. E., & Heil, J. A. (2011). Treatment of pediatric bipolar disorder: A review. *Minerva Psychiatry, 52*(1), 21–35.

Watson, S., Gallagher, P., Dougall, D., Porter, R., Moncrieff, J., Ferrier, I. N., & Young, A. H. (2014). Childhood trauma in bipolar disorder. *Australia and New Zealand Journal of Psychiatry, 48*, 564–570.

Youngstrom, E. A., & Duax, J. (2005). Evidence-based assessment of pediatric bipolar disorder, part I: Base rate and family history. *Journal of the American Academy of Child and Adolescent Psychiatry, 44*(7), 712–717.

Youngstrom, E. A., Findling, R. L., Youngstrom, J. K., & Calabrese, J. R. (2005). Toward an evidence-based assessment of pediatric bipolar disorder. *Review Journal of Clinical Child & Adolescent Psychology, 34*(3), 433–448.

14

Treatment of Bipolar Disorder

As with other mental health disorders discussed in this book, there is currently no cure for bipolar disorder (BD). However, people can recover through treatment and lead a normal life. Treatment focuses on controlling and preventing the symptoms. Medication in conjunction with some form of psychotherapy has been found to be the most effective in helping a young person manage his or her symptoms (Andreescu, Mulsant, & Emanuel, 2008). Family therapies have been found helpful in managing the daily problems of having a child with BD.

Medication

A common theme discussed throughout this book is the controversy of treating children and adolescents with medications developed and tested on adults. Medication, in the form of a mood stabilizer, has long been the first line of treatment for BD (Hirschfeld, 2005; Sachs, Printz, Kahn, Carpenter, & Docherty, 2000). Lithium was the first mood stabilizer approved by the US Food and Drug Administration (FDA). Lithium, which decreases abnormal brain activity, is a very effective medication for stabilizing the mood changes in BD. Additionally, antiseizure medications (also called anticonvulsants) commonly used to treat epilepsy and seizure disorders have been found effective for use as mood stabilizers. Two of the most commonly used antiseizure medications for treating BD are sodium valproate (Depakote) and carbamazepine (Tegretol). Depakote, Tegretol, and lithium have all been studied and found to effectively treat BD in children and adolescents (Hirschfeld, 2005; Sachs et al., 2000). In addition, Depakote has been approved by the FDA to treat seizure disorders in children as young as 10 years. Therefore, it may be less stigmatizing for a physician to treat a child with BD with Depakote rather than lithium. In addition to mood stabilizers and anticonvulsants,

Understanding the Mental Health Problems of Children and Adolescents. Kirstin Painter and Maria Scannapieco,
Oxford University Press (2021). © Oxford University Press. DOI: 10.1093/oso/9780190927844.003.0014

most recently there has been an increased focus on the effectiveness of atypical antipsychotics in managing bipolar symptoms, particularly symptoms of mania.

Medications used for treating BD have improved over the past 10 years, but everyone responds differently to them, and all medications have side effects. As with other types of medications discussed, it is important to remember that one must weigh the benefits against the risks of medications. Many of the side effects, including serious ones, will affect a very small portion of those taking it; however, the chance of side effects always exists. Some medications used for treating BD have been linked to serious problems; therefore, everyone taking them should be aware of the possible side effects, be monitored closely, and see a doctor regularly. Any problems with a medication should be immediately reported to the doctor. Table 14.1 provides an overview of the different class of medications used in treating BD. It is also very important to ask about and discuss negative interactions with other drugs. Consulting with a pharmacist about drugs contraindicated for concurrent usage with medications that a youth has been prescribed is very beneficial in heading off problems with drug interactions because pharmacists tend to be more knowledgeable about drug side effects than are doctors.

In addition to the side effects listed in Table 14.1, Depakote has been found to increase levels of the male hormone testosterone in some females and lead to a condition called polycystic ovarian syndrome (PCOS; Calabrese et al., 2005; Vainionpaa et al., 1999). PCOS can affect fertility and make the menstrual cycle become irregular. The symptoms of PCOS usually go away once a person stops taking Depakote. Pregnant females should not take Depakote because it has been linked to birth defects. Depakote, Tegretol, and other anticonvulsant medications come with an FDA warning stating that anyone taking these medications should be closely monitored for new or worsening symptoms of depression, suicidal thoughts or behaviors, or any unusual changes in mood or behavior.

Despite the possible side effects, children and teens with BD can get better with these medications. Families must weigh the risk versus the benefits of having their children take one of these medications. Caregivers have complained that medications cause their child to experience changes in their personalities and to be out of it or spaced out. At the same time, persons taking mood stabilizers complain that the medications make them feel slowed down, unproductive, and not themselves. They are used to the mania or hypomania and they like it. Feeling normal does not feel normal

Table 14.1 Different class of medications used for treating bipolar disorder

Brand name	Generic name	FDA approval for youth	Common side effects in children	Possible rare risk factors to monitor	Forms of medications
Lithium	Eskalith, Lithobid	Bipolar I 12 and older	Nausea Diarrhea Sedation Difficulty concentrating Trembling hands Increase thirst and urination Headache Weight gain Acne	Seizures Coma Convulsions Tardive Dyskinesia Hypothyroidism	Tablets, capsules, extended-release tablets, and liquids
Anticonvulsants: Developed to treat seizures, they have mood-stabilizing effect					
Depakote (Depakene)	Valproate	Off-label	Nausea Increased appetite Weight gain Sedation Increase in lipids (fats in the blood) Low blood platelet count Hair loss Tremor Vomiting	Pancreatitis Irreversible liver damage Hyperparathyroidism Diabetes	Tablets Delayed-release tables, and capsules

Lamictal	Lamotrigine	Off-labelPrevent depressive bipolar symptoms	Mild sedation Decreased concentration Headache Blurred vision Mild weight gain	Neutropenia (serious blood disorder) Stevens-Johnson syndrome (life-threatening allergic reaction) Suicidal thoughts	Tablet forms including chewable, disintegrating and extended release
Tegretol	Carbamazepine	Off-label	Sedation Ataxia (unsteady movements) Dizziness Blurred vision Nausea Vomiting Extreme exhaustion Memory problems Nystagmus (twitching of the eyes)	Irregular heart beat Loss of cells or platelets in blood Hypothyroidism or hyperparathyroidism Irreversible liver damage Neutropenia (serious blood disorder) Stevens-Johnson syndrome (life-threatening allergic reaction) Suicidal thoughts	Tablet forms including chewable and extended-release
Trileptal	Oxcarbazepine	Off-label	Dizziness Drowsiness Blurred or double vision Fatigue	Hyponatremia (disturbance of levels of salt in blood) Stevens-Johnson syndrome (life-threatening allergic reaction)	Tablet and oral suspension

(Continued)

Table 14.1 *Continued*

Brand name	Generic name	FDA approval for youth	Common side effects in children	Possible rare risk factors to monitor	Forms of medications
			Headaches Nausea Stomach ache Vomiting	Suicidal thoughts	

Antipsychotic medications approved for treating bipolar symptoms in children and adolescents

Brand name	Generic name	FDA approval for youth	Common side effects in children	Possible rare risk factors to monitor	Forms of medications
Risperdal	Risperidone	10 and over for treating	Drowsiness Dizziness Light-headedness Drooling Nausea Weight gain Tiredness Difficulty swallowing Muscle spasms Shaking (tremor) Mental/mood changes Interrupted breathing during sleep	Cerebrovascular events, including stroke Neuroleptic malignant syndrome (very rare, life-threatening reaction characterized by fever, altered mental status, muscle rigidity, and autonomic dysfunction Tardive dyskinesia (uncontrolled body movements) Hyperglycemia (high blood sugar)/ diabetes Hyperprolactinemia (higher than normal hormone prolactin which affect estrogen and testosterone)	Tablets: Oral solution Orally disintegrating tables

Orthostatic hypotension

Leukopenia, neutropenia and agranulocytosis (severe deficiency of types of white blood cells important to fighting infections)

Potential for cognitive and motor impairment

Seizures

Dysphagia (serious medical condition of difficulty swallowing)

Priapism (prolonged erection of the penis)

Disruption of body temperature regulation

Antiemetic Effect (important to management of nausea and vomiting)

Suicide

(continued)

Table 14.1 *Continued*

Brand name	Generic name	FDA approval for youth	Common side effects in children	Possible rare risk factors to monitor	Forms of medications
Zyprexa	Olanzapine	Acute symptoms of Bipolar I	Lack of energy Dry mouth Increased appetite Somnolence (sleepiness)	Hyperglycemia (high blood sugar)/ diabetes Increased cholesterol and triglycerides (type of fat) in blood	Orally Disintegrating Tablet Extended release Injectable
		13 and older	Tremor (shakes) Having hard or infrequent stools Dizziness Changes in behavior	Tardive dyskinesia (uncontrolled body movements)	
			Restlessness Headache Abdominal pain Pain in your arms or legs Tiredness	Drug reaction with eosinophilia and systemic symptoms(rare, potentially life-threatening, drug-induced hypersensitivity reaction) Neuroleptic malignant syndrome (very rare, life-threatening reaction characterized by fever, altered mental status, muscle rigidity, and autonomic dysfunction) Orthostatic hypotension (decreased blood pressure) Weight gain	

Abilify	Aripiprazole	Treats acute mania and mixed mania 10 and over	Somnolence (sleepiness) Insomnia Headache Nausea Vomiting Stuffy nose Fatigue Weight gain Increased or decreased appetite Uncontrolled movement Increased saliva or drooling Muscle stiffness	Hyperlipidemia (high concentration of fats or lipids in the blood) Hyperglycemia (high blood sugar)/diabetes Increased cholesterol and triglycerides (type of fat in blood) Tardive dyskinesia (uncontrolled body movements) Neuroleptic malignant syndrome (very rare, life-threatening reaction characterized by fever, altered mental status, muscle rigidity, and autonomic dysfunction) Orthostatic hypotension (decreased blood pressure) Low white blood cell count Seizures	Orally Disintegrating Tablet Injectable/Injection

(continued)

Table 14.1 *Continued*

Brand name	Generic name	FDA approval for youth	Common side effects in children	Possible rare risk factors to monitor	Forms of medications
				Weight gain Increased suicidal ideation (particularly when used in combination with Prozac	
Seroquel	Quetiapine	Acute mania 10 and over	Drowsiness Dizziness Fatigue Nausea Dry mouth Weight gain Increased appetite Vomiting	Hyperglycemia (high blood sugar)/diabetes Increased cholesterol and triglycerides in blood Tardive dyskinesia (uncontrolled body movements) Neuroleptic malignant syndrome (very rare, life-threatening reaction characterized by fever, altered mental status, muscle rigidity, and autonomic dysfunction) Hypertension (note: for adults hypotension) Weight gain Low white blood cell count	Tablet, Oral Injectable/Injection

| Saphris and Sycrest | Asenapine | Bipolar I 10–17 | Drowsiness Dizziness Light-headedness Weight gain | Extrapyramidal symptoms (EPS; muscle/nervous system problems) Dysphagia (serious medical condition of difficulty swallowing) Tardive dyskinesia (uncontrolled body movements) Neuroleptic malignant syndrome (very rare, life-threatening reaction characterized by fever, altered mental status, muscle rigidity, and autonomic dysfunction) Shaking (tremor), shuffling walk, stiff muscles, severe muscle spasms/cramping (such as twisting neck, arching back, eyes rolling up), mask-like expression of the face | Orally disintegrating tablet |

(*continued*)

Table 14.1 *Continued*

Brand name	Generic name	FDA approval for youth	Common side effects in children	Possible rare risk factors to monitor	Forms of medications
Lurasidone (Latuda)	Ziprasidone	Major depressive episodes for Bipolar I 10 and older	Nausea Weight gain Insomnia	Cerebrovascular adverse reactions Neuroleptic malignant syndrome Tardive dyskinesia Metabolic changes, hyperglycemia, dyslipidemia Weight gain Diabetes	Tablets

Information retrieved from FDA.gov.

to them. Because of this, it is not uncommon for persons to stop taking their medications in an effort to experience the high from mania, forgetting about the negative consequences that can result from poor decision-making, risk-taking, and other harmful behaviors. They also forget about the inevitable crash they will experience.

Each medication affects different people in different ways. Therefore, a psychiatrist may have to try out a couple of different medications before finding the most effective one for a particular person. In addition, antidepressant and/or antipsychotic medications are sometimes added to the medication regimen when a mood stabilizer is not enough to control depressive or psychotic symptoms (see Chapter 6 for a discussion of antidepressants and Chapter 16 for antipsychotic medications). It is important to note that a person with BD should never take an antidepressant without also taking a mood stabilizer. An antidepressant alone could result in a manic episode. It is also important to note that recent ongoing research through the National Institute of Mental Health (n.d.) is finding that adding an antidepressant to a mood stabilizer does not give any extra benefit.

Psychosocial Interventions

There is limited research in the literature on evidence-based practices or programs designed specifically for youth with BD. The majority of bipolar research focuses on adults. The limited existing research for youth experiencing BD has focused on cognitive-behavioral therapy (CBT), family-focused therapy (FFT), interpersonal and social rhythm therapy (IPSRT), and psychoeducation. All of these interventions share many of the same practices. They also use many of the same practices discussed in other chapters for treating illnesses such as anxiety disorders, depression, or attention deficit hyperactivity disorder.

Family-Focused Therapy

FFT was first developed for adults diagnosed with BD and their families and has since been adapted and is under evaluation for use with youth (Miklowitz & Goldstein, 1997; Miller, Solomon, Ryan, & Keitner, 2004;

Simoneau, Miklowitz, Richards, Saleem, & George, 1999). It is considered an adjunct to medication and not a replacement for medication. FFT is a time-limited treatment lasting for approximately 21 sessions. Sessions initially occur weekly and then titrate down to occur twice a month and finally monthly. Each session presents the theoretical underpinnings that families need to understand and cope (psychoeducation) and the skills to improve family communication and problem-solving (expressed emotion). As the focus of the first seven sessions of FFT, psychoeducation helps family members gain a better understanding of early-onset BD, what to expect with the illness, and available treatment options. Families learn to identify early warning signs of a manic or depressive episode so that they can intervene early, before the symptoms become worse. The remaining sessions focus on teaching the family new communication and problem-solving skills to enhance the overall quality of family interactions and to manage problems associated with the illness. The therapist teaches the family the new skills, and the family practices the skills in sessions. The therapist provides feedback to the family during the practice sessions. Between sessions, the family is given a homework assignment to track the times they use or attempt to use the new skills at home. After treatment ends, booster sessions are sometimes used as a way to help the family maintain the new skills.

Interpersonal and Social Rhythm Therapy

IPSRT is an evidence-based program (Frank, 2005). As with FFT, IPSRT is considered an adjunct to medication rather than a stand-alone treatment. It is a time-limited intervention focused on teaching youth skills to manage their illness and improve relationships. A key component of IPSRT is to develop and maintain a daily routine (social rhythm) that is based on individual biological and social rhythms, with specified times to sleep, do homework, and eat meals, for example. The theoretical underpinning of IPSRT is that maintaining a social rhythm will help protect against manic episodes. Therapists teach youth skills to manage stressful life events and stay on track with their social rhythm; they also emphasize the importance of and techniques for adhering to the prescribed medication regime.

Cognitive-Behavioral Therapy

CBT is the most extensively tested psychosocial treatment for depression. It is being used as an adjunct to medication for youth with BD (Pavuluri et al., 2004) and has been found to be effective in treating both children and adolescents experiencing depression. The focus of CBT is to change how one thinks and acts as a means of improving depression. This is based on the theory that depression is both caused and maintained by negative or irrational beliefs.

CBT is structured and time-limited, lasting anywhere from 6 to 12 weeks. The first goal of CBT is to help youth realize that they can control their own behaviors and therefore can change depression. The therapist works with the youth by teaching strategies to stop, confront, and change irrational and negative thought patterns.

Mood diaries or emotions charts are common tools used to assist young people to monitor thoughts, actions, physiological sensations, emotions, and events and to become aware of how these factors affect their depression. The therapist also teaches the youth problem-solving, coping, self-monitoring, relaxation, and social skills. Learning ways to relax in stressful situations helps the youth feel more competent and opens the door to trying out other skills. Homework is used as a strategy for increasing learning and integrating the skills being developed.

Case Studies

Tina

Tina is the 13-year-old who always made good grades, had lots of friends, and loved sports. Her behavior suddenly changed. She began having trouble sleeping, often pacing around the house throughout the night. She was unable to sleep more than 2 hours a night for several days, but she claimed not to feel tired.

At times her mood changed very quickly from overly happy to angry and irritable. She cursed at others for no known reason. She started talking rapidly about a lot of different things, but mainly she boasted about how much smarter and more popular she was than everyone else. During school, her behaviors were very disruptive. She would talk over the teacher about things not related to the class.

Her parents became concerned that she was using drugs. They did not know how to handle the situation. The final straw occurred when she stole their car and went for a ride even though she was not old enough to drive. The police stopped her for speeding. When they learned that she was not old enough to drive, they took her to the juvenile detention center. Her parents were able to convince the judge to drop the charges and allow them to take her to a hospital for drug and alcohol treatment.

When Tina was taken in for treatment, the doctor ordered a toxicology screening to determine what drugs she had been taking. Tina denied using drugs or alcohol, and her toxicology report came back negative for drugs and alcohol. She was transferred to the psychiatric adolescent unit of the hospital and, with parental consent, was started on Depakote against her will. Her parents did not want her to take the medication, but they did not know what else to do. After spending 3 weeks in the hospital, Tina was discharged and returned home to her normal life and school. She was given a follow-up appointment with her psychiatrist.

A few days after leaving the hospital, Tina told her parents that she was feeling good and did not need to take the Depakote. She stopped taking it. After a few days, she began experiencing rapid cycling of her moods and was again hospitalized. She was discharged with the same follow-up plan as for her last discharge, but was strongly counseled about the importance of staying on her medications.

Jack

When Jack was 7 years old, his parents noticed changes in his mood and behaviors over the course of several months. One minute, he would act silly and say silly things. He would make weird faces, laugh hysterically out of the clear blue, and run around the house. The next minute he would begin crying and tell his parents that he hated himself because he was ugly and stupid. He would apologize over and over for things that he perceived he did wrong but that were of no consequence. He went through periods of not needing sleep and exhibiting extreme levels of energy. During these times, he would start an activity and then move on to another activity without finishing the first. At other times, he would isolate himself in his room and not show any interest in playing video games or playing with friends. He would hit his baby sister, punch a wall, or exhibit other unprovoked aggressive behaviors. He told his parents that he did these things because the voices were telling him to do bad things.

Jack's parents became frustrated with his behavior, believing he was doing these things to get attention. Punishment did not seem to change his behaviors. One day, he choked his baby sister, bruising her neck. His mother called the police. The police said that they could not do anything to help because he was only 7 years old. They told her to call social services because he was a danger to his sister. Social services helped the parents find a residential facility, where Jack was admitted for long-term care. After 6 months in the treatment facility, Jack was discharged to return home. His behaviors improved significantly while in the facility. Each day, nurses gave him his medication and ensured that he swallowed it. He reached the top level of the facility's behavioral program, which allowed him to be discharged and return home.

Study Questions

1. What do these real-life scenarios have in common?
2. What are the differences?
3. Now that you know what happened to each of the youths, do you have any different thoughts on how you would have handled the situation if you were the families' social worker?

References

Andreescu, C., Mulsant, B. H., & Emanuel, J. E. (2008). Complementary and alternative medicine in the treatment of bipolar disorder: A review of the evidence. *Journal of Affective Disorders, 110*, 16.

Calabrese, J. R., Shelton, M. D., Rapport, D. J., Youngstrom, E. A., Jackson, K., Bilali, S., . . . Findling, R. L. (2005). A 20-month, double-blind, maintenance trial of lithium versus divalproex in rapid-cycling bipolar disorder. *American Journal of Psychiatry, 162*, 2152–2161.

Frank, E. (2005). *Treating bipolar disorder: A clinician's guide to interpersonal and social rhythm therapy*. New York: Guilford.

Hirschfeld, R. M. (2005). *Guideline watch: Practice guideline for the treatment of patients with bipolar disorder* (2nd ed.). Arlington, VA: American Psychiatric Association. Retrieved from http://psychiatryonline.org/pb/assets/raw/sitewide/practice_guidelines/guidelines/bipolar-watch.pdf

Miklowitz, D. J., & Goldstein, M. J. (1997). *Bipolar disorder: A family-focused treatment approach*. New York: Guilford.

Miller, I., Solomon, D. A., Ryan, C. E., & Keitner, G. I. (2004). Does adjunctive family therapy enhance recovery from bipolar I mood episodes? *Journal of Affective Disorders, 82*, 431–436.

National Institute of Mental Health. (n.d.). *Bipolar disorder.* Retrieved from www.nimh. nih.gov/health/topics/bipolar-disorder/index.shtml

Pavuluri, M. N., Graczyk, P. A., Henry, D. B., Carbray, J. A., Heidenrich, J., & Miklowitz, D. J. (2004). Child- and family-focused cognitive behavioral therapy for pediatric bipolar disorder: Development and preliminary results. *Journal of the American Academy of Child and Adolescent Psychiatry, 43*, 528–537.

Sachs, G. S., Printz, D. J., Kahn, D. A., Carpenter, D., & Docherty, J. P. (2000). The Expert Consensus Guideline Series: Medication treatment of bipolar disorder 2000, 1–104. New York: McGraw-Hill Healthcare Information Programs. Retrieved from http://www.senon-online.com/Documentation/telechargement/guidelines/guidelines%20TB%20Dep/Bipolar_2000.pdf

Simoneau, T. L., Miklowitz, D. J., Richards, J. A., Saleem, R., & George, E. L. (1999). Bipolar disorder and family communication: Effects of a psychoeducational treatment program. *Journal of Abnormal Psychology, 108*, 588–597.

Vainionpaa, L. K., Rattya, J., Knip, M., Tapanainen, J. S., Pakarinen, A. J., Lanning, P., . . . Isojarvi, J. I. (1999). Valproate-induced hyperandrogenism during pubertal maturation in girls with epilepsy. *Annals of Neurology, 45*, 444–450.

15

Schizophrenia Spectrum and First-Episode Psychosis

Schizophrenia is a serious mental illness that results in strange thinking, abnormal feelings, and/or odd behaviors. Psychosis is a symptom of schizophrenia that can result in the person interpreting reality in abnormal ways and have difficulty discerning real events from imaginary events. While psychosis can be a symptom of other mental health disorders (e.g., depression and bipolar disorder) or related to a physical health problem, for the purposes of this chapter we are specifically discussing schizophrenia spectrum disorders. In the United States, an estimated 100,000 adolescents and young adults experience first-episode psychosis (FEP) each year (Heinssen, Goldstein, & Azrin, 2014). Schizophrenia is one of the top 15 causes of disability. People who have schizophrenia often have co-occurring chronic medical conditions and other mental health disorders. They are at a higher risk of dying at a younger age than people without schizophrenia due to their co-occurring problems being undetected or undertreated, or from suicide.

Onset of schizophrenia in adolescents usually occurs between the ages of 13 and 18, though onset is considered rare before the age of 16. When schizophrenia does occur before at 16, it usually results in a more severe, chronic form of the disorder in adulthood (Vyas & Gogtay, 2012). Males have a higher prevalence rate than females (ratio of 1.4 to 1), and onset in males tends to emerge in late adolescence or the early twenties. For females, schizophrenia tends to emerge sometime in the twenties or thirties. Regardless of race or ethnicity, anyone can experience schizophrenia. Epidemiological studies show no difference in rates of schizophrenia based on race or ethnicity (US Department of Health and Human Services, 2001); however, studies have shown disparities in rates of diagnosis of schizophrenia based on race and ethnicity (Coleman et al., 2016; Georgia State University, 2010; Schwartz & Blankenship, 2014) and on psychiatric treatment received (Fleming, Barner,

Understanding the Mental Health Problems of Children and Adolescents. Kirstin Painter and Maria Scannapieco,
Oxford University Press (2021). © Oxford University Press. DOI: 10.1093/oso/9780190927844.003.0015

Brown, & Smith, 2011; Mallinger & Lamberti, 2007). These studies found that racial and ethnic minorities were more likely than whites to be diagnosed with schizophrenia but less likely to receive psychotropic medications or therapy. A study by Coleman and colleagues (2016) that looked at rates of diagnoses and treatment received by 7,523,956 patients supported previous studies in rates of diagnoses and receipt of medication. This points to the importance of cultural competence in assessment and treatment.

On television, people with schizophrenia are often depicted as homeless, walking around wearing too many layers of clothing and talking to themselves. This picture may be true for a very small population of people with schizophrenia who are not receiving treatment. Untreated schizophrenia can result in serious problems that interfere with all areas of a person's life and result in poverty, homelessness, legal problems, relationship difficulties, family conflicts, and difficulties at school or work. It is important for a person experiencing FEP to receive early treatment. The closer someone begins appropriate treatment following FEP, the greater their chances of recovery. Most people diagnosed with schizophrenia who receive appropriate and timely treatment can experience relief from their symptoms and lead full happy lives. For some people with schizophrenia, coping with symptoms and the ongoing need for intensive supports and services can be lifelong.

Causes

Schizophrenia affects an estimated 1 percent of the population. Most of what we know about schizophrenia has come from studies with adults. The exact causes of schizophrenia are not completely known; however, much progress in understanding schizophrenia has been made through genetic and brain research. Many years ago, ineffective mothering was thought to be the cause. Fortunately, because of research, ineffective mother is no longer blamed for causing schizophrenia. Current research suggests that schizophrenia is caused by many factors, including genes, brain chemistry, and environmental factors such as exposure to a virus, difficulties at birth, or prenatal malnutrition (US Department of Health and Human Services, n.d.).

Genes and Schizophrenia

Researchers believe that genetics play a role in the development of schizophrenia. Genetic risk factors have been found to extend to the molecular level in cells (Gandal et al., 2018). Although schizophrenia affects 1 percent or less of the general population, the risk increases to 10 percent for persons who have a parent or sibling with schizophrenia (Cannon et al., 2008; Regier et al., 1993). The highest risk of heritability (genetics) for schizophrenia occurs with identical twins (Cardno & Gottesman, 2000; Masi, Mucci, & Pari, 2006; Nicolson et al., 2000). When an identical twin develops schizophrenia, the other twin has an increased risk as high as 40–65 percent of also developing it. Adoption studies have helped inform scientists on causes of this disorder. Adopted children with a biological parent with schizophrenia have a higher risk of developing psychosis whether or not they live with the biological parent. If one of their adoptive parents, rather than a biological parent, has schizophrenia, they are at no more risk than the general population. Researchers have linked high levels of genetic mutations involving multiple genes and genetic malfunctioning that affects development of higher level brain functioning to schizophrenia (Walsh et al., 2008). Many research studies on the genetic connections to schizophrenia continue. It should be noted that there are people who have family members with schizophrenia who never develop it and other people who develop schizophrenia who do not have family members diagnosed with it.

Schizophrenia and the Brain

Research findings suggest that a chemical imbalance or the interactions of neurotransmitters, particularly the dopaminergic, serotonergic, and glutamatergic systems are involved in the pathology of schizophrenia. Insults to the brain prenatally or during puberty are other contributors to the development of schizophrenia. Prenatal insults may include viral infections, lack of oxygen at birth, starvation, or an untreated blood type incompatibility between a mother and fetus. Brain scans have shown that children who experience psychotic symptoms prior to puberty exhibit progressively abnormal brain development (Giedd et al., 1999; Rapoport et al., 1999; Thompson et al., 2001).

Researchers at the National Institute of Mental Health (NIMH) have been studying the brains of children with early-onset schizophrenia using high-resolution magnetic resonance imaging (MRI) scans (Giedd et al., 1999). The children in the study are evaluated by researchers every 2 years. These researchers hypothesize that an insult to the back of a child's brain contributes to the onset of schizophrenia. As they have followed children through the years, they have found evidence of significant shrinkage in brain tissue volume that starts in the back of the brain. The brain tissue continues to shrink as the disease progresses. These same researchers have found that healthy siblings of youth with schizophrenia show similar thinning, but this abnormality disappears as they age. Researchers have also found that the brains of children with schizophrenia share the same abnormalities as those of adults with schizophrenia (Gogtay et al., 2008). Home movies taken during childhood show that persons with adult-onset schizophrenia experienced uneven motor development in childhood, such as unusual crawling as children. This lends support to the idea that they may have had abnormalities in brain functioning during childhood, but the symptoms of schizophrenia did not become evident until they reached adulthood. Because a child's brain is constantly changing, it may take years before the effects of the brain insult are evident.

Signs and Symptoms

The age of onset and the developmental level of a person will affect how symptoms are experienced and their responsiveness to treatment. When schizophrenia emerges in adolescents, it can result in changes in the way they think or decisions they make, and they may experience distortions in how they experience their environment and how they relate to others. The symptoms of schizophrenia are typically harder to identify and interpret in adolescents than adults. As a result, adolescents with schizophrenia are often misdiagnosed with other mood, learning, or developmental disorders. For this reason, doctors must rule out these other medical conditions before diagnosing a patient with schizophrenia. Research suggests that persons who experience childhood onset of schizophrenia will have a different presentation of symptoms than those who experience onset as adults and adolescents. Children with schizophrenia may be even more seriously impaired. They are also more anxious and disruptive than were patients with adult-onset schizophrenia as children. However, the classifications of symptoms are the same regardless of age of onset. The symptoms of schizophrenia are classified as positive, negative, and cognitive (American Psychiatric Association [APA], 2013).

Positive Symptoms

Positive symptoms are thoughts, behaviors, or sensory perceptions experienced by a person with a mental illness that are not experienced by other persons. They are an exaggeration or a distortion of a person's normal functioning. Positive symptoms include hallucinations, delusions, thought disorders, and movement disorders. Psychotic symptoms usually appear later in the disease, most often between the ages of 16 and 30. Males tend to experience symptoms at an earlier age than females.

Hallucinations are distortions of reality that may come in the form of hearing, seeing, smelling, tasting, or feeling something that is not real; however, these sensations feel real to the person experiencing them. Hearing things that are not there (auditory hallucinations) is the most common type of hallucination. When someone experiences an auditory hallucination, he or she may hear voices or other sounds. Some people experience voices that say negative or demeaning things such as "you are a bad person" or "you cannot do anything right." *Command hallucinations* are experienced as one or more voices telling the person to do something such as "hit your sister" or "burn down the house." Because the voices are real to the person experiencing them, he or she may feel compelled to do what they say to do.

Delusions are beliefs in something that is not true. They are false beliefs about something despite having clear evidence to support otherwise, such as believing that the government is monitoring one's thoughts or controlling one's behavior. They can also cause a person to believe that he or she is someone or something else, such as a member of royalty or the most intelligent person in the world. Common types of delusions are listed in Table 15.1.

Thought disorders appear in the form of unusual ways of thinking. The person's thoughts may be disorganized and result in stopping speech in midsentence. It is not uncommon for someone experiencing a thought disorder to make up words or to take a long time to respond to a question.

Table 15.1 Common types of delusions

Type of delusions	Definition	Real-life example
Delusions of persecution	Belief, usually bizarre, that others are out to get you.	A patient believed that aliens had taken over the bodies of her family members and that they were trying to kill her.
Delusions of reference	A neutral event is believed to have a special and personal meaning	A patient believed the television was sending him, and only him, specific messages.
Delusions of grandeur	Belief that you are a famous or important figure or a belief that you have unusual powers, such as the ability to read minds.	A common delusion seen in many patients is a belief that he was Jesus Christ. One adult patient believed he was Jesus and needed to go to Israel. He purchased a plane ticket and took off.
Delusions of control	Belief that your thoughts or actions are being controlled by outside, alien forces.	One patient believed the government was stealing his thoughts

Negative Symptoms

Negative symptoms are thoughts, behaviors, or sensory perceptions experienced by the general population that are not experienced by a person with a mental illness. They disrupt a person's normal emotions or behaviors. For example, a person may neglect personal hygiene such as brushing teeth, taking baths, or changing into clean clothes. Isolation and disinterest in relationships often occur. Lacking motivation to do things, such as go to school or work, is also common. Negative symptoms may appear to be laziness, which can cause frustration in people who do not understand that these are symptoms of schizophrenia. The majority of antipsychotic medications do not treat the disorders' negative symptoms.

Cognitive Symptoms

Cognitive symptoms interfere with thought processes, resulting in problems understanding and using information. It is thought that a person with schizophrenia is born with these cognitive symptoms. If that is the case, a person will show signs of cognitive problems from the beginning of life but may not develop negative or positive symptoms until later in life. The ability to do well in school and other areas of life will be disrupted for these children because they cannot make sense of information and have trouble paying attention and remembering things. These symptoms are often attributed to other conditions, resulting in the lack of appropriate treatment.

Diagnosing Schizophrenia

Diagnosing schizophrenia can be difficult, particularly in young children and for someone who does not have experience in pediatric psychiatry. The first step in diagnosing schizophrenia should be a complete physical that includes toxicology screening and brain scans to rule out other possible explanations such as another medical condition or substance abuse. Once physical health problems and drug and alcohol abuse have been ruled out, a complete psychosocial history should be completed to investigate the onset of the youth's problems and the family's history of health/mental health problems, followed by a functional assessment of the youth to evaluate cognitive skills and daily functioning and a review of the youth's functioning at school.

A diagnosis of schizophrenia requires continuous signs of schizophrenia to have been present for at least 6 months, with at least two symptoms (positive, negative, and/or cognitive) lasting for at least 1 month (APA, 2013). The severity of the symptoms must cause serious impairment in a person's ability to function. In children and adolescents, the impairment in functioning may present as a failure to achieve age-appropriate levels of interpersonal or academic development. The *Diagnostic and Statistical Manual of Mental Disorders* (DSM) includes the following descriptive and course specifiers that are applicable after 12 months to all schizophrenia spectrum and other psychotic disorders:

- First episode, currently in acute episode (symptom criteria are fulfilled)
- First episode, currently in partial remission (symptom criteria are not fully fulfilled)
- First episode, currently in full remission (symptom criteria are not present)
- Multiple episodes, currently in acute episode
- Multiple episodes, currently in partial remission
- Multiple episodes, currently in full remission
- Continuous (subthreshold symptom periods being very brief relative to the overall course)
- Unspecified

In the DSM-5, a person needs at least one positive symptom: hallucinations, delusions, or disorganized language. Diagnosing schizophrenia has moved from categorizing symptoms as a subtype to a focus on measuring the severity of the dimensions of the disorder in each individual (Kupfer & Regier, 2011).

Schizophrenia in Children and Adolescents

Onset of schizophrenia is rare for children under the age of 12, affecting less than 1 percent (Hafner & Nowotny, 1995). As children move into adolescence, the prevalence increases. Researchers estimate that approximately 100,000 adolescents and young adults experience FEP each year. When it does occur, it can be difficult to recognize because it is so rare and because it emerges more slowly in children. Children normally do not experience a sudden onset of psychotic symptoms. The onset of symptoms is much slower in children. Research has shown that the earlier a person develops schizophrenia, the more severe the form of the disorder and the poorer the prognosis (Driver, Gogtay, & Rapoport, 2013). Prior to children experiencing psychosis, they often experience lags in motor and speech-language development and a decline in full-scale IQ. This phase of the disease is called the *prodromal phase*. These developmental disturbances result in the child having difficulties in school, social situations, and at home, but the lack of the psychotic symptoms makes it difficult to diagnose schizophrenia.

As the disease progresses, marked behavioral changes occur. Children may start talking about fears and ideas that are strange, saying things that do not make sense, clinging to parents, or seeming to withdraw and appear to be in their own world. They often have trouble discriminating between their dreams and reality or may confuse television or movies with reality. They often experience a loss of social skills and self-help skills. They become withdrawn and lose interest in having friends or being social. Children with schizophrenia are often mistakenly thought to have a disorder on the autism spectrum. About a third of children with schizophrenia have transient symptoms of an autism spectrum disorder (ASD), such as rocking, posturing, and arm flapping, and, like children with an ASD, they experience impairment across all life domains. Although diagnosing schizophrenia is difficult due to the similarity of its symptoms to those of autism, the disorders can be distinguished. Autism develops earlier in children. It is usually diagnosed by the time a child turns 3, whereas schizophrenia tends to develop when a child is 6 or 7 years old. Unlike a child with autism, a child with schizophrenia will experience hallucinations or delusions that persist for at least 6 months. Schizophrenia in children differs from adults in the sense that children's hallucinations and delusions are usually less elaborate.

Autism Spectrum Disorder

ASD is a complex neurodevelopmental disorder that has a wide variation in the type and severity of symptoms (APA, 2013). As with other disorders discussed in this book, the causes of ASD are not known; however, there is evidence to support that the cause is related to both genetic and environmental issues (NIMH, n.d). Risk factors for ASD include having a family member with ASD, having older parents, having a low birth weight, and co-occurring genetic conditions. ASD is not considered a serious mental illness or emotional disturbance by most in the mental health field. However, due to its shared genetic components and its high rates of co-occurrence and overlap in the presentation of symptoms with many mental, emotional, or behavioral disorders, we are including a brief discussion of ASD.

Symptoms for ASD develop in the first 2 years of life and can be reliably diagnosed by this age by a trained professional (Lord et al., 2006). People with ASD have difficulty with communication and interaction with other people, restricted interests, repetitive behaviors, and symptoms that affect the person's ability to function in school, work, and other areas of life (APA, 2013).

Social communication/interaction behaviors may include:

- Making little or inconsistent eye contact
- Having a tendency not to look at or listen to people
- Rarely sharing enjoyment of objects or activities by pointing at or showing things to others
- Failing to, or being slow to, respond to someone calling their name or to other verbal attempts to gain attention
- Having difficulties with the back and forth of conversation
- Often talking at length about a favorite subject without noticing that others are not interested or without giving others a chance to respond
- Having facial expressions, movements, and gestures that do not match what is being said

- Having an unusual tone of voice that may sound sing-song or flat and robot-like
- Having trouble understanding another person's point of view or being unable to predict or understand other people's actions

Restrictive/repetitive behaviors may include:

- Repeating certain behaviors or having unusual behaviors, such as repeating words or phrases (a behavior called *echolalia*)
- Having a lasting, intense interest in certain topics, such as numbers, details, or facts
- Having overly focused interests, such as with moving objects or with parts of objects
- Getting upset by slight changes in a routine
- Being more sensitive or less sensitive than other people to sensory input, such as light, noise, clothing, or temperature

Youth with ASD may or may not have intellectual or other impairments. Furthermore, a majority of youth with ASD (approximately 70 percent) also have a co-occurring psychiatric disorder (Rosen et al., 2018;). The DSM includes accompanying specifiers to identify co-occurring problems when making a diagnosis. These specifiers are

- With or without accompanying intellectual impairment
- With or without accompanying language impairment
- Associated with a known medical or genetic condition or environmental factor
- Associated with another neurodevelopmental, mental, or behavioral disorder
- With catatonia

Mental, emotional, and behavioral disorders that commonly co-occurs with ASD include anxiety disorders, mood disorders, attention deficit hyperactivity disorder (ADHD), oppositional defiant disorder (ODD), and obsessive-compulsive disorders (ODD). Co-occurrence of disorders complicates the ability to diagnosis accurately due to commonalities of symptoms between certain psychiatric disorders, the typical/atypical presentation of symptoms of other disorders in people with ASD, and differences in the cognitive levels of people with ASD. Multi-information and multimethod assessment, similar to the evidence-based assessment (EBA) discussed in Chapter 13, and the use of measures validated for ASD populations have been recommended for diagnosing ASD (e.g., Kerns et al., 2016; Mazefsky et al., 2010; Moskowitz et al., 2017). Table 15.2 identifies complicating information related to ASD as a result of co-occurrence with other mental health disorders or shared or overlapping commonalities of ASD with other disorders.

Table 15.2 Co-occurrence and/or symptom overlap of autism spectrum disorder (ASD) and other mental health disorders

Disorder	Co-occurrence estimates	Symptoms or problems related to ASD that overlap or share commonalities
Anxiety disorders	Anxiety (approximately 40 percent; van Steensel et al., 2011)	Social withdrawal Emotional dysregulation Anxiety related to separation anxiety
Obsessive-compulsive disorder		Repetitive behaviors
Depressive disorders	0.9–29 percent (Simonoff et al., 2008; Stewart et al., 2006).	Suicidal ideation/attempts Social isolation Sleep problems Atypical affect Cognitive rigidity
Bipolar disorder	0.7–1.9 percent (Levy et al., 2010).	Symptoms of depression: same as depressive disorders Symptoms of mania: Unusual thoughts and ideas in Irritability Decrease sleep Increased reactivity
ADHD	30–50 percent (Davis & Kollins, 2012)	Inattention hyperactivity-impulsivity Social impairments
Schizophrenia spectrum disorders	0–0.3 percent (Levy et al., 2010)	Catatonia Poor reality testing Social cognition deficits Emotional recognition deficits Sensory atypicalities could be mistaken for hallucinations Idiosyncratic thoughts could be mistaken for delusions Pragmatic speech could be mistaken for disordered speech (Eack et al., 2013; Starling & Dossetor, 2009)

Violence

The majority of persons with schizophrenia are not violent toward other persons (Swanson et al., 2006; Walsh, Buchanan, & Fahy, 2002). However, there is a prevailing belief that persons with schizophrenia are often violent. This is mostly due to the media. In television shows or movies, persons with schizophrenia often are portrayed as violent and unpredictable. The news media does not provide information about the majority of persons with schizophrenia who are doing well in life and those who have never been violent. Instead, it focuses on the very small minority of instances in which something tragic occurs. If a person with schizophrenia does become violent or dangerous, it often occurs as a result of psychosis. For instance, Mary believed an alien had invaded her mother's body and was out to harm her. Mary attacked her mother in an attempt to protect herself from the alien. Again, these instances are very rare. Persons with schizophrenia are more likely to harm themselves than to harm someone else. An estimated 10 percent of persons with schizophrenia commit suicide.

Tools for Assessing the Symptoms of Schizophrenia

There are some useful tools for measuring the positive and negative symptoms of schizophrenia. These instruments measure the severity of symptoms and help monitor the effectiveness of treatment.

The Positive and Negative Syndrome Scale

The Positive and Negative Syndrome Scale (PANSS; Kay, Fiszbein, & Opler, 1987) is probably the most well-known and utilized assessment tool for monitoring treatment effectiveness for schizophrenia. The PANSS is an easy to administer and highly reliable tool for measuring the symptoms of schizophrenia. It consists of 30 items that are rated on a 7-point Likert scale where a score of 1 means symptoms are absent and a score of 7 means that symptoms are extreme. Of the 30 items, 7 measure negative symptoms (PANSS-N). The remaining 23 items measure positive symptoms (PANSS-P).

The Four-Item Positive Symptoms Rating Scale and Brief Negative Symptom Assessment

The four-item Positive Symptoms Rating Scale (PSRS) and Brief Negative Symptom Assessment (BNSA) measure levels of positive and negative symptoms associated with schizophrenia (Alphs, Morlock, Coon, Van Willigenburg, & Panagides, 2010). Each of these instruments consists of four items. The PSRS is measured on a 7-point Likert scale. As with the PANSS, a score of 1 means that the symptom is not present and a score of 7 means that the symptoms are severe. The BNSA is measured on a 6-point Likert scale, with a score of 1 meaning that the symptoms are not present and a 6 meaning that the symptoms are severe. Positive symptoms measured include hallucinations, suspiciousness, unusual thought content, and conceptual disorganization. Negative symptoms measured by the BNSA include slow response time, blunted affect, reduced social drive, and poor hygiene.

Scale for the Assessment of Negative Symptoms

The Scale for the Assessment of Negative Symptoms (SANS; Andreasen, 1982, 1989) is a measurement instrument used in the field to assess the negative symptoms of schizophrenia. The SANS assesses across five areas of negative symptoms: affective blunting, impoverished thinking and cognition (alogia), lack of energy (avolition), disturbance of attention, and lack of interest or pleasure (anhedonia). The SANS is conducted on a 6-point scale, with 0 meaning that there are no negative symptoms and 5 indicating a severe level of the negative symptom.

Case Studies

Gus

Gus is a 10-year-old admitted to a psychiatric hospital after exhibiting aggressive behaviors at home and school. At school, Gus refused to stay in his seat and complete his work. When confronted by the teacher, he kicked over his desk and ran out of the school. He was picked up by police a few blocks away from the school and taken home. After the police left, Gus's behavior escalated. He destroyed his room. When his mother tried to calm him down, he ran into the kitchen, grabbed a large knife, and threatened to stab himself in the neck. His father restrained him and took the knife away. His parents drove him to the hospital, where he was evaluated by a psychiatrist. During the interview, Gus told the psychiatrist that he was seeing scary people. The psychiatrist admitted Gus to the children's unit for observation.

During his first few days on the unit, Gus was restrained and secluded multiple times for throwing chairs and doing other things that were threatening to other patients and staff. The psychiatrist started him on medications. The medications made Gus very drowsy. He spent many hours sleeping each day. After spending a week in the hospital, Gus was discharged to return home. He was given a follow-up appointment with another psychiatrist and returned to school.

Consider the following questions:

1. What symptoms was Gus experiencing?
2. Does he meet the criteria for schizophrenia? Explain. If he does, which type?
3. Based on your current knowledge, what interventions would you suggest? Do you believe that the appropriate intervention or treatment was provided?
4. Who should be included in the treatment planning and interventions?
5. What barriers might get in the way of effectively intervening?
6. What suggestions, thoughts, or ideas do you have for his family?

Erin

Erin is a 17-year-old in her junior year of high school. She was always an A student and very active in student government. She was the vice president of her class. Midway through her junior year, Erin suddenly stopped hanging out with friends. Her grades declined rapidly. Whereas she had always been very particular about wearing the latest fashions and would never leave the house without makeup, she began wearing sweats to school, and she stopped wearing makeup and attending to her personal hygiene, such as washing her hair. She said things to her parents that were very odd and sometimes started giggling for no reason. Her parents suspected that she was using drugs. She became very angry at her parents when they questioned her about the changes.

A few weeks after these notable changes in Erin's behavior, the school counselor, who was very concerned, contacted Erin's parents. Erin had turned in a test that had rambling sentences scribbled all over the page, and she had not answered the test questions. Her parents picked her up and took her to the hospital. A full medical evaluation was completed, including screening for drugs and alcohol. Nothing turned up. Her parents were questioned about any family history of mental illness. They both said there was no family history of mental illness. ,

Erin was admitted to the psychiatric unit of the hospital and was started on a regimen of antipsychotic medications. After a few weeks in the hospital, Erin did not show any improvement in her symptoms. She denied that anything was wrong and screamed at her parents to take her home.

How would you answer the following questions?

1. What symptoms was Erin experiencing?
2. Does she meet the criteria for schizophrenia? Explain. If she does, which type?
3. Based on your current knowledge, what interventions would you suggest? Do you believe that the appropriate intervention or treatment was provided?
4. Who should be included in the treatment planning and interventions?
5. What barriers might get in the way of effectively intervening?
6. What suggestions, thoughts, or ideas do you have for her family?

References

Alphs, L., Morlock, R., Coon, C., Van Willigenburg, A., & Panagides, J. (2010). The 4-Item Negative Symptom Assessment (NSA-4) Instrument: A simple tool for evaluating negative symptoms in schizophrenia following brief training. *Psychiatry, 7*(7), 26–32.

American Psychiatric Association (APA). (2013). *Diagnostic and statistical manual of mental disorders* (5th ed.). Washington, DC: Author.

Andreasen, N. C. (1982). Negative symptoms in schizophrenia: Definition and reliability. *Archives of General Psychiatry, 39,* 784–788.

Andreasen, N. C. (1989). The scale for the assessment of negative symptoms (SANS): Conceptual and theoretical foundations. *British Journal of Psychiatry Supplements, 7*, 49–58.

Cannon, T. D., Cadenhead, K., Cornblatt, B., Woods, S. W., Addington, J., Walker, E., . . . Heinssen, R. (2008). Prediction of psychosis in high-risk youth: A multi-site longitudinal study in North America. *Archives of General Psychiatry, 65*, 28–37.

Cardno, A. G., & Gottesman, I. I. (2000). Twin studies of schizophrenia: From bow-and-arrow concordances to Star Wars Mx and functional genomics. *American Journal of Medical Genetics, 97*, 12–17.

Coleman, K. J., Stewart, C., Waitzfelder, B. E., Zeber, J. E., Morales, L. S., Ahmed, A. T., . . . Simon, G. E. (2016). Racial-Ethnic Differences in Psychiatric Diagnoses and Treatment Across 11 Health Care Systems in the Mental Health Research Network. *Psychiatric Services, 67*(7), 749–757.

Driver, D. I., Gogtay, N., & Rapoport, J. L. (2013). Childhood onset schizophrenia and early onset schizophrenia spectrum disorders. *Child and Adolescent Psychiatric Clinics of North America, 22*, 539–555. doi:10.1016/j.chc.2013.04.001

Eack. S.M., Bahorika, A.L., Summer A.F. McKnight, S., Hogarty, S.S., Greenwald, D.P., Newhill, C.E., Phillips, M.L., Matcheri S. Keshavan, M.S., Minshewde, N.J. (2013). Commonalities in social and non-social cognitive impairments in adults with autism spectrum disorder and schizophrenia. Schizophrenia Research, 148, (1–3), 24–28.

Fleming, M., Barner, J. C., Brown, C. M., & Smith, T. (2011). Treatment disparities for major depressive disorder: Implications for pharmacists. *Journal of the American Pharmacological Association 51*(5), 605–612.

Gandal, M. J., Haney, J. R., Parikshak, N. N., Leppa, V., Ramaswami, G., Hartl, C., . . . White, K. P. (2018). Shared molecular neuropathology across major psychiatric disorders parallels polygenic overlap. CommonMind Consortium; PsychENCODE Consortium; iPSYCH-BROAD Working Group, Horvath S, Geschwind DH. *Science, 359*(6376), 693–697.

Georgia State University. (2016). Racial, ethnic differences found in psychiatric diagnoses, treatment, according to researchers. *ScienceDaily*, 2016, May 18. Retrieved from www.sciencedaily.com/releases/2016/05/160518094721.htm

Giedd, J. N., Blumenthal, J., Jeffries, N. O., Castellanos, F. X., Liu, H., Zijdenbos, A., . . . Rapoport, J. L. (1999). Brain development during childhood and adolescence: A longitudinal MRI study. *Nature Neuroscience, 2*, 861–863.

Gogtay, N., Lu, A., Leow, A. D., Klunder, A. D., Lee, A. D., Chavez, A., . . . Thompson, P. M. (2008). Three-dimensional brain growth abnormalities in childhood-onset schizophrenia visualized by using tensor-based morphometry. *Proceedings of the National Academy of Sciences of the United States of America, 105*(41), 15979–15984.

Hafner, H., & Nowotny, B. (1995). Epidemiology of early-onset schizophrenia. *European Archives of Psychiatry Clinics in Neuroscience, 245*, 80–92.

Heinssen, R. K., Goldstein, A. B., & Azrin, S. T. (2014). *Evidence-based treatments for first episode psychosis: Components of coordinated specialty care.* Bethesda, MD: National Institute of Mental Health. Retrieved from www.nimh.nih.gov/health/topics/schizophrenia/raise/

Kay, S. R., Fiszbein, A., & Opler, L. A. (1987). The positive and negative syndrome scale (PANSS) for schizophrenia. *Schizophrenia Bulletin, 13*, 261–276.

Kerns, C. M., Rump, K., Worley, J., Kratz, H., McVey, A., Herrington, J., & Miller, J. (2016). The differential diagnosis of anxiety disorders in cognitively-able youth with autism. *Cognitive and Behavioral Practice, 23*(4), 530–547.

Kupfer, D. J., & Regier, D. A. (2011). Neuroscience, clinical evidence, and the future of psychiatric classification in DSM-5. *American Journal of Psychiatry, 68*, 672–674.

Lord, C., Risi, S., DiLavore, P. S., Shulman, C., Thrum, A., & Pickles, A. (2006). Autism From 2 to 9 Years of Age. *Archives of General Psychiatry, 63*(6), 694–701.

Mallinger, J. B., & Lamberti, S. J. (2007). Racial differences in the use of adjunctive psychotropic medications for patients with schizophrenia. *Journal of Mental Health Policy and Economics, 10*(1), 15–22.

Mazefsky, C. A., Anderson, R., Conner, C. M., & Minshew, N. (2010). Child Behavior Checklist Scores for School-Aged Children with Autism: Preliminary Evidence of Patterns Suggesting the Need for Referral. *Journal of Psychopathology and Behavioral Assessment, 33*, 31–37.

Masi, G., Mucci, M., & Pari, C. (2006). Children with schizophrenia: Clinical picture and pharmacological treatment. *CNS Drugs, 20*, 841–866.

Moskowitz, J., Rosen, T., Lerner, M. D., & Levine, K. (2017). Assessment of Anxiety in Youth With Autism Spectrum Disorder. In Anxiety in Children and Adolescents with Autism Specturm Disorder, Evidence-Based Assessment and Treatment. In C. M. Kerns, P. Renno, E. A. Storch, P. C. Kendall, & J. J. Wood (Eds.), *Children and Adolescents with Autism Spectrum Disorder: Evidence-Based Assessment and Treatment* (pp. 79–104). Academic Press .

National Institute of Mental Health. (n.d.). Autism Spectrum Disorders. Retrieved 9/14/2020 from https://www.nimh.nih.gov/health/topics/autism-spectrum-disorders-asd/index.shtml

Nicolson, R., Lenane, M., Hamburger, S. D., Fernandez, T., Bedwell, J., & Rapoport, J. L. (2000). Lessons from childhood-onset schizophrenia. *Brain Research Review, 31*(2–3), 147–156.

Rapoport, J. L., Giedd, J. N., Blumenthal, J., Hamburger, S., Jeffries, N., Fernandez, T., . . . Evans, A. (1999). Progressive cortical change during adolescence in childhood-onset schizophrenia: A longitudinal magnetic resonance imaging study. *Archives of General Psychiatry, 56*, 649–654.

Regier, D. A., Narrow, W. E., Rae, D. S., Manderscheid, R. W., Locke, B. Z., & Goodwin, F. K. (1993). The de facto US mental and addictive disorders service system: Epidemiologic catchment area prospective 1-year prevalence rates of disorders and services. *Archives of General Psychiatry, 50*, 85–94.

Rosen, T. E., Mazefsky, C. A., Vasa, R. A., & Lerner, M. D. (2018). Co-occurring psychiatric conditions in autism spectrum disorder. *International Review of Psychiatry, 30*(1), 40–61.

Starling, J. & Dossetor, D. (2009). Pervasive developmental disorders and psychosis. Current Psychiatry Reports, 11(3):190–6.

Swanson, J. W., Swartz, M. S., Van Dorn, R. A., Elbogen, E., Wager, H. R., Rosenheck, R. A., . . . Lieberman, J. A. (2006). A national study of violent behavior in persons with schizophrenia. *Archives of General Psychiatry, 63*, 490–499.

Schwartz, R. C., & Blankenship, D. M. (2014). Racial disparities in psychotic disorder diagnosis: A review of empirical literature. *World Journal of Psychiatry, 4*, 133–140

Thompson, P. M., Vidal, C., Giedd, J. N., Gochman, P., Blumenthal, J., Nicolson, R., . . . Rapoport, J. L. (2001). Mapping adolescent brain change reveals dynamic wave of accelerated gray matter loss in very early-onset schizophrenia. *Proceedings of the National Academy of Sciences of the United States of America, 98*(20), 11650–11655.

US Department of Health and Human Services, National Institutes of Health, National Institute of Mental Health. (2019, July 11). Health Topics: Schizophrenia. Retrieved from https://www.nimh.nih.gov/health/topics/ schizophrenia/index.shtml

Vyas, N. S., & Gogtay, N. (2012). Treatment of early onset schizophrenia: Recent trends, challenges and future considerations. *Frontiers in Psychiatry, 3.* doi:10.3389/fpsyt.2012.00029

Walsh, E., Buchanan, A., & Fahy, T. (2002). Violence and schizophrenia: Examining the evidence. *British Journal of Psychiatry, 180,* 490–495.

Walsh, T., McClellan, J. M., McCarthy, S. E., Addington, A. M., Pierce, S. B., Cooper, G. M., . . . Sebat, J. (2008). Rare structural variants disrupt multiple genes in neurodevelopmental pathways in schizophrenia. *Science, 320*(5875), 539–543.

16

Treatment of Schizophrenia Spectrum Disorders and First-Episode Psychosis

Currently, there is no cure for schizophrenia, but hope exists in the research community that a cure will be discovered within the next decade. Additionally, it is predicted that schizophrenia can be prevented in persons with high-risk factors through further understanding of genes and brain chemistry. Unfortunately, we are not there yet. There is currently no sure way to prevent schizophrenia. However, people who possess risk factors for schizophrenia can minimize their symptoms or prevent them from getting worse by taking preventative measures such as reducing stress, getting adequate sleep, and avoiding drugs and alcohol. If symptoms do appear, early treatment may lessen the severity of the symptoms and improve the trajectory of the disorder. Effective treatment for early-onset schizophrenia includes a combination of medication and psychosocial, educational, and therapeutic interventions.

There has been a shift in the understanding of the trajectory of schizophrenia, from the belief that a person with schizophrenia will live with the symptoms for life to a focus on remission and recovery from the symptoms of schizophrenia (see, e.g., Emsley, Chiliza, Asmal, & Lehloenya, 2011; Liberman, Kopelowicz, Ventura, & Gutkind, 2002). Recovery has varying meanings in the literature. The term "remission" implies that a person is experiencing minimal or no positive, negative, or cognitive problems. The term "recovery" has been described as not only a significant remission of symptoms, but also the ability to function in society, both socially and vocationally (Liberman et al., 2002).

Studies evaluating the concepts of remission and recovery have varied widely in their findings, with anywhere from 17 to 88 percent of persons experiencing remission (Andreasen et al., 2005; De Hert et al., 2007; Emsley et al., 2011). The overall findings of these studies suggest that the differences

Understanding the Mental Health Problems of Children and Adolescents. Kirstin Painter and Maria Scannapieco,
Oxford University Press (2021). © Oxford University Press. DOI: 10.1093/oso/9780190927844.003.0016

between those who experience recovery and those who do not are based on the level of functioning prior to the onset of the illness, age of onset, proximity between first sign of symptoms and treatment, and gender. Thus, those who experienced remission or recovery had higher functioning prior to onset of the illness, onset of the disease after age 30, and treatment proximate to onset of symptoms; they were more likely to be female (Lambert, Karow, Leucht, Schimmelmann, & Naber, 2010). Those who experience early-onset schizophrenia are much less likely to achieve recovery than those with later onset. Most persons with schizophrenia will have to cope with these symptoms throughout life. Psychosocial interventions can help a family cope with the illness and help youth with activities of daily functioning, but they are not a substitute for medications.

An example of someone who experienced remission of symptoms and recovery to prior functioning is a young man diagnosed with schizophrenia who experienced his first psychotic episode in his mid-twenties. Prior to experiencing symptoms, he had a successful job, a girlfriend, and a close relationship with his parents. He experienced delusions that his parents were involved in the Oklahoma City bombing. He stayed in his room for days, making intricate maps and noting the ways that he believed his family was involved. He hardly slept and refused to eat. At the instigation of his family, he was committed to a hospital and required by court order to take medication. Several days after starting on the medication, he began questioning his thoughts, but he continued to believe them. After a few weeks on medication, he reported not knowing why he believed something so odd. He was discharged from the hospital and returned home to his family and his job.

Medication

Treatment for childhood schizophrenia is mostly based on research conducted with adults (Masi, Mucci, & Pari, 2006). Although antipsychotic medication is considered a first line of treatment for pediatric schizophrenia, there are few studies conducted with children and adolescents; however, existing studies suggest that antipsychotics can be effective in treating children and adolescents experiencing psychosis, and the earlier the medications are started following onset of psychosis, the more effective (Correll et al., 2011; Correll & De Hert, 2013). It can take as long as 6 months for a person to receive the full effects of antipsychotic medications (Lieberman et al., 2005).

The positive symptoms often go away within days of starting medication. Other symptoms, particularly negative symptoms, take far longer.

Since the 1950s, antipsychotic medications have vastly improved. Older (typical) medications such as haloperidol (Haldol) and fluphenazine (Prolixin) are used with decreasing frequency today. These older antipsychotics are effective in reducing hallucinations and delusions; however, they are not effective in treating the negative symptoms and they can cause debilitating side effects such as tardive dyskinesia (involuntary muscle movements) or muscle rigidity, spasms, tremors, and restlessness. These side effects, called *extrapyramidal side effects*, can become permanent.

The older antipsychotic medications have been mostly replaced by what are called new generation medications (atypical antipsychotics). Currently, five atypical antipsychotics are approved by the US Food and Drug Administration (FDA) for children and adolescents, with each medication approved for certain age ranges (see Table 16.1). The older medications are far less expensive than the new-generation medications, but the new atypical antipsychotics do not pose as significant a threat of extrapyramidal side effects as the older antipsychotics. On the other hand, like most medications, these new-generation medicines each comes with its own set of side effects (see Table 16.1). Throughout treatment with atypicals, it is extremely important to regularly monitor for weight and metabolic changes. It is estimated that as many as 62 percent of people with schizophrenia are overweight or obese, putting them at a high risk for cardiovascular morbidity and mortality (Ucok & Gaebel, 2008). In addition, persons with schizophrenia experience type II diabetes at nearly twice the rate of the general population.

The side effects of even the new-generation medications can be scary. However, they are the first line of treatment, and their benefits must be weighed against their risks. These newer medications are more effective in treating the psychotic symptoms (positive symptoms) than the older medications, and they also treat the negative symptoms. Additionally, some of them appear to be effective in improving depressive symptoms, memory, and mental functioning and reducing aggression and suicidal ideation. These new-generation antipsychotic medications have contributed greatly to the focus in the literature on remission and recovery. Each medication works in the brain a little differently from the others and different people respond to each of the medications differently. Antipsychotic medications need from 4 to 6 weeks to determine their effectiveness. If improvement is not seen within this time, a new antipsychotic medication should be tried. Often this can

Table 16.1 Atypical antipsychotics for children and adolescents

Brand name	Generic name	FDA approved age range	Common side effects in children	Possible risk factors to monitor	Forms of administration
Abilify	Aripiprazole	13–17	Somnolence (sleepiness) Insomnia Headache Nausea Vomiting Stuffy nose	Hyperglycemia (high blood sugar)/ diabetes	Orally disintegrating tablet Injectable/Injection
				Increased cholesterol and triglycerides (type of fat in blood	
				Tardive dyskinesia (uncontrolled body movements)	
			Fatigue Weight gain Increased or decreased appetite	Neuroleptic malignant syndrome (very rare, life-threatening reaction characterized by fever, altered mental status, muscle rigidity, and autonomic dysfunction)	
				Orthostatic hypotension (decreased blood pressure)	
			Uncontrolled movement Increased saliva or drooling Muscle stiffness	Low white blood cell count	
				Seizures	
				Weight gain	
				Increased suicidal ideation (particularly when used in combination with Prozac)	
Zyprexa	Olanzapine	13–17	Lack of energy Dry mouth Increased appetite Somnolence (sleepiness) Tremor (shakes)	Hyperglycemia (high blood sugar)/ diabetes	Orally disintegrating tablet
				Increased cholesterol and triglycerides (type of fat) in blood	Extended release Injectable
				Tardive dyskinesia (uncontrolled body movements)	

Invega	Paliperidone	12–17	Somnolence (sleepiness)	Hyperglycemia (high blood sugar)/	Tablets
			Akathisia (movement	diabetes	
			disorder that makes it	Increased cholesterol and	
			hard to stay still)	triglycerides in blood	
			Tremor	Tardive dyskinesia (uncontrolled	
			Dystonia (movement	body movements)	
			disorder in which		
			muscles contract		
			uncontrollably)		

Having hard or
infrequent stools
Dizziness
Changes in behavior
Restlessness

Headache
Abdominal pain
Pain in arms or legs
Tiredness

Drug reaction with eosinophilia and
systemic symptoms (rare, potentially
life-threatening, drug-induced
hypersensitivity reaction)

Neuroleptic malignant syndrome
(very rare, life-threatening reaction
characterized by fever, altered
mental status, muscle rigidity, and
autonomic dysfunction)

Orthostatic hypotension (decreased
blood pressure)
Weight gain
Hyperlipidemia (high concentration
of fats or lipids in the blood)

Table 16.1 *Continued*

Brand name	Generic name	FDA approved age range	Common side effects in children	Possible risk factors to monitor	Forms of administration
			Muscle rigidity Anxiety Weight gain Tachycardia (excessively fast heart rate)	Neuroleptic malignant syndrome (very rare, life–threatening reaction characterized by fever, altered mental status, muscle rigidity, and autonomic dysfunction)	
Seroquel	Quetiapine	13–17	Drowsiness Dizziness Fatigue Nausea Dry mouth Weight gain Increased appetite Vomiting	Hyperglycemia (high blood sugar)/ diabetes Increased cholesterol and triglycerides in blood Tardive dyskinesia (uncontrolled body movements) Neuroleptic malignant syndrome (very rare, life–threatening reaction characterized by fever, altered mental status, muscle rigidity, and autonomic dysfunction) Hypertension (note: for adults hypotension) Weight gain Low white blood cell count	Tablet, oral Injectable/Injection

Risperdal	Risperidone	10–17	Drowsiness Dizziness Light-headedness Drooling	Cerebrovascular events, including stroke	Tablets Oral solution Orally disintegrating tables
			Nausea Weight gain Tiredness Difficulty swallowing Muscle spasms	Neuroleptic malignant syndrome (very rare, life-threatening reaction characterized by fever, altered mental status, muscle rigidity, and autonomic dysfunction) Tardive dyskinesia (uncontrolled body movements)	
			Shaking (tremor) Mental/mood changes Interrupted breathing during sleep	Hyperglycemia (high blood sugar)/diabetes Hyperprolactinemia (higher than normal hormone prolactin, which affect estrogen and testosterone) Orthostatic hypotension Leukopenia, neutropenia and agranulocytosis (severe deficiency of types of white blood cells important to fighting infections)	

(Continued)

Table 16.1 *Continued*

Brand name	Generic name	FDA approved age range	Common side effects in children	Possible risk factors to monitor	Forms of administration
				Potential for cognitive and motor impairment	
				Seizures	
				Dysphagia (serious medical condition of difficulty swallowing)	
				Priapism (prolonged erection of the penis)	
				Disruption of body temperature regulation	
				Antiemetic effect (important to management of nausea and vomiting)	
				Suicide	

All information in chart retrieved from FDA.gov.

result in what seems to families like a long trial-and-error process to determine which medication will be most effective for an individual. Studies are currently under way to determine which of the atypical medications is most effective in treating specific symptoms.

It is also important for persons to follow their medication plan and not stop taking their medication without a psychiatrist's direction. The side effects of the new-generation medications are often related to medication discontinuation. One factor consistent with all such medications is that every time a person discontinues medication without a doctor's advice, it becomes more difficult for him or her to get back to the level of functioning achieved before stopping (Andreasen, Liu, Ziebell, Vora, & Ho, 2013). Because of the side effects and the way that the psychotropic medications make them feel, people do not want to take these medications. It is not uncommon for people to *cheek* their medicine, meaning that they hold it between their gums and cheek and pretend to take it, but instead spit it out when no one is looking.

Psychosocial Interventions

Some of the interventions designed for adults with schizophrenia and some of the interventions designed for treatment of other mental health problems in youth have been adapted to treat childhood schizophrenia (Burns & Hoagwood, 2002; Burns, Hoagwood, & Mrazek, 1999). As described in Chapter 2, wraparound service is considered a promising practice for supporting and improving the lives of youth experiencing severe emotional or behavioral problems and their caregivers. Wraparound is not a specific treatment for schizophrenia; however, its focus on each family's individual needs, strengths, and desires can be an effective model for working with children diagnosed with schizophrenia and their families. Through the incorporation of formal (including evidence-based practices and programs) and informal services and community supports, families can receive the support and strength they need.

Although medications treat the symptoms, it does not help the youth and family with the day-to-day struggles of dealing with schizophrenia. Other psychosocial interventions are needed to help cope with the disease. Supportive therapies in conjunction with medication can be helpful in improving activities of daily living such as money management, grooming, and social adjustment and in supporting caregivers. Psychosocial education teaches the youth, caregivers, and other family members about schizo-phrenia, its trajectory, and available treatments. Through education, families can learn to identify the early signs of problems so that they can seek help before symptoms exacerbate. Education can also help families understand the importance of medication and the detrimental effects of discontinuing a medication without psychiatrist supervision or the effects of not taking a medication as prescribed. Families can also learn to watch for side effects that need attention from the psychiatrist.

Cognitive-Behavioral Therapy

CBT in conjunction with medication has been found to be helpful in teaching needed skills such as problem-solving and stress reduction to help persons cope with their illnesses (Hogarty et al., 2002). Training in social skills and daily living skills can help youth to function better in school and participate in daily activities. Research has found that persons with early-onset schiz-ophrenia experience high levels of impairment in attaining educational or occupational goals and financial independence as adults.

Multisystemic Therapy-Psychiatric

Multisystemic therapy-psychiatric (MST-P) is an adaptation of the tradi-tional multisystemic therapy model discussed in Chapter 12 (Henggeler et al., 1999; Henggeler, Schoenwald, Rowland, & Cunningham, 2002; Rowland & Westlake, 2006). MST-P is on National Registry of Evidence-Based Practices and Programs published by the Substance Abuse and Mental Health Services Administration (SAMHSA, 2014) for the treatment of youth with behavioral and mental health problems. The goal of MST-P is to keep children who are at risk of psychiatric hospitalization in their home and com-munity. Like traditional MST, MST-P utilizes a social ecological approach, focusing treatment on the youth, caregivers, school, or other environments contributing to problems; however, it has been adapted to specifically treat youth with serious behavioral and mental health problems rather than ju-venile offenders. MST-P integrates evidence-based psychiatric interventions into the MST model.

The MST-P team is slightly different from the traditional clinical MST team. It includes a part-time psychiatrist and a crisis caseworker in addition to the full-time doctoral-level supervisor and four master's-level therapists. The therapists receive specialized mental health training in addition to the 5-day MST training. Rather than being the sole provider of treatment, they coordinate with the psychiatrist. Multisystemic treatment consultation is provided by both an MST expert consultant and an MST expert psychiatrist.

Coordinated Specialty Care for First-Episode Psychosis

Coordinated specialty care (CSC) is a recovery-oriented, 2- to 3-year, evidence-based treatment program targeted at youth and young adults aged 15 through 25 experiencing first-episode psychosis (FEP) (Heinssen, Goldstein, & Azrin, 2014). The goal of CSC is to identify people experiencing FEP and initiate treatment as quickly as possible, so an important component of a CSC program is active outreach and engagement. A CSC program consists of a multidisciplinary team trained in FEP that provides services based on the needs and preferences of the client. Services include case management, medication management, primary care coordination, crisis intervention, therapy, supported employment or education, family education and support, substance abuse treatment, and transition of care. One member of the team is designated as the primary care manager. As in wraparound and MST, the client, his or her family members, and the multidisciplinary team work together to develop an individualized treatment plan. Services are provided in the home, community, and in clinic settings.

In 2008, the National Institute for Mental Health (NIMH) funded the Recovery After an Initial Schizophrenia Episode (RAISE) (Heinssen et al., 2014). Through RAISE, the NIMH funded two research projects of CSC, one project was called RAISE Early Treatment Program (RAISE-ETP) and the second project was called Recovery After an Initial Schizophrenia Episode Implementation and Evaluation Study (RAISE-IES). Through the RAISE-ETP study, the NIMH found that people receiving early treatment through CSC stayed in treatment longer and experienced improvement in psychosis, relationships, and quality of life compared to people receiving typical treatment. The people who received CSC also were more involved in school or work. RAISE-IES project examined the administrative factors related to establishing a CSC program. Researchers also examined the clinical aspects of CSC and factors related to clients' and their families' satisfaction with services. Researchers examined client's symptoms and functioning across a span of 2 years and found promising outcomes. Not only did mental health symptoms improve, but people receiving CSC also experienced impoved educational and social outcomes. In addition, the people who received CSC felt positively about the services because they were treated with respect and caring and the services they received were effective. As part of RAISE-IEX, tools and manuals were developed for use by others wanting to start a CSC program. Those materials are available at https://www.nimh.nih.gov/health/topics/schizophrenia/raise/coordinated-specialty-care-for-first-episode-psychosis-manual-i-outreach-and-recruitment.shtml. There is no cost to use the materials.

Case Studies

Gus

Gus is the 10-year-old who was admitted to a psychiatric hospital after exhibiting aggressive behaviors at home and school. While in the hospital he was restrained and secluded multiple times for verbally and physically aggressive behaviors. He complained of seeing scary people. The psychiatrist diagnosed him with psychotic disorder not otherwise specified because Gus did not meet the criteria for a diagnosis of schizophrenia. The psychiatrist started Gus on antipsychotic medications. The medications made Gus very drowsy. He spent many hours sleeping each day. After spending a week in the hospital, he was discharged to return home. He was given a follow-up appointment with another psychiatrist and returned to school.

Gus could not keep his eyes open. He slept for hours. When awake, he seemed very drowsy and not completely coherent. He was not aggressive, but he also could not function. His mother took him to his psychiatric appointment. Unlike the psychiatrist who treated Gus in the hospital, this psychiatrist ordered a full medical evaluation and completed an in-depth psychosocial evaluation. During the interview, Gus disclosed that he was being sexually abused by a teenage neighbor. The psychiatrist took Gus off the antipsychotic medication, started him on paroxetine (Paxil) to help with anxiety, and referred him to a therapist who specialized in working with abused children. After 6 months, Gus was doing well in school and at home.

Erin

Erin is the 17-year-old who experienced serious changes in school functioning, peer relationships, and personal hygiene and began exhibiting odd behaviors such as giggling for no known reason. The school counselor contacted Erin's parents because Erin turned in a test that had rambling sentences scribbled all over the page, and she had not answered the test questions. Her parents picked her up and took her to the hospital. A full medical evaluation was completed. Screening for drugs and alcohol was negative.

Erin was admitted to the psychiatric unit of the hospital. After completing an in-depth psychiatric evaluation, the psychiatrist determined that Erin was hearing voices. Because Erin had not been having symptoms for at least 6 months, she diagnosed Erin with schizophreniform. The symptoms for schizophreniform are the same as those for schizophrenia, but there is no requirement for 6 months of symptoms. Erin was started on an antipsychotic medication. After a few weeks in the hospital, she was still not experiencing any improvement in symptoms. The psychiatrist was concerned that Erin was not improving. She began to suspect that Erin was not taking her medications. She asked the nurse to watch Erin swallow the pills and to check her mouth to be sure that she had swallowed them. After a few days, Erin's behaviors improved. She maintained an odd affect, but she denied hearing voices. Erin was discharged to her home after spending a month in the hospital.

Erin was not able to function in the classroom. She was referred to the school psychologist for testing. The psychologist recommended that Erin be considered to have an emotional disturbance and transferred to a special education class with other youth with emotional or behavioral problems. A meeting was held with Erin, her parents, the school counselor, the psychologist, a special education teacher, and her current teachers. Everyone but Erin agreed that she should be transferred to special education.

A few weeks after being discharged from the hospital, Erin's symptoms returned. She had stopped taking her medications. Her parents could not control her. She was taken back to the hospital. The doctor felt that Erin needed long-term care so she was transferred to the state psychiatric hospital, where she stayed for nearly 3 months. When she was discharged to her home, Erin never returned to school. She continued to go off and on her medications and was rehospitalized several times. She was diagnosed with schizophrenia and referred to the local community health center so that she could receive case management services in addition to psychiatrist services. The case manager helped Erin apply for Social Security Disability Insurance so that she could get disability checks to help support her and so that she could qualify for Medicaid. Erin continued to live with her parents.

Study Questions

1. What do these real- life scenarios have in common?
2. What are the differences?
3. Now that you know what happened to each of the youths, do you have any different thoughts on how you would have handled the situation if you were the families' social worker?

References

Andreasen, N. C., Carpenter, W. T., Jr., Kane, J. M., Lasser, R. A., Marder, S. R., & Weinberger, D. R. (2005). Remission in schizophrenia: Proposed criteria and rationale for consensus. *American Journal of Psychiatry, 162*, 441–449.

Andreasen, N. C., Liu, D., Ziebell, S., Vora, A., & Ho, B. C. (2013). Relapse duration, treatment intensity, and brain tissue loss in schizophrenia: A prospective longitudinal MRI study. *American Journal of Psychiatry, 170*, 609–615.

Burns, B. J., & Hoagwood, K. (Eds.). (2002). *Community treatment for youth: Evidence-based interventions for severe emotional and behavioral disorders.* New York: Oxford University Press.

Burns, B. J., Hoagwood, K., & Mrazek, P. J. (1999). Effective treatment for mental disorders in children and adolescents. *Clinical Child and Family Psychology Review, 2*, 199–254.

Correll, C. U., Canas, F., Levy, P., Montes, J-M., Fagiolini, A., Papageorgiou, G., Rossi, A., Sturlason, R., & Zink, M. (2011). Individualizing antipsychotic treatment selection in schizophrenia: characteristics of empirically derived patient subgroups. *European Psychiatry, 26*(1 Suppl 1), 3–16.

Correll, C. U., & De Hert, M. (2013). Antipsychotics for acute schizophrenia: making choices. *Lancet, 382* (9896), 919–920.

De Hert, M., van Winkel, R., Wampers, M., Kane, J., van Os, J., & Peuskens, J. (2007). Remission criteria for schizophrenia: Evaluation in a large naturalistic cohort. *Schizophrenia Research, 92*(1–3), 68–73.

Emsley, R., Chiliza, B., Asmal, L., & Lehloenya, K. (2011). The concepts of remission and recovery in schizophrenia. *Current Opinion in Psychiatry, 24,* 114–121.

Heinssen, R. K., Goldstein, A. B., & Azrin, S. T. (2014). *Evidence-based treatments for first episode psychosis: Components of coordinated specialty care.* Bethesda, MD: National Institute of Mental Health. Retrieved from www.nimh.nih.gov/health/topics/schizophrenia/raise/nimh-white-paper-csc-for-fep_147096.pdf

Henggeler, S. W., Rowland, M. D., Randall, J., Ward, D. M., Pickrel, S. G., Cunningham, P. B., . . . Santos, A. B. (1999). Home-based multisystemic therapy as an alternative to the hospitalization of youths in psychiatric crisis: Clinical outcomes. *Journal of the American Academy of Child and Adolescent Psychiatry, 38,* 1331–1339.

Henggeler, S. W., Schoenwald, S. K., Rowland, M. D., & Cunningham, P. B. (2002). *Serious emotional disturbance in children and adolescents: Multisystemic therapy.* New York: Guilford.

Hogarty, G. E., Flesher, S., Ulrich, R., Carter, M., Greenwald, D., Poque-Geile, M., . . . Zoretich, R. (2002). Cognitive enhancement therapy for schizophrenia: Effects of a 2-year randomized trial on cognition and behavior. *Archives of General Psychiatry, 200,* 866–876.

Lambert, M., Karow, A., Leucht, S., Schimmelmann, B. G., & Naber, D. (2010). Remission in schizophrenia: Validity, frequency, predictors, and patients' perspective 5 years later. *Dialogues in Clinical Neuroscience, 12,* 393–407.

Liberman, R. P., Kopelowicz, A., Ventura, J., & Gutkind, D. (2002). Operational criteria and factors related to recovery from schizophrenia. *International Review of Psychiatry, 14,* 256–272.

Lieberman, J. A., Stroup, T. S., McEvoy, J. P., Swartz, M. S., Rosenheck, R. A., Perkins, D. O., . . . Hsaio, J. K. (2005). Effectiveness of antipsychotic drugs in patients with chronic schizophrenia. *New England Journal of Medicine, 353,* 1209–1223.

Masi, G., Mucci, M., & Pari, C. (2006). Children with schizophrenia: Clinical picture and pharmacological treatment. *CNS Drugs, 20,* 841–866.

Rowland, M. D., & Westlake, L. A. (2006). *Mental health multisystemic therapy psychiatry resource book.* Mount Pleasant, SC: MST Services.

Substance Abuse and Mental Health Services Administration. (2014). National registry of evidence-based programs and practices. Retrieved from http://www.nrepp.samhsa.gov/Index.aspx

Ucok, A., & Gaebel, W. (2008). Side effects of atypical antipsychotics: A brief overview. *World Psychiatry, 7,* 58–62.

17

Substance Abuse Co-Occurrence with Mental Health Issues

This chapter considers substance use and abuse (including pain relievers or opioids) and present diagnostic criteria and discusses substance use disorder (SUD) co-occurring with mental health conditions (co-occurring disorders or COD). The types of drugs most used by children and adolescents is presented, and the chapter concludes with a discussion of the evidence-based interventions for COD, mental illness, and substance abuse. The world of substance abuse is always changing, and it is difficult for the field to keep up: presented in this chapter is the current state of knowledge, but social workers need to play an active role in keeping current with trends in drugs of abuse.

Adolescents use alcohol and other drugs for many reasons, including curiosity, to feel good, to reduce stress, and to feel grown up or to fit in. It is difficult to know which adolescent will experiment and stop and which will develop serious problems. Teenagers at risk for developing serious alcohol and drug problems include

- Those with a family history of substance abuse
- Those who are depressed
- Those who have low self-esteem
- Those who feel that they don't fit in or are out of the mainstream

Substance use and abuse, which includes alcohol and drugs, is an important health and social problem among adolescents and young adults. Substance abuse disorders are among the most common disorders in adolescents and commonly co-occur with a wide range of psychiatric disorders. One-third of youth with a SUD also have co-occurring

Understanding the Mental Health Problems of Children and Adolescents. Kirstin Painter and Maria Scannapieco, Oxford University Press (2021). © Oxford University Press. DOI: 10.1093/oso/9780190927844.003.0017

mental health issues (Substance Abuse and Mental Health Services Administration [SAMHSA], 2018). Adolescents and young adults with mental health conditions have higher rates of substance abuse-related disorders than do adolescents and young adults in the general population (Anthony, Taylor, & Raffo, 2011).

SUDs are associated with maladaptive use, abuse, or dependency that results in adverse social, behavioral, psychological, and physiological consequences for the child or adolescent. For youth, consequences are most frequently expressed as deterioration in peer and family relationships, decline in school attendance and academic functioning, higher levels of negative affect (depression and anxiety), and involvement in antisocial behaviors (Jordan, Scannapieco, & Vandiver, 2009).

Substance Use in the General Population

It is important to explore the use of alcohol and other drugs with youth, particularly those with mental health issues, because substance use will exacerbate the risk of health and behavioral issues. Adolescence is a time of experimentation, and some usage of alcohol and other drugs should be expected. To get a sense of what is normal usage across the youth population, we will review statistics across age, gender, and race.

According to the Substance Abuse and Mental Health Services Administration (SAMHSA) (Center for Behavioral Health Statistics and Quality [CBHSQ], 2018) more than half of Americans aged 12 or older (51.8 percent) reported being current drinkers of alcohol in the 2016 survey. Table 17.1 provides a breakdown by age, sex, and racial/ethnic group for youth who reported being current users of alcohol (SAMHSA, 2011a; CBHSQ, 2018).

In 2016, 10.6 percent of youth aged 12–17 were current illicit drug users. Table 17.2 provides a breakdown of illicit drug use reported by these youth by substance, sex, and racial/ethnic group.

Given the percentages of current alcohol and drug users shown in Tables 17.1 and 17.2, it is important to understand the continuum of usage and be able to distinguish between use and abuse of alcohol and other drugs.

Table 17.1 Percentage of youth reporting current usage of alcohol

By age	%
12–17	9.2
18–25	57.1
By sex, age 12–17	
Male	13.7
Female	13.5
By racial/ethnic group, age 12–17	
Asian	4.8
Black	10.8
American Indian/Alaska Native	11.1
Youth reporting two or more races	13.0
Hispanic	13.9
White	14.9

Continuum of Alcohol and Drug Use

Adolescents who use drugs or alcohol can be characterized along a continuum. Levels of use are generally identified as use, abuse, and dependence. For many youth and adolescents, some alcohol and drug use is normal and should be expected. Developmentally, youth are experimenting with adult-like behaviors, and substance use will not generally lead to addiction. Use of drugs or alcohol by an adolescent to experiment or socialize and in moderation is usually considered substance use rather than substance abuse. For adolescents who have a mental illness and are on medication, however, even small amounts of alcohol or other drugs may cause physical, emotional, or social problems. So how much is too much? According to the *Diagnostic and Statistical Manual of Mental Disorders V* (American Psychiatric Association, 2013) abuse and dependence are assessed by specific criteria. Abuse of alcohol or drugs includes at least one of the following factors in the last 12 months:

Table 17.2 Percentage of youth aged 12–25 reporting current use of illicit drugs

By substance	%
Marijuana	7.4
Psychotherapeutic drugs (nonmedical use); includes pain relievers, tranquilizer, stimulants, and sedatives.	3.0
Inhalants (nonmedical use)	1.1
Hallucinogens	0.9
Cocaine	0.2
By sex	
Male[a]	10.4
Female[a]	9.8
By racial/ethnic group (ages 12 or older)	
Asian	3.5
Native Hawaiian or other Pacific Islander	5.4
American Indian	12.5
Alaska Native	12.1
Black	10.7
Hispanic	8.1
White	9.1

[a]Males were more likely than females to be current marijuana users (8.3% vs. 6.4%), whereas females were more likely than males to be current users of psychotherapeutic drugs (3.7% vs. 2.3%) and current nonmedical users of pain relievers (3.0% vs. 2.0%).

From CBHSQ (2018).

- Recurrent substance use resulting in failure to fulfill obligations at work, home, or school
- Recurrent substance use in situations that are physically hazardous;
- Recurrent substance-related legal problems
- Continued substance use despite having persistent or recurrent social or interpersonal problems caused by or exacerbated by the substance

Dependence, also referred to as *addiction,* is a pattern of use that results in three or more of the following symptoms in a 12-month period:

- *Tolerance*, or needing more of the drug or alcohol to get high
- *Withdrawal*, in the form of physical symptoms that occur when alcohol or other drugs are not used, such as tremors, nausea, sweating, and shakiness
- Substance taken in larger amounts and over a longer period than intended
- Persistent desire or unsuccessful efforts to cut down or control substance use
- A great deal of time spent in activities related to obtaining the substance, using the substance, or recovering from its effects
- Important social, occupational, or recreational activities eliminated or reduced because of substance use
- Continued substance use despite knowledge of persistent or recurrent physical or psychological problems caused or exacerbated by the substance

Assessment

There is significant overlap in the symptoms and behaviors of adolescents who are misusing drugs or alcohol with those of other mental health conditions. Identification and assessment need to be accurate and comprehensive to ensure correct treatment. The assessment involves efficient identification of substance use and related problems, psychiatric co-occurrence, and psychosocial problems. The first phase of the assessment should be the identification of an SUD. Because it is often not possible or desirable to have an adolescent take a physical test, such as a urinalysis or blood test, to identify substance use, a brief screening instrument can be used. Once it becomes clear that the adolescent has a SUD, a more comprehensive assessment of problem severity needs to be conducted.

A *screening tool* is a brief self-report or interview focused on the youth's behavior, thoughts, and feelings. It usually takes 5–15 minutes to administer and is scored to determine if the youth is within a range that indicates the likelihood of having a substance abuse problem. There are many screening instruments available, and some examples of standardized self-report screening tools are presented here. Comprehensive assessment will be discussed in a later section.

Brief Screening Instruments

A specialized six-item screen in the public domain, *Car, Relax, Alone, Forget, Friends, Trouble (CRAFFT)*, is designed to be administered verbally during a routine interview to address both alcohol and drug use. (For more information, see http://www.projectcork.org/clinical_tools/pdf/CRAFFT.pdf.) Some sample questions include

- Have you ever ridden in a car driven by someone (including yourself) who was high or using alcohol or drugs?
- Do you ever forget things you did while using alcohol or drugs?
- Do your family or friends ever tell you that you should cut down on your drinking or drug use?

The *Rutgers Alcohol Problem Index* (http://adai.washington.edu/instruments/pdf/Rutgers_Alcohol_Problem_Index_210.pdf) is an 18-item screening tool that assesses adolescent problem drinking and related negative consequences (White & Labouvie, 1989). Each of the sample items listed below is used to assess the frequency of the behavior in relationship to alcohol use during the past 3 years:

- Had withdrawal symptoms; that is, felt sick because you stopped or cut down on drinking?
- Suddenly found yourself in a place that you could not remember getting to?
- Felt that you needed more alcohol than you used to in order to get the same effect?

The *Michigan Alcohol Screening Test* (https://outcometracker.org/library/MAST.pdf) contains 25 items that provide a general measure of problem severity. Three sample questions are:

- Do you feel you are a normal drinker (with "normal" meaning drinking as much or less than most other people)?
- Have you ever awakened the morning after drinking the night before and found that you could not remember a part of the evening?
- Does any near relative or close friend ever worry or complain about your drinking?

Comprehensive Assessment

The outcome of the brief screening determines the need for a more comprehensive assessment. The comprehensive assessment explores the extent and nature of the substance involvement, psychosocial issues, and co-occurring mental health disorders. It is important to consider developmental domains such as cognitive, emotional, physical, and social. This assessment provides the more extensive information needed to determine the most appropriate intervention. Included in the determination of the intervention are treatment setting (e.g., inpatient or outpatient); type of intervention (e.g., family therapy, medications, or group therapy); and intensity, frequency, and type of contacts with therapist or resources. Specialized training is required to administer both comprehensive and brief screening tools. The following are some examples of comprehensive assessments:

- The Global Appraisal of Individual Needs (GAIN) is a semi-structured interview that measures recent and lifetime functioning in several areas, including substance use, legal and school functioning, and psychiatric symptoms. The comprehensiveness and multidimensionality of the GAIN require a relatively long administration time and lengthy and detailed training. (For more information, see http://www.gaincc.org.)
- The Teen Addiction Severity Index (T-ASI) is a semi-structured interview that consists of seven content areas: chemical use, school status, employment-support status, family relationships, legal status, peer-social relationships, and psychiatric status. Adolescent and interviewer severity ratings are elicited on a 5-point scale for each content area. (More information is available from http://pubs.niaaa.nih.gov/publications/AssessingAlcohol/InstrumentPDFs/70_T-ASI.pdf.)
- The Personal Experience Inventory (PEI) is a self-administered, multiscale questionnaire. It consists of several scales that measure drug use problem severity, psychosocial risk, and response distortion tendencies. Supplemental problem screens measure eating disorders, suicide potential, physical/sexual abuse, and parental history of drug abuse. (More information is available at http://www.wpspublish.com/store/p/2905/personal-experience-inventory-pei.)

Indicators of Substance Abuse and
Mental Health Disorders

Often an adolescent's behavior or appearance can provide signs of a substance abuse or mental health disorder. Adolescents experiencing depression, bulimia, or early stages of substance use may be actively trying to conceal their activity from adults. Research has shown that these problems are often difficult for caregivers and other adults to identify (Levitt, Saka, Romanelli, & Hoagwood, 2007; Moore, Guarino, & Marsh, 2014). The National Institute of Mental Health and SAMHSA developed a toolkit (http://store.samhsa.gov/shin/content/SMA12-4700/SMA12-4700.pdf) to help human service organizations identify signs that indicate the need to take action and address mental health or substance use conditions in children and adolescents. The following action signs are identified:

- Feeling very sad or withdrawn for more than 2 weeks
- Seriously trying to harm or kill oneself, or making plans to do so
- Sudden overwhelming fear for no reason, sometimes with a racing heart or fast breathing
- School related-truancy, failing classes, drop out, loss of scholarship
- Involvement in many fights, using a weapon, or wanting to badly hurt others
- Severe out-of-control behavior that can hurt oneself or others
- Not eating, throwing up, or using laxatives to lose weight
- Intense worries or fears that get in the way of daily activities
- Extreme difficulty concentrating or staying still that puts one in physical danger or causes school failure
- Repeated use of drugs or alcohol
- Severe mood swings that cause problems in relationships
- Drastic changes in behavior or personality

As reported (Jordan et al., 2009; Moore et al., 2014), indicators of substance-induced disorders for adolescents include but are not limited to physical signs (e.g., fatigue, repeated health complaints, red and glazed eyes, and lasting cough), emotional signs (e.g., personality change, irritability, irresponsible behavior, sudden mood changes, low self-esteem, poor judgment, and depression), family issues (e.g., disintegration of relationships with family and friends, starting arguments, breaking rules, and withdrawing from

Box 17.1 General signs of alcohol or drug use

Home

- Loss of interest in family activities
- Disrespect for family rules
- Verbal or physical abuse
- Disappearance of valuable items or money
- Not telling where they are going
- Constant excuses for behavior

School

- Sudden drop in grades
- Truancy or always being late to school
- Loss of interest in learning
- Poor work performance
- Defiance of authority
- Reduced memory and attention span
- Poor attitude toward sports or other extracurricular activities

Physical and emotional signs

- Different friends
- Smell of alcohol or marijuana on breath or body
- Unexplainable mood swings and behavior
- Overreaction to criticism or rebelliousness
- Negativity, argumentativeness, paranoia or confusion, destructiveness, or anxiety
- Feeling overly tired or being hyperactive
- Drastic weight gain or loss
- Cheating or stealing

family activities), school problems (e.g., drop in grades, change in attitude about school, many absences, truancy, and discipline problems), and social problems (e.g., engaging in criminal activities, theft, or vandalism; changes in dress style or appearance; and new friends who share similar signs).

Signs of substance use must be considered in the context of the adolescent's development and situation. Many indicators are normal adolescent behaviors, but if the youth is exhibiting several over a period of time, it is important to assess substance use. Some other general signs of alcohol or drug use are listed in Box 17.1.

Commonly Used Drugs and Alcohol

In addition to understanding the signs and symptoms of substance use, you should know the different types of drugs, how to identify them, and their health effects. Also important is knowing their street names or slang terms and how they are administered so you can communicate with the adolescent. As shown in Table 17.3, substances can generally be categorized into seven areas: alcohol, cannabinoids, stimulants, opiates, club drugs, dissociative drugs, and other. Adolescents are also increasingly abusing prescription drugs.

Prescription Drug Use Among Adolescents

Prescription drugs are the fastest growing drug problem in the United States (SAMHSA, 2015). Many adolescents are under the misconception that prescription drugs are safer than street or illicit drugs. The use of psychotherapeutic drugs makes up a larger part of the overall US drug problem than was true in the 1990s. After alcohol and marijuana, prescription and over-the-counter drugs are among the most commonly abused drugs by twelfth graders (National Institute on Drug Abuse, n.d.), partly because there is an increase in prescription drugs overall and partly because use of illicit drugs is down. Young people seem less concerned about using prescription drugs because of their legitimate widespread use. Additionally, adolescents and young adults are aware of only the positive benefits and not the dangers of using prescription drugs for nonmedical reasons.

Prescription drug abuse occurs when someone takes a medication prescribed for someone else or takes his or her own prescribed medication in a dosage other than that prescribed. Young people often abuse prescription drugs belonging to friends or relatives to get high, treat pain, or help them study or stay alert longer. Often teens will use the drug in a different form or dosage to get high quicker. Most prescription drugs come in pill form. Young adults who abuse prescription drugs may crush the pill and then swallow, sniff, or inject it, which may cause serious side effects or addiction. For example, when oxycodone (OxyContin) is crushed and inhaled, a 12-hour dose hits the central nervous system all at once, which increases the risk of addiction and overdose (National Institute on Drug Abuse, 2014).

Table 17.3 Characteristics of commonly abused alcohol and drugs

Category	Street name	Administered	Acute effects	Health risk
Alcohol				
Liquor, beer, and wine		Swallowed	Euphoria, mild stimulation, relaxation, lowered inhibitions, slurred speech, nausea, loss of coordination	Increased risk of injuries, violence, fetal damage, depression, hypertension, liver and heart disease, addiction
Cannabinoids				
Marijuana	Blunt, dope, ganja, grass, herb, joint, bud, Mary Jane, pot, reefer, green, weed	Smoked, swallowed	Euphoria, relaxation, slowed reaction time, distorted sensory perception, impaired balance and coordination, increased heart rate and appetite, anxiety, panic attacks, psychosis	Cough, frequent respiratory infections, possible mental health decline, addiction
Hashish	Boom, gangster, hash, hash oil, hemp	Smoked or swallowed	Euphoria, relaxation, slowed reaction time, distorted sensory perception, impaired balance and coordination, increased heart rate and appetite, anxiety, panic attacks, psychosis	Cough, frequent respiratory infections, possible mental health decline, addiction
Opioids				
Heroin	Smack, horse, brown sugar, dope, H, junk, skag, skunk, white horse, China white, cheese (with over-the-counter cold medicine and antihistamine)	Injected, smoked, snorted	Euphoria, drowsiness, impaired coordination, dizziness, confusion, nausea, sedation, feeling of heaviness in the body, slowed or arrested breathing	Constipation, endocarditis, hepatitis, HIV, addiction, fatal overdose

Table 17.3 *Continued*

Category	Street name	Administered	Acute effects	Health risk
Pain relievers (opioids)	Hydrocodone (e.g., Vicodin), oxycodone (e.g., OxyContin)	Swallowed, snorted, injected	Euphoria, drowsiness, impaired coordination, dizziness, confusion, nausea, sedation, feeling of heaviness in the body, slowed or arrested breathing	Constipation, headaches, irregular heart best, overdose, death
Opium	Big O, black stuff, block, gum, hop	Swallowed, smoked	Euphoria, drowsiness, impaired coordination, dizziness, confusion, nausea, sedation, feeling of heaviness in the body, slowed or arrested breathing	Constipation, endocarditis, hepatitis, HIV, addiction, fatal overdose
Stimulants				
Cocaine	Blow, bump, C, candy, Charlie, coke, crack, flake, rock, snow, toot	Snorted, smoked, injected	Increased heart rate, blood pressure, body temperature, and metabolism; feelings of exhilaration; increased energy and mental alertness; tremors; reduced appetite; irritability; anxiety; panic; paranoia; violent behavior; psychosis	Nasal damage from snorting, weight loss, insomnia, cardiac or cardiovascular complications, stroke, seizures, addiction

(*Continued*)

Table 17.3 *Continued*

Category	Street name	Administered	Acute effects	Health risk
Amphetamines	Bennies, black beauties, crosses, hearts, LA turnaround, speed, truck drivers, uppers	Swallowed, snorted, smoked, injected	Increased heart rate, blood pressure, body temperature, and metabolism; feelings of exhilaration; increased energy and mental alertness; tremors; reduced appetite; irritability; anxiety; panic; paranoia; violent behavior; psychosis	Weight loss, insomnia, cardiac or cardiovascular complications, stroke, seizures, addiction
Methamphetamines	Meth, ice, crank, chalk, crystal, fire, glass, go fast, speed	Swallowed, snorted, smoked, injected	Increased heart rate, blood pressure, body temperature, and metabolism; feelings of exhilaration; increased energy and mental alertness; tremors; reduced appetite; irritability; anxiety; panic; paranoia; violent behavior; psychosis	Severe dental problems, weight loss, insomnia, cardiac or cardiovascular complications, stroke, seizures, addiction
Club Drugs				
MDMA (methylenedioxy-methamphetamine)	Ecstasy, Adam, clarity, Eve, lover's speed, peace, uppers	Swallowed, snorted, injected	Mild hallucinogenic effects, increased tactile sensitivity, empathic feelings, lowered inhibition, anxiety, chills, sweating, teeth clenching, muscle cramping	Sleep disturbances, depression, impaired memory, hyperthermia, addiction

Table 17.3 *Continued*

Category	Street name	Administered	Acute effects	Health risk
Flunitrazepam (associated with sexual assault)	Rohypnol, forget- me pill, Mexican Valium, R2, roach, Roche, roofies, roofinol, rape, rophies	Swallowed, snorted	Mild hallucinogenic effects, increased tactile sensitivity, empathic feelings, lowered inhibition, anxiety, chills, sweating, teeth clenching, muscle cramping, sedation, muscle relaxation, confusion, memory loss, dizziness, impaired coordination	Addiction
GHB (gamma-hydroxybutyric acid; associated with sexual assault)	G, Georgia home boy, grievous bodily harm, liquid ecstasy, soap, scoop, goop, liquid x	Swallowed	Mild hallucinogenic effects, increased tactile sensitivity, empathic feelings, lowered inhibition, anxiety, chills, sweating, teeth clenching, muscle cramping	Unconsciousness, seizures, coma
Dissociative drugs				
Ketamine	Ketalar SV, cat Valium, K, Special K, vitamin K	Injected, snorted, smoked	Feelings of being separate from one's body and environment, impaired motor function, impaired memory, delirium, respiratory depression and arrest, death	Anxiety, tremors, numbness, memory loss, nausea
PCP and analogs	Phencyclidine, angel dust, boat, hog, love boat, peace pill	Swallowed, smoked, injected	Psychosis, aggression, violence, slurred speech, loss of coordination, hallucinations, feelings of being separate from one's body and environment, impaired motor function, impaired memory, delirium, respiratory depression and arrest, death	Anxiety, tremors, numbness, memory loss, nausea

Table 17.4 Characteristics of commonly abused prescription drugs

Category	Commercial and street names	Administered	Acute effects	Health risk
Depressants				
Barbiturates	Amytal, Nembutal, Seconal, Phenobarbital; barbs, reds, red birds, tooies, yellows	Injected, swallowed	Euphoria, unusual excitement, fever, sedation, reduced anxiety, feelings of well-being, lowered inhibitions, slurred speech, poor concentration, confusion, dizziness, impaired coordination and memory	Lowered blood pressure, slowed breathing, tolerance, withdrawal, addiction, increased risk of respiratory distress and death when combined with alcohol
Benzodiazepines	Ativan, Halcion, Librium, Valium, Xanax; candy, downers, sleeping pills, tranks	Swallowed	Sedation, reduced anxiety, feelings of well-being, lowered inhibitions, slurred speech, poor concentration, confusion, dizziness, impaired coordination and memory	Addiction, worsening of some breathing problems, possible birth defects for pregnant women, in the elderly may lead to falling
Sleep medication	Ambien, Sonata, Lunesta; forget-me pill, Mexican Valium, R2, Roche, roofies, roofinaol, rope, rophies	Swallowed, snorted	Sedation, reduced anxiety, feelings of well-being, lowered inhibitions, slurred speech, poor concentration, confusion, dizziness, impaired coordination and memory	Burning or tingling in the hands, arms, feet, or legs; changes in appetite, difficulty keeping balance, dizziness, daytime drowsiness, mental slowing or problems with attention or memory

Table 17.4 *Continued*

Category	Commercial and street names	Administered	Acute effects	Health risk
Opioids/morphine				
Codeine	Empirin with Codeine, Fiorinal with Codeine, Robitussin A-C, Tylenol with Codeine; Captain Cody, schoolboy	Injected, swallowed	Pain relief, euphoria, drowsiness, sedation, weakness, dizziness, nausea, impaired coordination, confusion, dry mouth, itching, sweating, clammy skin, constipation	Slowed or arrested breathing, lowered pulse and blood pressure, tolerance, addiction, unconsciousness, coma, death (risk of death increased when combined with alcohol or other central nervous system depressants)
Morphine	Roxanol, Duramorph; Miss Emma, monkey, white stuff	Injected, swallowed, smoked	Pain relief, euphoria, drowsiness, sedation, weakness, dizziness, nausea, impaired coordination, confusion, dry mouth, itching, sweating, clammy skin, constipation	Slowed or arrested breathing, lowered pulse and blood pressure, tolerance, addiction, unconsciousness, coma, death (risk of death increased when combined with alcohol or other central nervous system depressants)
Methadone	Methadose, Dolophine; fizzies, amidone	Swallowed, injected	Significant overdose risk when used improperly, pain relief, euphoria, drowsiness, sedation, weakness, dizziness, nausea, impaired coordination, confusion, dry mouth, itching, sweating, clammy skin, constipation	Slowed or arrested breathing, lowered pulse and blood pressure, tolerance, addiction, unconsciousness, coma, death (risk of death increased when combined with alcohol or other central nervous system depressants)

(Continued)

Table 17.4 *Continued*

Category	Commercial and street names	Administered	Acute effects	Health risk
Fentanyl and analogs	Actiq, Duragesic, Sublimaze; Apache, China girl, China white, dance fever, friend, goodfella, jackpot, murder 8, TNT, Tango and Cash	Injected, smoked, snorted	80 to 100 times more potent analgesic than morphine; pain relief, euphoria, drowsiness, sedation, weakness, dizziness, nausea, impaired coordination, confusion, dry mouth, itching, sweating, clammy skin, constipation	Slowed or arrested breathing, lowered pulse and blood pressure, tolerance, addiction, unconsciousness, coma, death (risk of death increased when combined with alcohol or other central nervous system depressants)
Other opioid pain relievers				
Oxycodone HCL, Hydrocodone Bitartrate, Hydromorphone, Oxymorphone, Meperidine, Propoxyphene	Tylox, Oxycontin, Percodan, Percocet, Vicodin, Lortab, Demerol; Oxy, O.C., oxycotton, kicker, hillbilly, percs, smack, smurfs, footballs, stop signs, blue heaven, blues, Mrs. O	Chewed, swallowed, snorted, injected, suppositories	Muscle relaxation, high abuse potential, pain relief, euphoria, drowsiness, sedation, weakness, dizziness, nausea, impaired coordination, confusion, dry mouth, itching, sweating, clammy skin, constipation	Slowed or arrested breathing, lowered pulse and blood pressure, tolerance, addiction, unconsciousness, coma, death (risk of death increased when combined with alcohol or other central nervous system depressants)

Table 17.4 *Continued*

Category	Commercial and street names	Administered	Acute effects	Health risk
Stimulants				
Amphetamines	Biphetamine, Dexedrine, Adderall; bennies, black beauties, crosses, hearts, LA turnaround, speed, truck drivers, uppers	Injected, swallowed, smoked, snorted	Feelings of exhilaration, increased energy, mental alertness	Increased heart rate, blood pressure, and metabolism; reduced appetite; weight loss; nervousness; insomnia; seizures; heart attack; stroke; rapid breathing; tremor; loss of coordination; irritability; panic; hallucinations; impulsive behavior; addiction
Methylphenidate	Concerta, Ritalin; JIF, MPH, R-ball, Skippy, the smart drug, Vitamin R	Injected, swallowed, snorted	Feelings of exhilaration, increased energy, mental alertness	Increased or decreased blood pressure, increased heart rate and metabolism, reduced appetite, weight loss, digestive problems, nervousness, insomnia, seizures, heart attack, stroke
Other compounds				
Dextromethorphan (DXM)	Found in some cough and cold medicines; Robotripping, Robo, Triple C	Swallowed	Euphoria, slurred speech	Increased heart rate and blood pressure, dizziness, nausea, vomiting, confusion, paranoia, distorted visual perceptions, impaired motor function

Commonly Abused Prescription Drugs

Similar to illicit drugs, prescription drugs that are abused fall into categories: depressants, opioids and morphine derivatives, stimulants, and other compounds (Table 17.4).

Treatment of Co-Occurring Disorders

Treatment of mental illness along with a SUD is a relatively new field, and evidence-based practices developed specifically for clients with CODs are limited. Therefore it is important to consider evidence-based practices developed solely for either mental health or substance abuse. The current state of the science highlights the need for evidence-based thinking in making both programmatic and clinical decisions in the treatment of people with CODs (SAMHSA, 2014).

At the *treatment level*, interventions that have their own evidence to support them as evidence-based practices are frequently a part of a comprehensive and integrated response to persons with CODs. These interventions, described previously in this book, include

- Psychopharmacological interventions (e.g., desipramine and buproprion for people with cocaine use disorders and depression; Kranzler & Ciraulo, 2005). Of note, medication-assisted treatment for opioid misuse among young people is only at 3 percent (Knopf, 2018).
- Motivational interventions (e.g., motivational enhancement therapy; Miller & Rollnick, 2013)
- Cognitive-behavioral interventions (e.g., contingency management; Godley et al., 2014, 2017; Higgins, Silverman, & Heil, 2007; Roth, Brunette, & Green, 2005)

At the *program level*, three models have an evidence base for producing positive clinical outcomes for persons with CODs: the modified therapeutic community (MTC), integrated dual disorders treatment, and assertive community treatment. The MTC (De Leon, 1993; De Leon, Sacks, Staines, & McKendrick, 2000; Sacks, Banks, McKendrick, & Sacks, 2008) for persons with CODs is a 12- to 18-month residential treatment program because youth with SUDs often benefit from a highly structured environment

(Levy, 2019). Developed for individuals with co-occurring SUDs and mental disorders, the MTC is a structured and active program based on community-as-method (i.e., the community is the treatment agent) and mutual peer self-help. It is a comprehensive treatment model that adapts the traditional therapeutic community in response to the psychiatric symptoms, cognitive impairments, and reduced level of functioning of the client with co-occurring disorders. Treatment encompasses four stages (admission, primary treatment, live-in reentry, and live-out reentry) that correspond to stages within the recovery process. The staged format allows gradual progress and rewards improvement with increased independence and responsibility. Goals, objectives, and expected outcomes are established for each stage and are integrated in an individual treatment plan with goals specific to each client. Staff members function as role models, rational authorities, and guides (Center for Substance Abuse Treatment, 2007).

Research has strongly indicated that, to recover fully, a person with a COD needs treatment for both problems. *Integrated dual disorder treatments* provide assistance for each condition, helping people recover from both in one setting and at the same time.

Key to integrated dual disorder treatment is the inclusion of assistance beyond standard therapy or medication, such as assertive outreach, job and housing assistance, family counseling, and even money and relationship management. This personalized treatment is viewed as long term and can begin at any stage of recovery. A strengths-based approach is at the foundation of integrated treatment (SAMHSA, 2014).

Assertive community treatment is designed as a service delivery model in which a team of professionals assumes responsibility for providing the specific mix of services that each person needs at the appropriate frequency and intensity and for the appropriate length of time. Team members are available 24 hours a day, 7 days a week. Services are provided in the community in places and situations where problems arise, rather than in an office or clinic setting. Interventions are integrated through collaboration among team members.

References

American Psychiatric Association. (2013). *Diagnostic and statistical manual of mental disorders* (5th ed.). Washington, DC: Author.

Anthony, E. K., Taylor, S. A., & Raffo, Z. (2011). Early intervention for substance abuse among youth and young adults with mental health conditions: An exploration of community mental health practices. *Administration and Policy in Mental Health and Mental Health Services Research, 38*, 131–141. doi:10.1007/s10488-010-0308-x

Center for Behavioral Health Statistics and Quality (CBHSQ). (2018). *2017 National Survey on Drug Use and Health: Detailed Tables.* Rockville, MD: Substance Abuse and Mental Health Services Administration.

Center for Substance Abuse Treatment. (2007). *Understanding evidence-based practices for co-occurring disorders* (COCE Overview Paper 5, DHHS Publication No. SMA 07-4278). Rockville, MD: Substance Abuse and Mental Health Services Administration.

De Leon, G. (1993). Modified therapeutic communities for co-occurring substance abuse and psychiatric disorders. In J. Solomon, S. Zimberg, & E. Shollar (Eds.), *Dual diagnosis: Evaluation, treatment, training, and program development* (pp. 137–156). New York: Plenum.

De Leon, G., Sacks, S., Staines, G., & McKendrick, K. (2000). Modified therapeutic community for homeless mentally ill chemical abusers: Treatment outcomes. *American Journal of Drug and Alcohol Abuse, 26*, 461–480.

Godley, S. H., Hunter, B. D., Fernández-Artamendi, S., Smith, J. E., Meyers, R. J., & Godley, M. D. (2014). A comparison of treatment outcomes for Adolescent Community Reinforcement Approach participants with and without co-occurring disorders. *Journal of Substance Abuse Treatment, 46*, 463–471. doi:10.1016/j.jsat.2013.10.013

Godley, M. D., Passetti, L. L., Subramaniam, G. A., Funk, R. R., Smith, J. E., & Meyers, R. J. (2017). Adolescent community reinforcement approach implementation and treatment outcomes for youth with opioid problem use. *Drug and Alcohol Dependence, 174*, 9–16. doi:10.1016/j.druglacdep.2016.12.029

Higgins, S. T., Silverman, K., & Heil, S. H. (Eds.). (2007). *Contingency management in substance abuse treatment.* New York: Guilford.

Jordan, C., Scannapieco, M., & Vandiver, V. L. (2009). Health promotion strategies for the mental health needs of children and families. In V. L. Vandiver (Ed.), *Integrating health promotion and mental health: An introduction to policies, principles, and practices* (pp. 283–310). New York: Oxford University Press.

Knopf, A. (2018). Buprenorphine for adolescents and young adults: Recommendations based on data. *Alcoholism & Drug Abuse Weekly, 30*(11), 1–4. Retrieved from https://doi:10.1002/adaw.31890

Kranzler, H. R., & Ciraulo, D. A. (Eds.). (2005). *Clinical manual of addiction psychopharmacology.* Arlington, VA: American Psychiatric Publishing.

Levitt, J. M., Saka, N., Romanelli, L. H., & Hoagwood, K. (2007). Early identification of mental health problems in schools: The status of instrumentation. *Journal of School Psychology, 45*, 163–191.

Levy, S. (2019). Youth and the opioid epidemic. *Pediatrics, 143*(2), e20182752. doi:10.1542/peds.2018-2752

Miller, W. R., & Rollnick, S. (2013). *Motivational interviewing: Helping people change.* (3rd ed.). New York: Guilford.

Moore, S. K., Guarino, H., & Marsh, L. A. (2014). "This is not who I want to be:" Experiences of opioid-dependent youth before, and during, combined buprenorphine and behavioral treatment. *Substance use & Misuse, 49*(3), 303–314. doi:10.3109/10826084.2013.832328

National Institute on Drug Abuse. (n.d.). Topics in brief: Prescription drug abuse. Retrieved from http://www.drugabuse.gov/publications/term/163/TopicsInBrief

National Institute on Drug Abuse. (2014). NIDA for teens. Retrieved from http://teens.drugabuse.gov/facts/facts_mj1.php

Roth, R. M., Brunette, M. F., & Green, A. I. (2005). Treatment of substance use disorder in schizophrenia: A unifying neurobiological mechanism? *Current Psychiatry Reports, 7*, 283–291.

Sacks, S., Banks, S., McKendrick, K., & Sacks, J. Y. (2008). Modified therapeutic community for co-occurring disorders: A summary of four studies. *Journal of Substance Abuse Treatment, 34*, 112–122.

Substance Abuse and Mental Health Services Administration (SAMHSA). (2011a). *Identifying mental health and substance use problems of children and adolescents: A guide for child-serving organizations* (HHS Publication No. SMA *12–4670*). Rockville, MD: Author.

Substance Abuse and Mental Health Services Administration (SAMHSA). (2014). National registry of evidence-based programs and practices. Retrieved from http://www.nrepp.samhsa.gov/Index.aspx

Substance Abuse and Mental Health Services Administration (SAMHSA). (2015). Specific populations and prescription drug misuse and abuse. Retrieved from https://www.samshsa.gov/prescription-drug-misuse-abuse/specific-populationsyouth-young-adult

Substance Abuse and Mental Health Services Administration (SAMHSA). (2018). *Key substance use and mental health indicators in the United States: Results from the 2107 National Survey on Drug Use and Health* (HHS Publication No. SMA 18-5068, NSDUH Series H-53). Rockville, MD: Center for Behavioral Health Statistics and Quality, Substance Abuse and Mental Health Services Administration. Retrieved from https://www.samhsa.gov/data/

White, H. R., & Labouvie, E. W. (1989). Towards the assessment of adolescent problem drinking. *Journal of Studies on Alcohol, 50*, 30–37.

18

Children and Adolescents with Mental Illness and the Education System

School is an important aspect of all youths' and children's lives. They spend most of each school day in the classroom. It is often not until the child enters the school system that mental health issues are discovered. Schoolteachers, social workers, nurses, and other personnel are in an exceptional position to identify child mental health and substance abuse issues because they are in sustained contact and often have a trusting relationship with children. Schools also provide a safe and expected place to address behaviors resulting from mental health issues. At the end of the chapter, we will share several evidence-informed interventions designed for use in schools, supporting the importance of the school setting for the struggling child or adolescent.

School can be a challenging place for children experiencing emotional or behavioral problems. If a child is not in the most appropriate setting and receiving the most appropriate supports, there can be serious, life-long consequences. The caregivers of these children can also find the school system challenging, particularly if they do not understand their children's rights and how to advocate for their children's needs. What are the educational system's obligations for dealing with children who have a mental health problem?

There are two federal laws that protect children with disabilities. The first is the Individuals with Disabilities Education Act (IDEA; 2004). This act sets achievement standards and provides guidance to schools on how to help students achieve these standards. The IDEA requires the educational system to ensure that eligible children with disabilities, including mental health disabilities, receive the same educational opportunities as children without disabilities.

The second federal provision is included in Section 504 of the Rehabilitation Act of 1973. This is a federal civil rights law that prohibits

Understanding the Mental Health Problems of Children and Adolescents. Kirstin Painter and Maria Scannapieco,
Oxford University Press (2021). © Oxford University Press. DOI: 10.1093/oso/9780190927844.003.0018

discrimination against people with disabilities. Under this law, children with disabilities are afforded the right to the same educational programs and experiences as nondisabled children. To ensure this, schools must make necessary accommodations to allow children with disabilities the same opportunities as other children. All children with a disability are covered by Section 504. To be covered under IDEA, a child must meet certain eligibility criteria.

Individuals with Disabilities Education Act

The IDEA requires that special education and related services be made available free of charge to every eligible child with a disability (aged 3–21), including preschoolers. These services are specially designed to address the child's individual needs associated with the disability—in this case, emotional disturbance, as defined by IDEA (and further specified by states). In recent school years, more than 490,000 children and youth received these services to address their individual needs related to emotional disturbance.

Each year, more than 6 million children from 3 to 21 years old receive special education and related services. Of those, nearly 1 in 12 children receive the services because of an emotional disturbance. The IDEA spells out the requirement for schools to provide services to children when their disability interferes with their ability to learn. State educational laws define how children should be identified and served under IDEA. The federal government provides state funds to help pay for accommodations that are needed to help a child with special needs receive an appropriate education in the least restrictive situation. If states do not comply with IDEA, they stand to lose those federal funds.

The first step for a child to receive special education services under IDEA is a complete evaluation by qualified school professionals to determine if the child has a mental health problem covered under the state's educational plan and if that problem is interfering with the child's ability to learn in a regular classroom setting. This evaluation is provided free of charge in public schools.

Once the evaluation is completed, the caregiver(s) and school personnel meet to review the results and determine whether special educational supports and services are needed, and if so, what types of supports and services are appropriate. If the family disagrees with the findings of the evaluation or the recommendations, they can request an independent evaluation by qualified professionals who do not work for the school.

Definition of a Child with a Disability Under IDEA

There are various disability categories under which a child may be found eligible for special education and related services:

- Autism
- Deafness
- Deaf-blindness
- Developmental delay
- Emotional disturbance
- Hearing impairment
- Intellectual disability
- Multiple disabilities
- Orthopedic impairment
- Other health impairment
- Specific learning disability
- Speech or language impairment
- Traumatic brain injury
- Visual impairment including blindness

If a student is deemed eligible, and the family agrees to special education accommodations, school personnel including teachers and counselors have a face-to-face meeting with the family and any other persons the family would like to participate. It can be helpful for the family to have a family advocate who understands IDEA attend the meeting with them. Together, the team should develop an individualized educational program (IEP) that spells out educational goals, short-term objectives, and services or accommodations to be provided through the school. Accommodations may include alterations in assignments, changes in expectations for the child to receive a passing grade, modification to the environment to reduce distractions or temptations, or an individualized behavior plan.

A meeting should be held with the team at least once a year to review the goals, objectives, and services; determine if they are meeting the needs of the child; and set new goals and objectives. Meetings can be requested earlier if the plan needs to be changed to better meet the child's educational needs. In addition to an annual IEP meeting, the child should be re-evaluated at least once every 3 years and no more than once a year to determine continued eligibility and to address any new needs. If a family does not feel that the child's needs are being met, or if the child's rights are being violated, the family can request due process.

Emotional and Behavioral Problems

When children with emotional or behavioral problems exhibit behaviors that interfere with their ability to learn or with the ability of other children around them to learn, a *behavioral intervention plan* should be put in place. An assessment should be conducted to determine the type of behavior and its frequency and duration, as well as the situations under which it does or does not occur. The behavioral plan is then developed to prevent the problem behavior from occurring. A common strategy is to use a token system that allows the child to earn tokens when the problem behavior does not occur and lose tokens when it does. The child can accrue tokens that can be used to purchase a privilege or reward. The reward must be something that is important to the specific child, and it must be delivered in increments based on the child's age and maturity level. For instance, a first-grader should not have to wait a month before earning a reward.

Intervention Strategies

Schools afford professionals who work in the school system a unique opportunity to intervene with children who have experienced mental health issues. Prior to entering school, children may have experienced abuse for years. Parents may not have had any prior assistance with learning new and effective ways of child rearing or support in overcoming the many challenges of raising children with limited resources. The school can begin to provide the needed positive and secure relationships with peers and adults and the social support and connection to other forms of social support for the family. Teachers can provide opportunities for personal development, thus fostering accomplishment, and boosting the child's self-esteem and feelings of mastery. They can help children build self-confidence and navigate the process of developing peer relationships.

All schools have children at risk of mental health issues or children with a mental health issue. These children often have difficulty learning, and, consequently, it is difficult for the classroom teacher to manage their behaviors. Additionally, many children, particularly in large urban areas, are in foster or kinship care and require special attention from school personnel, Child Protective Services, and other mental health workers. In a time of drastic budget cuts to both educational and mental health systems, building alliances to address the intervention needs of children identified as having mental health issues is critical to the mission of the school system, the education of children, and the mission of mental health agencies, as well as the safety and well-being of the child. The school social worker and other mental health professionals must be at the forefront of coordinating alliances and working with other social service agencies in addressing the needs of school-aged children.

School-based interventions can take many forms. Partnering with mental health agencies to establish programs will help to ensure that children at risk are properly identified. Often local mental health agencies are in a better position to be aware of community resources.

Children who receive intervention services through school-based alliances have been found to improve their school performance and their attendance and to have fewer behavior problems (US Department of Health and Human Services, 2008). Social workers interested in building school-based alliances may want to refer to the elements of building an effective alliance using an approach based on the identified problem that the alliance has chosen:

1. *Direct services to at-risk children and families.* These may include interventions such as home visits, individual or group counseling, mentoring, support groups, social events, and tutoring. Examples include
   a. After-school programs focusing on social, recreational, educational or therapeutic issues
   b. Problem-solving, assertiveness training, or conflict resolution programs
   c. Mentoring programs using adults for educational and social development

    d. Services for special needs children that focus on developmental and educational screening and advocacy for services such as transportation

2. *Development of resource guides for school personnel.* Mental health agencies often have directories of community services relevant to the needs of at-risk children in the school setting. Through the collaboration, a resource guide specific to the needs of school personnel can be developed that addresses appropriate referral sources for families and children at risk of maltreatment.

Evidence-Informed Interventions

There are many evidence-informed school-based interventions directed at improving children's and adolescents' mental health. The following interventions selected from the National Registry of Evidence-Based Programs and Practices (Substance Abuse and Mental Health Services Administration [SAMHSA], 2014) are associated with middle childhood and adolescence:

- *All Stars* is a school-based program for middle school students (11–14 years) that is designed to prevent and delay the onset of high-risk behaviors such as drug use, violence, and premature sexual activity.
- *American Indian Life Skills Development/Zuni Life Skills Development.* Suicide is the second leading cause of death among American Indians from 15 to 24 years old, according to the Centers for Disease Control and Prevention (2014). The estimated rate of completed suicides among American Indians in this age group is about three times higher than that among comparably aged US youth overall (37.4 vs. 11.4 per 100,000, respectively).
- The *Anti-Defamation League (ADL) Peer Training Program* is an anti-bias and diversity training program intended for use in middle and high schools. The program prepares select students to be peer trainers.
- *Building Assets–Reducing Risks* (BARR) is a multifaceted school-based prevention program designed to decrease the incidence of substance abuse (tobacco, alcohol, and other drugs), academic failure, truancy, and disciplinary incidents among ninth-grade youth.

- *Care, Assess, Respond, Empower* (CARE), formerly called Counselors CARE (C-CARE) and Measure of Adolescent Potential for Suicide (MAPS), is a high-school-based suicide prevention program targeting high-risk youth.
- *Coping and Support Training* (CAST) is a high school-based suicide prevention program targeting youth from 14 to 19 years old that delivers life skills training and social support in a small group format (6–8 students per group).
- The *Challenging Horizons Program* (CHP) is a school-based set of interventions for middle or junior high school students with attention deficit hyperactivity disorder. Building on behavioral and cognitive theories about the nature of the disorder, CHP aims to provide a safe learning environment enhanced by supportive counseling relationships between students and staff.
- The *Children of Divorce Intervention Program* (CODIP) is a school-based preventive intervention delivered to groups of children from ages 5 to 14 who are dealing with the challenges of parental separation and divorce.
- The *Cognitive Behavioral Intervention for Trauma in Schools* (CBITS) program is a school-based group and individual intervention designed to reduce symptoms of posttraumatic stress disorder, depression, and behavioral problems; improve peer and parent support; and enhance coping skills among students exposed to traumatic life events, such as community and school violence, physical abuse, domestic violence, accidents, and natural disasters.
- The Columbia University *TeenScreen Program* identifies middle and high school youth in need of mental health services due to risk for suicide and undetected mental illness. The program's main objective is to assist in the early identification of problems that might not otherwise come to the attention of professionals.
- *Fourth R: Skills for Youth Relationships* is a curriculum for eighth- and ninth-grade students that is designed to promote healthy and safe behaviors related to dating, bullying, sexuality, and substance use.
- *Interpersonal Psychotherapy for Depressed Adolescents* (IPT-A) is a short-term, manual-driven outpatient treatment intervention that focuses on the current interpersonal problems of adolescents (aged 12–18 years) with mild to moderate depression.

- *Keepin' It REAL* is a multicultural, school-based substance use prevention program for students from 12 to 14 years old. It uses a 10-lesson curriculum taught by trained classroom teachers in 45-minute sessions over 10 weeks, with booster sessions delivered in the following school year.
- *The Leadership Program's Violence Prevention Project* (VPP) is a school-based intervention for early and middle adolescents. It is designed to prevent conflict and violence by improving conflict resolution skills, altering norms about using aggression and violence (including lowering tolerance for violence), and improving behavior in the school and community.
- *Linking Education and Awareness of Depression and Suicide (LEAD): For Youth* is a curriculum for high school students in ninth through twelfth grades that is designed to increase knowledge of depression and suicide, modify perceptions of depression and suicide, increase knowledge of suicide prevention resources, and improve intentions to engage in help-seeking behaviors.
- *LifeSkills Training* (LST) is a school-based program that aims to prevent alcohol, tobacco, and marijuana use and violence by targeting the major social and psychological factors that promote the initiation of substance use and other risky behaviors.
- The *Michigan Model for Health* is a comprehensive and sequential health education curriculum that aims to give students aged 5–19 years (grades K–12) the knowledge and skills needed to practice and maintain healthy behaviors and lifestyles.
- The *Model Adolescent Suicide Prevention Program* (MASPP) is a public health-oriented suicidal behavior prevention and intervention program originally developed for a small American Indian tribe in rural New Mexico to target high rates of suicide among its adolescents and young adults.
- *Nurturing Parenting Programs* (NPP) are family-based programs for the prevention and treatment of child abuse and neglect. The programs were developed to help families who have been identified by child welfare agencies for past child abuse and neglect or who are at high risk for child abuse and neglect.
- *Peaceful Alternatives to Tough Situations* (PATTS) is a school-based aggression management program designed to help students

increase positive conflict resolution skills, increase the ability to forgive transgressions, and reduce aggressive behavior.

- The *PreVenture Programme: Personality-Targeted Interventions for Adolescent Substance Misuse* is a school-based program designed to prevent alcohol and drug misuse among 13- to 15-year-old students.
- *Project ALERT* is a school-based prevention program for middle or junior high school students that focuses on alcohol, tobacco, and marijuana use. It seeks to prevent adolescent nonusers from experimenting with these drugs and to prevent youth who are already experimenting from becoming more regular users or abusers.
- *Reconnecting Youth (RY): A Peer Group Approach to Building Life Skills* is a school-based prevention program for students from ages 14 to 19 that teaches skills to build resiliency against risk factors and control early signs of substance abuse and emotional distress.
- *Responding in Peaceful and Positive Ways* (RiPP) is a school-based violence prevention program for middle school students. It is designed to be implemented along with a peer mediation program. Students practice using a social-cognitive problem-solving model to identify and choose nonviolent strategies for dealing with conflict.
- The *Safe & Civil Schools Positive Behavioral Interventions and Supports (PBIS) Model* is a multicomponent, multitiered, comprehensive approach to school-wide improvement. Integrating applied behavior analysis, research on effective schools, and systems change management theory, the intervention is an application of positive behavior support (PBS), a set of strategies or procedures designed to improve behavior by employing positive and systematic techniques.
- The *SANKOFA Youth Violence Prevention Program* is a strengths-based, culturally tailored preventive intervention for African American adolescents from 13 to 19. The goal of this school-based intervention is to equip youth with the knowledge, attitudes, skills, confidence, and motivation to minimize their risk for involvement in violence, victimization owing to violence, and other negative behaviors, such as alcohol and other drug use.
- *Say It Straight* (SIS) is a communication training program designed to help students and adults develop empowering communication skills and behaviors and increase self-awareness, self-efficacy, and personal and social responsibility.

- *Second Step* is a classroom-based social skills program for children from 4 to 14 years of age that teaches socioemotional skills aimed at reducing impulsive and aggressive behavior while increasing social competence.
- *SOS Signs of Suicide* is a 2-day secondary school-based intervention that includes screening and education. Students are screened for depression and suicide risk and referred for professional help as indicated.
- *Stay on Track* is a school-based substance abuse prevention curriculum conducted over a 3-year period with students in grades six through eight. The intervention is designed to help students assess the risks associated with substance abuse; enhance decision-making, goal-setting, communication, and resistance strategies; improve antidrug normative beliefs and attitudes; and reduce substance use.
- *Storytelling for Empowerment* is a school-based bilingual (English and Spanish) intervention for teenagers at risk for substance abuse, HIV, and other problem behaviors due to living in impoverished communities with high availability of drugs and limited health care services.
- *Students Taking a Right Stand* (STARS) Nashville Student Assistance Program (SAP) is based on an employee assistance model and provides comprehensive school-based prevention services for students in kindergarten through twelfth grade.
- *Teaching Kids to Cope* (TKC) is a cognitive-behavioral health education program, based on stress and coping theory, for adolescents aged 12–18 with depressive symptomatology and/or suicidal ideation. This group treatment program teaches adolescents a range of skills designed to improve their coping with stressful life events and decrease their depressive symptoms.
- *Teenage Health Teaching Modules* (THTM), a school-based health curriculum for students in grades six to twelve, attempts to improve students' immediate and long-term health by influencing their knowledge, attitudes, and behaviors regarding critical adolescent health content areas, including alcohol, tobacco, and other drug use; injury and violence prevention; and mental and emotional health.
- *Too Good for Drugs* (TGFD) is a school-based prevention program for kindergarten through twelfth grade that builds on students' resiliency by teaching them how to be socially competent and autonomous problem-solvers.
- *Too Good for Violence* (TGFV) is a school-based violence prevention and character education program for students in kindergarten through

twelfth grade. It is designed to enhance pro-social behaviors and skills and improve protective factors related to conflict and violence.

- *Trauma-Focused Coping* (TFC), sometimes called *multimodality trauma treatment,* is a school-based group intervention for children and adolescents in grades four through twelve who have been exposed to a traumatic stressor (e.g., disaster, violence, murder, suicide, fire, or accident).

Collaborations between school social workers and mental health workers are necessary to effectively intervene in the problems surrounding mental health issues and their impact on education. Working together in a common effort for a common purpose will allow for both effective and efficient uses of resources. Alliances between the school system and the mental health system will move us forward in addressing the prevention and treatment needs of children and families who are at risk of mental health issues. Through creativity, trust, and dedication, school social workers can bring about collaborations that make a difference in the lives of children and families.

References

Individuals with Disabilities Education Act. (2004). 20 USC.A. §§ 1400–1485.

Rehabilitation Act of 1973 (1973). Pub. L. 93–112, 87 Stat. 355 (codified as 29 USC. § 701).

Substance Abuse and Mental Health Services Administration (SAMHSA). (2014). National registry of evidence-based programs and practices. Retrieved from http://www.nrepp.samhsa.gov/Index.aspx

US Department of Health and Human Services, Children's Bureau. (2008). *School-based child maltreatment programs: Synthesis of lessons learned.* Washington, DC: Author.

Mental Health Resources for Working with Children and Adolescents

Adverse Childhood Experiences (ACEs)
https://www.cdc.gov/violenceprevention/childabuseandneglect/acestudy/index.html?CDC_AA_refVal=https%3A%2F%2Fwww.cdc.gov%2Fviolenceprevention%2Facestudy%2Findex.html

Adolescent and Teen Health Topics
http://www.cdc.gov/HealthyYouth/healthtopics/index.htm

Adolescent Development
http://fcs.osu.edu/family-life/teens-and-young-adults/parenting-adolescents
http://www.umm.edu/ency/article/002003.htm
https://ufhealth.org/adolescent-development

Adolescent Growth and Development
http://www.ext.vt.edu/topics/family/child-development/index.html

Adolescent Health and Development
http://www.who.int/maternal_child_adolescent/topics/adolescence/second-decade/en/

Brain
http://www.nimh.nih.gov/health/educational-resources/brain-basics/brain-basics.shtml

Child and Adolescent Development
http://www.themediaproject.com/facts/development/index.htm

Child and Teen Health
http://www.nlm.nih.gov/medlineplus/childandteenhealth.html
Diagnostic and Statistical Manual of Mental Disorders (DSM)
http://www.psychiatry.org/psychiatrists/practice/dsm/dsm-5/online-assessment-measures

Evidence-Based Practices

   Parent-Child Interaction Therapy: www.pcit.org
   Functional Family Therapy: https://www.fftllc.com
   Multisystemic Therapy: www.mstservices.com
   Multidimensional Treatment Foster Care: https://www.cibhs.org/multidimensional-treatment-foster-care-mtfc

Girl Power: National Public Education Campaign
https://www.ncjrs.gov/App/publications/abstract.aspx?ID=172442

Girls' Health
http://girlshealth.gov

Health Insurance Portability and Accountability Act of 1996 (HIPAA)

https://www.hhs.gov/sites/default/files/ocr/privacy/hipaa/understanding/consumers/
consumer_rights.pdf
https://www.hhs.gov/sites/default/files/ocr/privacy/hipaa/understanding/consumers/
privacy-security-electronic-records.pdf
https://www.hhs.gov/sites/default/files/ocr/privacy/hipaa/understanding/consumers/
sharing-family-friends.pdf
https://www.hhs.gov/hipaa/for-individuals/faq/index.html
https://www.youtube.com/watch?v=bonloqeOrAg&feature=youtu.be

Interdepartmental Serious Mental Illness Coordinating Committee (ISMICC)
https://www.congress.gov/bill/114th-congress/house-bill/2646
https://www.samhsa.gov/ismicc

Mental Health
http://www.samhsa.gov/treatment
National Adolescent Health Information Center
http://nahic.ucsf.edu/

Normal Adolescent Development
http://life.familyeducation.com/puberty/growth-and-development/36357.html
http://www.aacap.org/AACAP/Families_and_Youth/Facts_for_Families/Home.aspx

Positive Youth Development
http://www.acf.hhs.gov/sites/default/files/fysb/whatispyd20120829.pdf

Public Health Data Systems
   Youth Risk Behavior Surveillance System (YRBSS). The YRBSS is a national survey
      conducted by the US Centers for Disease Control (CDC). It monitors health risk
      behaviors including tobacco use, substance abuse, unintentional injuries and vi-
      olence, and sexual behaviors that contribute to unintended pregnancy and STDs.
      For information, statistics, trend reports, and much more, visit https://www.cdc.
      gov/healthyyouth/data/yrbs/overview.htm
   National Survey of Children's Health (NSCH). The NSCH is a national survey funded
      by the Department of Health and Human Services, Maternal and Child Health
      Bureau (MCHB) of the Health Resources and Services Administration (HRSA).
      NSCH examines the health of children, including those with special needs, with
      an emphasis on well-being, such as medical homes, family interactions, parental
      health, school and after-school experiences, and safe neighborhoods. The survey
      also collects information on the presence of a mental or behavioral problem. To
      obtain more information, publications, data, survey questions, and more, visit
      https://www.cdc.gov/nchs/slaits/nsch.htm.

School Health Policies and Programs Study (SHPPS). The SHPPS is a national survey conducted through the Division of Adolescent and School Health, National Center for HIV/AIDS, Viral Hepatitis, STD, and TB Prevention, Center for Disease Control and Prevention. The SHPPS assesses school health policies and practices at the state, district, school, and classroom levels. Collected data include mental health and social service policies. More information on SHPPS can be found at https://www.cdc.gov/healthyyouth/data/shpps/index.htm

National Health and Nutrition Examination Survey (NHANES). The NHANES is conducted through the National Center for Health Statistics at the CDC. The NHANES assesses health and nutritional status through interviews and physical examinations. Collected data cover a number of conditions, including depression and anxiety, symptoms of covered conditions, concerns associated with mental health and substance abuse, and mental health service use and need. Complete information on NHANES can be found at https://www.cdc.gov/nchs/nhanes/about_nhanes.htm

National Health Interview Survey (NHIS). The NHIS collects data on both adult's and children's mental health and mental disorders. For adults, this includes serious psychological distress and feelings of depression and anxiety. For children, this includes the presence of attention deficit hyperactivity disorder and autism spectrum disorder. The NHIS also examines mental health service use and whether individuals have unmet mental health needs. For more information on the NHIS, including data and statistics, visit https://www.cdc.gov/nchs/nhis/nhis_products.htm

Behavioral Risk Factor Surveillance System (BRFSS). The BRFSS is a national survey conducted by the CDC, National Center for Chronic Disease Prevention and Health Promotion, Division of Population Health. The BRFSS collects information on health risk behaviors, preventative practices, and health care access. Questions include recent mentally unhealthy days, anxiety and depressive disorders, mental illness and stigma, and psychological distress. Visit https://www.cdc.gov/brfss/index.html

Stages of Adolescent Development
http://www.childdevelopmentinfo.com/development/teens_stages.shtml

Suicide Prevention
https://suicidepreventionlifeline.org/wp-content/uploads/2016/08/Lifeline-Policy-for-Helping-Callers-at-Imminent-Risk-of-Suicide.pdf
https://suicidepreventionlifeline.org/wp-content/uploads/2016/08/Suicide-Risk-Assessment-Standards-1.pdf
https://suicidepreventionlifeline.org/wp-content/uploads/2016/09/SLTB-IR-Article-2014.pdf
https://suicidepreventionlifeline.org/wp-content/uploads/2016/09/Lifeline-Follow-Up-Guidance1214.pdf
https://suicidepreventionlifeline.org/wpcontent/uploads/2018/09/lifeline_socialmedia_toolkit.pdf
National Suicide Prevention Lifeline 1-800-273-8255

Teen Development
http://www.nlm.nih.gov/medlineplus/teendevelopment.html
http://kidshealth.org/teen

Teen Health Center
http://teenshealth.org/teen

Teen Mental Health
http://www.nlm.nih.gov/medlineplus/teenmentalhealth.html

Teens' Page
http://www.nlm.nih.gov/medlineplus/teenspage.html

Teenage Health
http://healthfinder.gov/HealthTopics/Population/pre-teens-and-teens
Youth Development Links
http://ncfy.acf.hhs.gov
Trauma-Informed Care
The National Child Traumatic Stress Network
https://www.nctsn.org/trauma-informed-care
National Council for Behavioral Health
https://www.nctsn.org/trauma-informed-care
Substance Use/Misuse and Youth
https://www.nctsn.org/trauma-informed-care
National Center on Substance Abuse and Child Welfare
https://ncsacw.samhsa.gov

Index